Sports Medicine Imaging

Guest Editor

MICHAEL J. TUITE, MD

RADIOLOGIC CLINICS
OF NORTH AMERICA

www.radiologic.theclinics.com

Consulting Editor
FRANK H. MILLER, MD

November 2010 • Volume 48 • Number 6

SAUNDERS an imprint of ELSEVIER, Inc.

W.B. SAUNDERS COMPANY
A Division of Elsevier Inc.

1600 John F. Kennedy Boulevard ● Suite 1800 ● Philadelphia, Pennsylvania 19103-2899

http://www.theclinics.com

RADIOLOGIC CLINICS OF NORTH AMERICA Volume 48, Number 6
November 2010 ISSN 0033-8389, ISBN 13: 978-1-4377-2596-4

Editor: Barton Dudlick
Developmental Editor: Donald Mumford

Radiologic Clinics of North America (ISSN 0033-8389) is published bimonthly by Elsevier Inc., 360 Park Avenue South, New York, NY 10010-1710. Months of issue are January, March, May, July, September, and November. Periodicals postage paid at New York, NY and additional mailing offices. Subscription prices are USD 386 per year for US individuals, USD 610 per year for US institutions, USD 185 per year for US students and residents, USD 450 per year for Canadian individuals, USD 766 per year for Canadian institutions, USD 556 per year for international individuals, USD 766 per year for international institutions, and USD 266 per year for Canadian and foreign students/residents. To receive student and resident rate, orders must be accompanied by name of affiliated institution, date of term and the signature of program/residency coordinatior on institution letterhead. Orders will be billed at individual rate until proof of status is received. Foreign air speed delivery is included in all *Clinics* subscription prices. All prices are subject to change without notice. **POSTMASTER:** Send address changes to *Radiologic Clinics of North America*, Elsevier Health Sciences Division, Subscription Customer Service, 3251 Riverport Lane, Maryland Heights, MO63043. **Customer Service: Telephone: 1-800-654-2452** (U.S. and Canada); **1-314-447-8871** (outside U.S. and Canada). **Fax: 1-314-447-8029. E-mail: journalscustomerservice-usa@ elsevier.com** (for print support); **journalsonlinesupport-usa@elsevier.com** (for online support).

Reprints. For copies of 100 or more of articles in this publication, please contact the Commercial Reprints Department, Elsevier Inc., 360 Park Avenue South, New York, New York 10010-1710. Tel.: (+1) 212-633-3812; Fax: (+1) 212-462-1935; E-mail: reprints@elsevier.com.

Radiologic Clinics of North America also published in Greek Paschalidis Medical Publications, Athens, Greece.

Radiologic Clinics of North America is covered in *MEDLINE/PubMed (Index Medicus), EMBASE/Excerpta Medica, Current Contents/Life Sciences, Current Contents/Clinical Medicine, RSNA Index to Imaging Literature, BIOSIS, Science Citation Index,* and *ISI/BIOMED*.

Printed and bound in the United Kingdom
Transferred to Digital Print 2011

Contributors

CONSULTING EDITOR

FRANK H. MILLER, MD
Professor of Radiology; Chief, Body Imaging
Section and Fellowship Program and GI
Radiology; and Medical Director MRI, Department
of Radiology, Northwestern University Feinberg
School of Medicine, Chicago, Illinois

GUEST EDITOR

MICHAEL J. TUITE, MD
Professor of Radiology and Chief, Musculoskeletal
Division, Department of Radiology, University
of Wisconsin Medical School and University
of Wisconsin Health, Madison, Wisconsin

AUTHORS

BENNETT A. ALFORD, MD
Professor of Radiology and Orthopaedic Surgery,
Department of Radiology, Division of
Musculoskeletal Imaging, University of Virginia
Health Sciences Center, Charlottesville, Virginia

MARK W. ANDERSON, MD
Professor of Radiology and Orthopaedic Surgery,
Department of Radiology; Chief, Division of
Musculoskeletal Imaging, University of Virginia
Health Sciences Center, Charlottesville, Virginia

DONNA G. BLANKENBAKER, MD
Musculoskeletal Division, Department
of Radiology, University of Wisconsin School of
Medicine and Public Health, Madison, Wisconsin

CAROL A. BOLES, MD
Associate Professor, Department of Radiology,
Wake Forest University Baptist Medical Center,
Winston-Salem, North Carolina

KIRKLAND W. DAVIS, MD
Associate Professor of Radiology, Department
of Radiology, University of Wisconsin Hospital
and Clinics, University of Wisconsin School of
Medicine and Public Health, Madison, Wisconsin

LUKE H. DEADY, MD
Clinical Fellow, Division of Musculoskeletal
Radiology, Department of Medical Imaging,
University of Toronto Health Network, Toronto
Western Hospital, Toronto, Ontario, Canada;
Staff Radiologist, Department of Medical Imaging,
Royal Prince Alfred Hospital, Camperdown,
New South Wales, Australia

ARTHUR A. DE SMET, MD
Musculoskeletal Division, Department
of Radiology, University of Wisconsin School
of Medicine and Public Health, Madison,
Wisconsin

CRISTIN FERGUSON, MD
Assistant Professor, Department of Orthopedic
Surgery, Wake Forest University Baptist Medical
Center, Winston-Salem, North Carolina

BRADLEY A. MAXFIELD, MD
Associate Professor of Radiology, Chief
of Pediatric Radiology, Section of Pediatric
Radiology, Department of Radiology, University
of Wisconsin School of Medicine and Public
Health, Madison, Wisconsin

WILLIAM C. MEYERS, MD, MBA
Chairman, Department of Surgery, Drexel
University College of Medicine, Philadelphia,
Pennsylvania

FRANK E. MULLENS, MD, MPH
Clinical Fellow, Department of Radiology,
Musculoskeletal Division, Thomas Jefferson
University Hospital, Philadelphia, Pennsylvania

ARTHUR H. NEWBERG, MD
Chief of Musculoskeletal Imaging, Department of
Radiology, New England Baptist Hospital; Professor
of Radiology and Orthopedics, Tufts University
School of Medicine, Boston, Massachusetts

JOEL S. NEWMAN, MD
Chairman, Department of Radiology, New England
Baptist Hospital; Clinical Professor of Radiology,
Tufts University School of Medicine, Boston,
Massachusetts

DAVID SALONEN, MD
Associate Professor, Division of Musculoskeletal
Radiology, Department of Medical Imaging,
University of Toronto University Health Network,
Toronto Western Hospital, Toronto, Ontario,
Canada

MICHAEL J. TUITE, MD
Professor of Radiology and Chief, Musculoskeletal
Division, Department of Radiology,
University of Wisconsin Medical School,
University of Wisconsin Health,
Madison, Wisconsin

ADAM C. ZOGA, MD
Associate Professor of Radiology,
Director of Musculoskeletal MRI,
Thomas Jefferson University, Philadelphia,
Pennsylvania

Contents

Joel S. Newman and Arthur H. Newberg

Basketball injuries are most prevalent in the lower extremity, especially at the ankle and knee. Most basketball injuries are orthopedic in nature and commonly include ligament sprains, musculotendinous strains, and overuse injuries including stress fractures. By virtue of its excellent contrast resolution and depiction of the soft tissues and trabecular bone, magnetic resonance imaging has become the principal modality for evaluating many basketball injuries. In this article, commonly encountered basketball injuries and their imaging appearances are described. The epidemiology of basketball injuries across various age groups and levels of competition and between genders are reviewed.

Luke H. Deady and David Salonen

Skiing and snowboarding are ever increasing in popularity, with participation across a wide patient demographic. This article focuses on common skiing and snowboarding injuries, with an emphasis on unique mechanisms of injury and discusses the contribution of equipment design to evolving patterns of injury. Knowledge of mechanisms of injury and injury patterns allows a targeted approach to the interpretation of imaging modalities in this patient population.

Michael J. Tuite

Injuries in triathletes are common and are mostly overuse injuries. Rotator cuff tendinitis is the most common complaint from swimming, but the incidence of tendinopathy and rotator cuff tears on magnetic resonance imaging is comparable in triathletes without and with shoulder pain. Cycling injuries are mainly to the knee, including patellar tendinosis, iliotibial band syndrome, and patellofemoral stress syndrome, and to the Achilles tendon and the cervical and lumbar spine. Running is associated with most injuries in triathletes, during both training and racing, causing the athlete to discontinue the triathlon. In addition to knee injuries from running, triathletes may also develop foot and ankle, lower leg, and hip injuries similar to single-sport distance runners. Some injuries in triathletes may be mainly symptomatic during one of the three sports but are exacerbated by one or both of the other disciplines.

Mark W. Anderson and Bennett A. Alford

Injuries to the shoulder and elbow are common in athletes involved in sporting activities that require overhead motion of the arm. An understanding of the forces involved in the throwing motion, the anatomic structures most at risk, and the magnetic resonance imaging appearances of the most common associated injuries can help to improve diagnostic accuracy when interpreting imaging studies in these patients.

Hip injuries are common in athletes, and there is an extensive differential diagnosis of potential causes. This article reviews the anatomy of the hip, and discusses the imaging findings of hip pathology in athletes including skeletal, intraarticular, and extra-articular abnormalities. The role of radiography, computed tomography (CT), magnetic resonance (MR) imaging, MR arthrography, CT arthrography, and sonography in evaluating each condition is discussed.

Many athletes struggle with groin pain for years without ever receiving a clear diagnosis or being offered an effective treatment plan. Confusion among treatment providers can also frequently lead to suboptimal surgeries for presumed hernias or nerve entrapment syndromes. Imaging, and in particular magnetic resonance (MR) imaging, should play a primary role in the workup, diagnosis, and treatment of athletic pubalgia. This review outlines standard of care, cutting-edge MR imaging techniques for athletic pubalgia, and reviews the spectrum of imaging findings that are encountered in this patient group.

With increasing youth participation in organized sports, more injuries in this age group are being treated by primary care and sports medicine physicians. Overuse injuries are much more common now than in past decades, with Little League shoulder, Little League elbow, and gymnast wrist being particular concerns. Rotator cuff tears and glenoid labral injuries, once thought to be rare in this age group, are also more common now. Osteochondritis dissecans of the elbow is relatively common and typically fares poorly without surgery. Wrist abnormalities that occur nowadays include triangular fibrocartilage tears. Tendonitis, which is now observed frequently in clinical practice in this age group, rarely requires imaging.

Injuries to pediatric athletes, which are becoming increasingly common, take the form of acute injuries and chronic overuse injuries. Acute injuries of the lower extremity include avulsions of the pelvic apophyses, muscle-tendon injuries, transient dislocation of the patella, ankle sprains, and acute tears of the anterior cruciate ligament and menisci. Magnetic resonance (MR) imaging of the latter 2 injuries should approach the accuracy of MR imaging of the adult knee. Chronic overuse injuries of the lower extremity in this age group include stress fractures, which are most common in the tibia; ankle impingement syndromes; osteochondritis dissecans of the knee and osteochondral lesions of the talus; and traction apophysitis, most commonly presenting as Osgood-Schlatter disease and Sinding-Larsen-Johannson disease, affecting the patellar tendon. Imaging findings of all these lesions are characteristic, and allow radiologists to assist their clinical colleagues in diagnosing and treating pediatric athletic injuries.

Acute spinal injuries are fortunately rare in pediatric sports but can be catastrophic. Imaging is integral to the diagnosis and care of spinal trauma. Plain radiographs and CT are critical for detecting vertebral fracture, and MR imaging is an essential adjunct for evaluating muscular, ligamentous, and spinal cord injury. Back pain is a common complaint among athletes of all ages. The growing spine has unique weaknesses that result in a higher rate of detectable radiologic abnormalities. Disk pathology is less common in children, and is often uniquely associated with fracture of the ring apophyses. Spondylolysis is far more prevalent in youth athletes than in their adult counterparts, requiring a different approach to imaging for assessment of adolescent back pain.

Over time, women have become more extensively involved in athletic programs. The female athlete presents a unique challenge to sports medicine in general. Although specific types of injuries are the same as in the male athlete, the female athlete is at higher risk for some of these injuries. Injuries may be sport specific, but gender-related injuries are also related to morphologic and physiologic differences between the male and female athlete. This article reviews some of the differences between the male and female athlete and focuses on a few prominent injuries or risks related specifically to the woman athlete.

GOAL STATEMENT

The goal of the *Radiologic Clinics of North America* is to keep practicing radiologists and radiology residents up to date with current clinical practice in radiology by providing timely articles reviewing the state of the art in patient care.

ACCREDITATION

The *Radiologic Clinics of North America* is planned and implemented in accordance with the Essential Areas and Policies of the Accreditation Council for Continuing Medical Education (ACCME) through the joint sponsorship of the University of Virginia School of Medicine and Elsevier. The University of Virginia School of Medicine is accredited by the ACCME to provide continuing medical education for physicians.

The University of Virginia School of Medicine designates this educational activity for a maximum of 15 *AMA PRA Category 1 Credits*™ for each issue, 90 credits per year. Physicians should only claim credit commensurate with the extent of their participation in the activity.

The American Medical Association has determined that physicians not licensed in the US who participate in this CME activity are eligible for a maximum of *15 AMA PRA Category 1 Credits*™ for each issue, 90 credits per year.

Credit can be earned by reading the text material, taking the CME examination online at http://www.theclinics.com/home/cme, and completing the evaluation. After taking the test, you will be required to review any and all incorrect answers. Following completion of the test and evaluation, your credit will be awarded and you may print your certificate.

FACULTY DISCLOSURE/CONFLICT OF INTEREST

The University of Virginia School of Medicine, as an ACCME accredited provider, endorses and strives to comply with the Accreditation Council for Continuing Medical Education (ACCME) Standards of Commercial Support, Commonwealth of Virginia statutes, University of Virginia policies and procedures, and associated federal and private regulations and guidelines on the need for disclosure and monitoring of proprietary and financial interests that may affect the scientific integrity and balance of content delivered in continuing medical education activities under our auspices.

The University of Virginia School of Medicine requires that all CME activities accredited through this institution be developed independently and be scientifically rigorous, balanced and objective in the presentation/discussion of its content, theories and practices.

All authors/editors participating in an accredited CME activity are expected to disclose to the readers relevant financial relationships with commercial entities occurring within the past 12 months (such as grants or research support, employee, consultant, stock holder, member of speakers bureau, etc.). The University of Virginia School of Medicine will employ appropriate mechanisms to resolve potential conflicts of interest to maintain the standards of fair and balanced education to the reader. Questions about specific strategies can be directed to the Office of Continuing Medical Education, University of Virginia School of Medicine, Charlottesville, Virginia.

The faculty and staff of the University of Virginia Office of Continuing Medical Education have no financial affiliations to disclose.

The authors/editors listed below have identified no financial or professional relationships for themselves or their spouse/partner:
Bennett A. Alford, MD; Mark W. Anderson, MD; Donna G. Blankenbaker, MD; Carol A. Boles, MD; Arthur A. De Smet, MD; Luke H. Deady, MD; Barton Dudlick, (Acquisitions Editor); Theodore E. Keats, MD, (Test Author); Bradley A. Maxfield, MD; William C. Meyers, MD, MBA; Frank H. Miller, MD (Consulting Editor); Frank E. Mullens, MD, MPH; Arthur H. Newberg, MD; Michael J. Tuite, MD (Guest Editor); and Adam C. Zoga, MD.

The authors/editors listed below have identified the following financial or professional relationships for themselves or their spouse/partner:
Kirkland W. Davis, MD is an industry funded research/investigator for Endocare, Inc.
Cristin Ferguson, MD is a consultant for BC Genesis.
Joel S. Newman, MD has served on the Advisory Committee/Board of ONI Medical Corp., and serves on the Advisory Committee/Board of InSight Corporation.
David Salonen, MD is a consultant for Centocor Inc., Abbott Laboratories, and Janssen Pharmaceuticals.

Disclosure of Discussion of Non-FDA Approved Uses for Pharmaceutical Products and/or Medical Devices.
The University of Virginia School of Medicine, as an ACCME provider, requires that all faculty presenters identify and disclose any off-label uses for pharmaceutical and medical device products. The University of Virginia School of Medicine recommends that each physician fully review all the available data on new products or procedures prior to clinical use.

TO ENROLL

To enroll in the Radiologic Clinics of North America Continuing Medical Education program, call customer service at 1-800-654-2452 or sign up online at http://www.theclinics.com/home/cme. The CME program is available to subscribers for an additional annual fee USD 245.

Radiologic Clinics of North America

THE CLINICS ARE NOW AVAILABLE ONLINE!

Access your subscription at:
www.theclinics.com

Preface
Sports Medicine Imaging

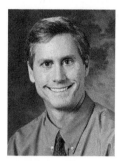

Michael J. Tuite, MD
Guest Editor

This issue of *Radiologic Clinics of North America* is dedicated to selected topics in sports medicine imaging. Imaging of sports injuries continues to grow and is driven mainly by two factors. The first is that more people are participating in athletics, particularly women, who have had more opportunities for organized team sports since the passing of Title IX.[1] Although only about 10% of American adults get some form of regular exercise, 60–70% of Americans at least occasionally play a sport.[2] In addition, the baby boomer generation grew up participating in more organized sporting activities, and as they have gotten older, many continue to play these sports.[3]

The second factor is that, although athletic activities are associated with many health benefits, they can also lead to musculoskeletal injuries. This is particularly true in those who play sports aggressively, and in older individuals. In older athletes, aging tendons and joints are more vulnerable to injury. A study by the US Consumer Product Safety Commission found that an estimated 6 million people 65 years of age and older were treated in US hospital emergency rooms for sports-related injuries in 2006.[3] This represents a 54% increase from 1990 to 1996 and is larger than the 8% increase in the over-65 population. Overuse injuries are also common, with one in seven Americans suffering from a musculoskeletal impairment, many of which are caused by, or symptomatic when attempting, athletic activities.[4] Overall, 70% of people report having a sports-related injury at some point in their life, and these injuries account for 15% of all visits to family physicians.[5]

Sports-related injuries are also increasing in children and adolescents. This is probably because of the increased emphasis on trying to excel in a single sport, leading many kids to play one sport year round.[6] Performing the same athletic activity without an off-season places a significant strain on the growing musculoskeletal system.

Multiple articles and textbooks have been written on sports medicine imaging. We have decided to try something a little different and have divided this issue into three groups of articles. In the first portion, we will present the imaging of injuries seen in three sports that have not received a lot of attention in the imaging literature: basketball, skiing/snowboarding, and triathlons. In the second group of articles, we discuss three conditions with recent advances: the overhead throwing athlete shoulder and elbow, athletic hip injuries, and athletic pubalgia. Finally, the last group of articles looks at pediatric sports-related upper extremity, lower extremity, and spine injuries, as well as special considerations in the female athlete.

We are fortunate to bring together an excellent group of authors for this issue. Joel Newman and Arthur Newberg of New England Baptist Hospital and Tufts University School of Medicine share their knowledge of imaging basketball injuries from their years of association with the team orthopedist for the Boston Celtics.

Radiol Clin N Am 48 (2010) xi–xii
doi:10.1016/j.rcl.2010.10.002

Luke Deady and Davis Salonen from the University of Toronto share their experiences imaging skiers and snowboarders north of the border. I present the imaging of injuries seen in triathletes, including injuries seen in those training for their first sprint triathlon, up to racers in the Wisconsin Ironman Triathlon World Championship Qualifier event.

Mark Anderson and Bennet Alford of the University of Virginia discuss the recent advances in understanding the mechanism of injury in the throwing shoulder and elbow. Donna Blankenbaker of the University of Wisconsin shares her extensive experience with MR arthrography and ultrasound of the athletic hip. The "Father of Athletic Pubalgia Imaging," Adam Zoga, and his colleagues, Frank Mullens of Thomas Jefferson University and William Meyers of Drexel University, present an excellent summary of the "sports hernia."

Kirk Davis of the University of Wisconsin then details in two articles pediatric upper and lower extremity injuries. Brad Maxfield, Chief of Pediatric Radiology at the American Family Children's Hospital and the University of Wisconsin, discusses pediatric sports-related spine injuries. Finally, Carol Boles and Cristin Ferguson of Wake Forest Bowman Gray Medical Center describe the special features to look for when imaging female athletes.

As the volume of sports-related injuries continues to increase, it becomes increasingly important for the practicing radiologist to be able to recognize their imaging findings. We hope that this issue of *Radiologic Clinics of North America*

helps you in interpreting these imaging studies, while also being enjoyable to read.

Michael J. Tuite, MD
Musculoskeletal Division Department of Radiology
University of Wisconsin Medical School
and UW Health
MC 3252
600 Highland Avenue
Madison, WI 53792, USA

E-mail address:
mjtuite@wisc.edu

REFERENCES

1. Templeton KJ, Hame SL, Hannafin JA, et al. Sports injuries in women: sex- and gender-based differences in etiology and prevention. Instr Course Lect 2008;57: 539–52.
2. AAOS. Sports and Exercise: People reporting leisure-time physical activitiy. In: AAOS Online Fact Sheet. Available at: http://orthoinfo.aaos.org/topic.cfm?topic=A00324. Accessed June 15, 2010.
3. AAOS. Stay active: safe at any age. In: AAOS Online Fact Sheet. Available at: http://orthoinfo.aaos.org/topic.cfm?topic=A00102. Accessed June 15, 2010.
4. Praemer A, Furner S, Rice DP. Musculoskeletal conditions in the United States. Rosemont (IL): American Academy of Orthopedic Surgeons; 1999.
5. Shrier I. Approach to injuries in active people. Can Fam Physician 2006;52:727–31.
6. Kerssemakers SP, Fotiadou AN, de Jonge MC, et al. Sport injuries in the paediatric and adolescent patient: a growing problem. Pediatr Radiol 2009;39:471–84.

Basketball Injuries

Joel S. Newman, MD[a,b],*, Arthur H. Newberg, MD[a,b]

KEYWORDS
- Magnetic resonance imaging • Basketball injuries
- Ankle sprain • Stress fracture • Musculotendinous strain

The popularity of basketball not only in the United States but also worldwide has led to a greater focus on associated injuries and on ways to prevent these injuries through appropriate conditioning.[1–3] Basketball is relatively unique among both professional and collegiate athletics in that both men and women compete in the sport. This fact has been further enhanced by the rise of the Women's National Basketball Association (WNBA) and by the increasing popularity of both men's and women's college basketball among the general public.

Although basketball is not considered to be a contact sport, injuries are surprisingly frequent, whether in high school competition, at the collegiate level, or in adult professional players.[4–7] Some injury patterns are seen in players of all ages and in both men and women. Other injuries have a predilection for a specific age group or gender.[1,8] Although the primary focus of this article is on orthopedic injuries, it should be emphasized that there are several nonorthopedic injuries commonly encountered in basketball players as well.

IMAGING TECHNIQUES

Most acute periarticular injuries, including suspected ligament sprains, are initially evaluated with conventional radiography. Magnetic resonance (MR) imaging is typically used when there is suspicion of internal derangement at the knee, such as meniscal or ligament tear (**Figs. 1 and 2**), chondral injury, or osseous contusion, at the shoulder for suspected rotator cuff tear, and at the ankle when osteochondral injury is suspected. The early diagnosis and grading of musculotendinous strain is also accomplished via targeted MR imaging (**Fig. 3**).[9] In basketball players, muscle injuries at the anterior abdominal wall/groin and lower extremities are approached in this manner. MR imaging has largely supplanted radionuclide bone scintigraphy for the diagnosis of osseous stress injury, and should be used when stress injury is suspected and radiographs are negative.

Computed tomography (CT) has a supplementary role in the setting of athletic injury but is recommended for the assessment of fracture healing, particularly in the foot, and can be readily performed with fixation hardware in place. Two-dimensional multiplanar reformations of helically acquired data are now routinely performed, and 3-dimensional models may be useful for operative planning. CT may also be helpful to confirm suspected osseous avulsions, given its ability to detect small avulsed cortical fragments.

In some chronic or recalcitrant periarticular injuries, MR arthrography may be indicated. Distension of the joint with a dilute solution of gadolinium in saline optimizes the visualization of the labral and capsular supporting structures at the shoulder and labral and chondral structures at the hip. MR arthrography is particularly useful in the setting of glenohumeral instability[10] and in the detection of labral tears at the hip (**Fig. 4**).[11]

In the United States, the use of ultrasonography in the musculoskeletal system is more limited because of radiologist preference for MR imaging and limited operator training in this application. Nevertheless, ultrasonography is a useful adjunct for the evaluation of tendon and other soft tissue injuries and for image-guided interventions in the musculoskeletal system.[12]

[a] Department of Radiology, New England Baptist Hospital, 125 Parker Hill Avenue, Boston, MA 02120, USA
[b] Tufts University School of Medicine, Boston, 145 Harrison Boston, MA 02111, USA
* Corresponding author. Department of Radiology, New England Baptist Hospital, 125 Parker Hill Avenue, Boston, MA 02120.
E-mail address: jnewman@caregroup.harvard.edu

Radiol Clin N Am 48 (2010) 1095–1111
doi:10.1016/j.rcl.2010.07.007

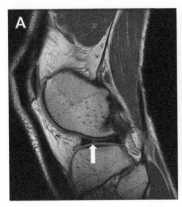 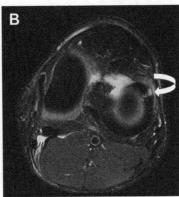

Fig. 1. Complex lateral meniscus tear in a 24-year-old professional basketball player. (*A*) Sagittal proton-density (PD) and (*B*) axial PD fat-saturated images demonstrate a complex radial tear of the lateral meniscus (*arrow*). The tear can be clearly seen on the axial sequence extending to the periphery (*curved arrow*).

EPIDEMIOLOGY OF BASKETBALL INJURIES

Longitudinal studies of professional, collegiate, and high school basketball players over multiple consecutive seasons elucidate several important features of injuries sustained while playing the sport. In general, injuries are significantly more common during competition rather than during practice.[4] The ankle is the most frequently injured anatomic site.[5,7] There are both commonalities and differences in injury patterns between male and female players.[1,2,8,13] Despite basketball not being considered a contact sport, injuries are frequently sustained during contact between players.[14] Moreover, the incidence of injuries in basketball players is quite high relative to other sporting activities.[2]

In basketball, lower extremity injuries predominate, with the ankle, specifically ankle sprains, representing the most common injury.[5,7] In a recently published series reviewing injuries in high school basketball players in the United States, 39.7% of all injuries were at the ankle or foot.[4] Knee and back injuries are also relatively prevalent; injuries at the hip and groin occur less frequently.[7] In the upper extremity, hand and wrist injuries are most commonly encountered.[4,5]

ANKLE AND FOOT
Ankle Sprains

Ankle sprains are the most common acute injury sustained in basketball players.[5,7] In a 2-year prospective study of female Greek professionals, there were 1.12 sprains per 1000 exposure hours with players missing an average of 7.01 practice or game sessions for each injury. Most injuries occurred within the 3-point line.[15] Nelson and colleagues[16] described the incidence of ankle injury in high school athletes in the United States with a rate of 7.74 injuries per 10,000 exposures. In a series reported by Deitch and colleagues[8] comparing injuries in the National Basketball Association (NBA) and the WNBA, lateral ankle sprains were the most common injury diagnosis (13.7% of injuries) in both leagues. A 10-year prospective study spanning the NBA seasons from 1988–1989 to 1997–1998 described 942 ankle sprains, 9.4% of all injuries.[7]

Lateral ankle sprains predominate over medial sprains,[17] and some investigators refer to ankle sprain as exclusively an injury of the lateral ligament complex.[18] Lateral sprains generally result from an inversion injury with the foot in slight plantar flexion, such as when one player steps

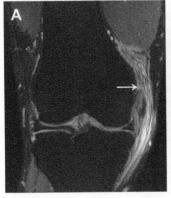 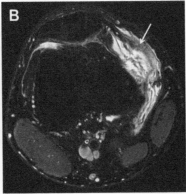

Fig. 2. Medial collateral ligament (MCL) sprain and medial patellofemoral ligament tear in a 25-year-old professional basketball player. (*A*) Coronal PD fat-saturated image demonstrates MCL sprain. There is indistinctness of MCL fibers and marked adjacent soft tissue edema (*arrow*). (*B*) Axial T2 fat-saturated image demonstrates that the medial patellofemoral ligament is torn and there is marked soft tissue edema (*arrow*).

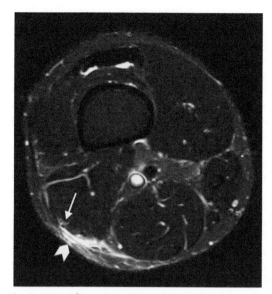

Fig. 3. Biceps femoris musculotendinous strain in a 39-year-old professional basketball player. Axial T2 fat-saturated image shows edema in the biceps muscle (*arrow*) and fluid adjacent to the muscle in the surrounding soft tissues, representing a small hematoma (*arrowhead*).

on the foot of another player, rolling the ankle inward, or when the player lands awkwardly, twisting the ankle. Cutting, turning, or pushing off awkwardly may also result in ankle sprain. The

anterior talofibular ligament is most commonly injured followed by the calcaneofibular ligament (**Fig. 5**). Eversion injury is much less common, occurring secondary to either dorsiflexion with eversion or external rotation of the foot. Nevertheless, eversion injuries may be relatively serious because the deltoid ligament, anterior tibiofibular ligament, and interosseous membrane may be involved with the disruption of ankle mortise.[17,19]

A basketball player who has sustained an ankle sprain is evaluated at the time of the injury. Clinically minor injuries may require no further evaluation. More significant injuries may warrant radiographic evaluation of the ankle with anteroposterior, oblique (mortise), and lateral views. Radiographs may reveal fracture or joint malalignment accompanying more severe sprains[18] and may also reveal osseous injuries remote from the ankle, including navicular avulsions and avulsion fractures of the base of the fifth metatarsal.[20]

Although clinical examination alone may suffice for the confirmation of ligament deficiency,[18] MR imaging may be useful in cases of major or chronic ankle sprains with recalcitrant symptoms. MR imaging depicts ligament integrity[21] and may

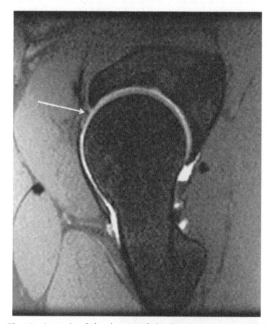

Fig. 4. Anterior labral tear of the hip in a 40-year-old professional basketball player. T1 fat-saturated oblique axial sequence from an MR arthrogram shows a tear at the base of the anterior labrum (*arrow*).

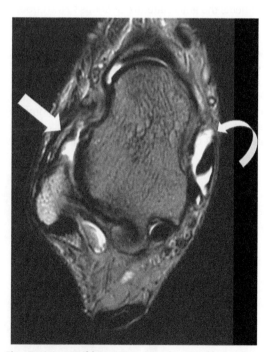

Fig. 5. Acute ankle sprain. Anterior talofibular ligament (ATFL) injury in a 24-year-old professional basketball player. Axial T2-weighted image demonstrates an abnormal ATFL. The ligament is thick and distal fibers are indistinct (*arrow*), consistent with an ankle sprain. Incidentally noted is fluid in the posterior tibialis tendon sheath (*curved arrow*).

also detect concomitant injuries that are radiographically occult, including chondral or osteochondral injuries of the talar dome (Fig. 6).[22] Moreover, there are several common acute injuries of the ankle and hindfoot that may present with symptoms of lateral ankle sprain, including fractures of the anterolateral process of the calcaneus, os trigonum fractures, and tear of the superior peroneal retinaculum (SPR) with peroneal tendon subluxation.[20] Both of these conditions as well as osseous contusions should be readily apparent on MR imaging.

Acute Foot Injuries

As described by McDermott,[20] several significant injuries to the foot, in addition to those already described, may also present with symptoms of ankle sprain. These injuries include avulsion fractures of the navicular and/or base of the fifth-ray metatarsal. Another often overlooked injury is the avulsion at the origin of the extensor digitorum brevis muscle from the lateral calcaneus.

Fractures of the anterolateral process of the calcaneus typically occur with the foot abducted and plantar flexed. This mechanism puts tension on the bifurcate ligament, which normally connects the anterolateral calcaneus to the cuboid and navicular.[20] These fractures may be difficult to identify on conventional radiographs, and attention should be directed to this location on MR imaging or CT in all individuals with a history of ankle and foot trauma (Fig. 7). Healing of anterolateral process fractures may be protracted.[23] In the authors' experience, CT with multiplanar image reformation is the most accurate modality for the assessment of healing of these fractures.

Tears of the SPR may occur during acute dorsiflexion with strong contraction of the peroneal muscles to prevent further dorsiflexion. This combination of events may lead to the tear of the fibular retinacular attachment. A small fragment of the bone may be avulsed at the SPR attachment on the fibula (so-called flake sign). Once the SPR is avulsed, the peroneal tendons may dislocate anteriorly.[20]

Avulsion fractures of the base of the fifth metatarsal occur secondary to inversion stress. As described by McDermott,[20] an injury of this type may be sustained in basketball when a player rebounding the ball lands on the foot of another player. The rebounding player experiences an inversion sprain with contraction of the peroneus brevis muscle. This sequence of events results in an avulsion of the peroneus brevis attachment at the base of the fifth metatarsal.

Overuse Injuries at the Ankle, Foot, and Lower Leg

Overuse injuries of the ankle, foot, and lower leg include osseous stress injuries, shin splints, and soft tissue injuries. Bone scintigraphy has been traditionally used for the diagnosis of osseous stress fracture, particularly when radiographic results are negative. MR imaging has largely supplanted bone scan for the diagnosis of early stress injury, particularly in the competitive athlete (Fig. 8). In addition, the excellent contrast resolution of MR imaging makes it the imaging modality of choice for the evaluation of soft tissue injury, including musculotendinous strain,[9] ligament injury, and other traumatic and inflammatory conditions involving the soft tissues.

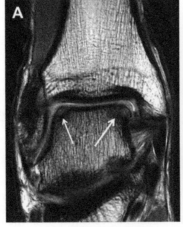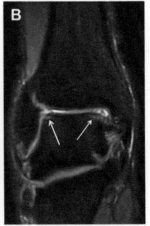

Fig. 6. Osteochondral injury of the right talar dome in a 32-year-old professional basketball player. (A) Coronal PD high-resolution and (B) coronal PD fat-saturated images. There are areas on both the medial and lateral talar dome demonstrating cartilage defects with mild underlying osseous edema (arrows).

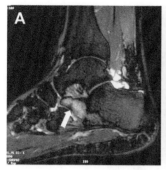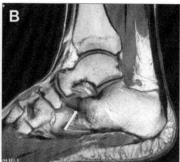

Fig. 7. Anterior lateral calcaneal process fracture in a 19-year-old division I female college basketball player. (*A*) Sagittal short-tau inversion recovery (STIR) image of the right ankle demonstrates intense osseous edema of the anterior lateral process of the calcaneus (*arrow*). (*B*) Sagittal T1 image demonstrates low signal intensity of the anterior lateral process with a fracture line seen as a wavy line of low signal intensity (*arrow*).

Osseous stress fractures occurring below the knee in the basketball player frequently involve the tibia or the distal fibula, the latter most common approximately 5 cm proximal to the tip of the lateral malleolus. Stress fractures may also be observed, albeit less commonly, in the tarsal navicular, calcaneus, metatarsals, and cuneiforms (**Fig. 9**).[24] On bone scan, stress fractures manifest as increased radiotracer uptake; on MR imaging, a low signal intensity fracture line is observed and there may be considerable osseous or perosseous edema surrounding the fracture on fluid-sensitive sequences.

Fractures in trabecular bone, such as the calcaneus, may show intraosseous sclerosis on radiographs with healing but no significant extraosseous callus. Metatarsal stress fractures often manifest as exuberant callus with healing. Navicular stress injury is notoriously difficult to diagnose

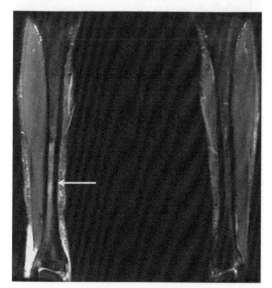

Fig. 8. Stress of the reaction tibia in a 21-year-old basketball player. Coronal STIR image demonstrates osseous edema in the medullary cavity of the right tibia (*arrow*). No actual fracture is seen. An evolving stress injury is thought to be represented.

on radiographs. Typically, these fractures are oriented in the sagittal plane, and propagate in proximal to distal and dorsal to plantar[25] directions with no significant callus (**Fig. 10**). Both MR imaging and CT are useful for diagnosing navicular stress fracture (**Fig. 11**); CT is used to monitor healing.

One particularly problematic foot injury in basketball players, which may result from overuse, is the Jones fracture. The Jones fracture is located at the diaphyseal-metaphyseal junction of the proximal fifth metatarsal and results from the abnormal loading of the lateral foot when the heel is elevated and the metatarsophalangeal (MTP) joints are hyperextended (**Fig. 12**). There may be a considerable time lag between onset of symptoms and radiographic changes.[24]

Jones fractures may be slow to heal, with a high rate of nonunion when treated nonoperatively. Fernandez Fairen and colleagues[26] performed a prospective nonrandomized study of basketball players with fractures of the proximal one-third of the shaft of the fifth-ray metatarsal. Approximately half of the cases were acute fractures and half represented stress fractures. All 9 stress fractures were treated with compression screw fixation; all healed within 8 to 14 weeks. Four of the 8 acute fractures were treated nonoperatively; half went on to nonunion after 12 weeks and required internal fixation (**Fig. 13**).

Given the exquisite sensitivity of MR imaging for the detection of bone marrow edema, this technique may play a role in identifying early stress changes resulting from altered biomechanics (**Fig. 14**). This observation is particularly significant in the metatarsals, as shown by one investigator who performed preseason MR imaging examinations on members of a National Collegiate Athletic Association (NCAA) men's team with subsequent follow-up.[27] The early detection of stress reaction in a metatarsal on MR imaging may allow for early intervention (ie, rest, orthotic support), preventing subsequent fracture.

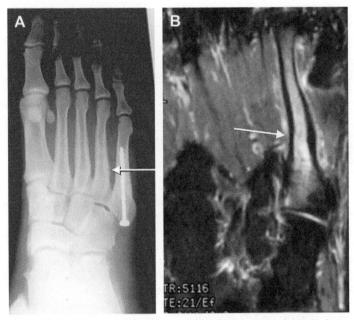

Fig. 9. Stress fracture in the fourth metatarsal in a 26-year-old professional basketball player. (*A*) Internal oblique radiograph of the right foot demonstrates cortical thickening and a fracture of the fourth metatarsal shaft. (*Arrow*) The old Jones fracture with open reduction internal fixation should be noted. (*B*) Axial STIR image demonstrates the fourth metatarsal osseous edema and periosseous soft tissue edema (*arrow*).

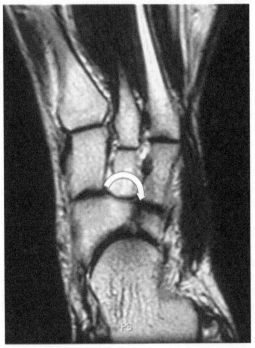

Fig. 10. Tarsal navicular stress fracture in a 19-year-old division I female basketball player. Axial T2 image demonstrates a fracture line in the middle third of the tarsal navicular consistent with a stress fracture (*curved arrow*).

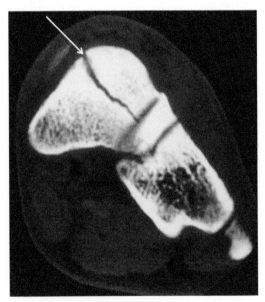

Fig. 11. Tarsal navicular stress fracture in a 23-year-old professional basketball player. Coronal CT demonstrates an oblique acute fracture through the navicular (*arrow*). The patient's fracture healed with nonoperative treatment.

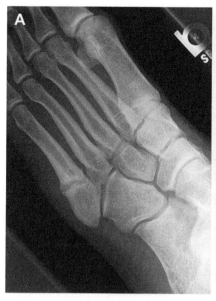
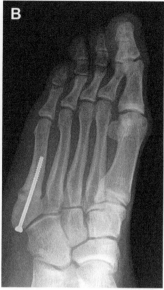

Fig. 12. Jones fracture in a 28-year-old professional basketball player. (*A*) Internal oblique radiograph of the left foot demonstrates a chronic un-united Jones fracture of the proximal fifth metatarsal shaft. The fracture line is clearly seen with some peripheral callous and sclerosis along the fracture margins. (*B*) Postoperative radiograph demonstrating screw placement within the fifth metatarsal.

Several soft tissue conditions in the lower leg and foot of basketball players may result from overuse. In the lower leg, these include musculotendinous strain and contusion, muscle herniation, and tendinosis (**Fig. 15**).[24] Achilles tendinosis may be both insertional and noninsertional in location. At the ankle and hindfoot, plantar fasciitis is not uncommon (**Fig. 16**) and anterior ankle impingement may be a sequela of chronic lateral ankle sprains with ligament injury. At the forefoot, sesamoid and MTP joint injuries, synovitis, and adventitial bursa formation may be observed.[20]

KNEE

Given the nature of the game of basketball with jumping, intermittent sprints, and frequent stops and starts, it is no surprise that knee injuries, both acute and those caused by overuse, are quite common. A study of young elite basketball players by the Australian Institute of Sport over a 6-year period revealed that 18.8% of all injuries were at the knee followed by 16.6% at the ankle. Although ankle sprains were the most common injury diagnosis, the multiplicity of injuries at the knee contributed to the higher incidence at that location.[28]

MR imaging of the Asymptomatic Knee

Several studies have focused on MR imaging findings at the knee in active but asymptomatic basketball players. These findings illustrate the daily wear and tear on the knee that is sustained in competitive basketball. In a study of asymptomatic collegiate basketball players by Major and

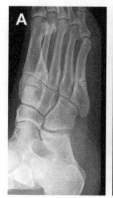
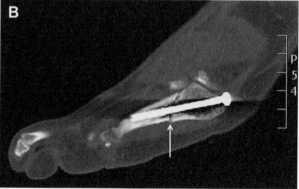

Fig. 13. Jones fracture in a 21-year-old basketball player. (*A*) Internal oblique radiograph of the right foot. There is a typical proximal diaphyseal fracture. (*B*) Sagittal reconstructed CT scan 2.5 months postoperatively, demonstrating the screw placement and persistence of the fracture line (*arrow*). The fracture subsequently healed.

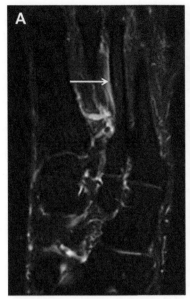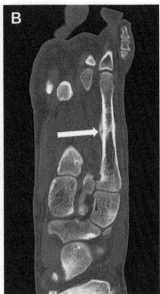

Fig. 14. Stress fracture in the third metatarsal in a 30-year-old professional basketball player. (*A*) Axial STIR image of the forefoot demonstrates minimal periosteal high signal intensity along the shaft of the third metatarsal (*arrow*). A fracture was not demonstrated at this time. (*B*) Coronal reformatted CT image 6 weeks later demonstrates a healing stress fracture with periosteal new bone formation (*arrow*).

Helms,[29] 74% had at least one abnormal finding. Most common abnormalities included bone marrow edema (41%), articular cartilage abnormality (41%), joint effusion (35%), and patellar tendon signal abnormality (24%) (**Fig. 17**). There were no meniscal tears. Kaplan and colleagues[30] described asymptomatic articular cartilage lesions in 47.5% of players who had passed their preseason physical examination. Lesions in the patellofemoral cartilage were more commonly

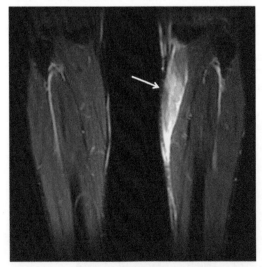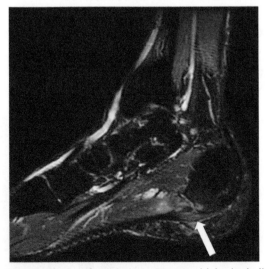

Fig. 15. Gastrocnemius contusion in a 26-year-old professional basketball player. Coronal STIR image demonstrates high signal intensity edema in the proximal gastrocnemius muscle (*arrow*). There is a feathered appearance in the medial head of the gastrocnemius.

Fig. 16. Plantar fasciitis in a 21-year-old basketball player. Sagittal STIR image demonstrates thickening and indistinctness of the proximal plantar fascia (*arrow*). There is mild soft tissue edema and minimal osseous edema of the inferior aspect of the calcaneus (*arrow*).

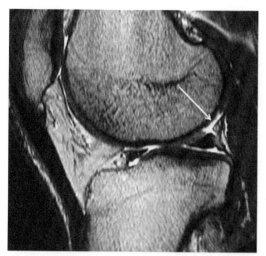

Fig. 17. Asymptomatic chondral defect in the left knee in a 29-year-old professional basketball player. Sagittal T2 weighted image demonstrates a focal full-thickness chondral defect of the posterior lateral femoral condyle (*arrow*).

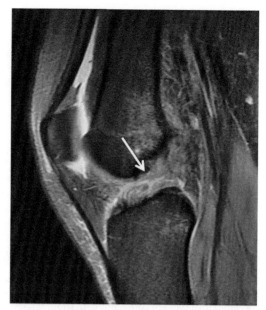

Fig. 18. Acute tear of the ACL in a 19-year-old division I female basketball player. Sagittal STIR sequence through the injured knee demonstrates disruption of ACL fibers (*arrow*). The remaining ACL fibers are amorphous and wavy with areas of discontinuity. Other sequences demonstrated the associated bone contusions in the lateral femoral condyle and lateral tibial plateau. (*Courtesy of* Diane English, MD, Brighton, MA)

observed than those in the femorotibial joint. Elevated intrameniscal signal was documented in 20%, chiefly in the medial meniscus.

Acute Knee Ligament Injuries

Anterior cruciate ligament (ACL) tears are a severe injury resulting in significant loss of playing time and lengthy rehabilitation after surgical repair. From an epidemiologic standpoint, ACL injury in basketball players shows a strong female predilection; this is not the case with many other orthopedic injuries, which affect men and women more equally.[6,13,31] In a meta-analysis of incidence of ACL injury as a function of gender and sport, the female to male ratio was 3.5:1 in basketball, 2.67:1 in soccer, and 1:1 in alpine skiing.[32] In a review of injuries sustained in collegiate women's basketball at the University of Connecticut, women experienced ACL injuries at 2 to 4 times the rate of male basketball players (**Fig. 18**).[33]

A study performed by the International Olympic Committee attributed the increased risk of ACL injury in female athletes to the following risk factors: an elevated risk in the preovulatory phase of the menstrual cycle, decreased intercondylar notch width on radiographs, and a predisposition to increased knee abduction on landing in female athletes.[34] The role of intercondylar notch width as a risk factor for ACL injury in women has been disputed by other investigators. In an 11-year prospective study of male athletes, notch width was not a predictor of subsequent ACL injury.[35]

The mechanism of injury to the ACL in basketball is more commonly noncontact as compared with football in which contact between players typically results in ACL tear. In basketball, deceleration and/or sudden change in direction may cause abnormal rotation of the tibia, resulting in ACL injury.[36] Krosshaug and colleagues[37] studied the mechanism of ACL tear in 39 basketball players via a video analysis of each injury. Of the 39 injuries, 11 involved contact; the remainder were noncontact injuries. Mean flexion angle was higher in female players, and valgus knee collapse also occurred more frequently in women.

Although many competitive basketball players return to action after ACL reconstruction, in others the injury is career ending. A recent study reviewed the performance outcomes of ACL reconstruction in NBA players. Twenty-two percent of players did not return to competition. Of the individuals who returned, 44% experienced a significant decrease in player efficiency rating, which is compiled based on data such as games played, field goal percentage, and turnovers per game.[38]

In contrast to ACL tears, injuries to the posterior cruciate ligament (PCL) are exceedingly rare in basketball. Treatment for isolated PCL tears is generally nonoperative (**Fig. 19**). Surgical repair

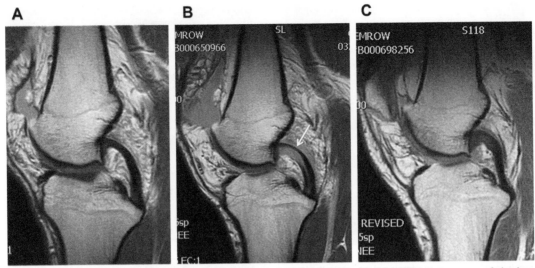

Fig. 19. Recurrent PCL strain in a 32-year-old professional basketball player. (*A*) Sagittal PD image of the knee demonstrates a normal PCL. (*B*) Sagittal PD image 1 year later shows a thickened PCL with increased signal intensity within the ligament consistent with strain related to a hyperextension injury (*arrow*). (*C*) At a follow-up scan 3 months later, sagittal PD image shows healing of the PCL strain with some residual proximal thickening and slight increase in signal intensity.

of the PCL may be pursued in the setting of multiple ligament injury.[39]

Overuse Injuries

Overuse injuries at the knee predominate at the extensor apparatus. Some investigators consider the entity jumper's knee to apply to tendinosis occurring anywhere along the extensor mechanism from quadriceps tendon to the tibial tubercle and not exclusively to that involving the proximal patellar tendon (Fig. 20).[40] In a 10-year prospective study of injury and illness in the NBA, patellofemoral inflammation accounted for 8.1% of orthopedic injuries, second only to ankle sprains, and resulted in 803 missed days. The investigator concluded, "patellofemoral inflammation may be the 'silent endemic' among basketball players."[7]

Injuries to the extensor mechanism, including the patellofemoral joint, in basketball appear to result from the eccentric muscle contraction inherent in sudden decelerations and jumping. These mechanisms may lead to microscopic tendon tear, especially in the proximal patellar tendon. Similarly, excessive force generated across the patellofemoral articulation may result in overuse injury, particularly in individuals with underlying joint malalignment. Severe and long-standing abnormal stress may even lead to patellar or quadriceps tendon rupture or patellar stress fractures.[40]

MR imaging in the axial and sagittal planes readily depicts injuries to the extensor mechanism and patellofemoral joint. Patellar tendinosis manifests as abnormal thickening and elevated signal in the proximal patellar tendon.[41,42] In the distal

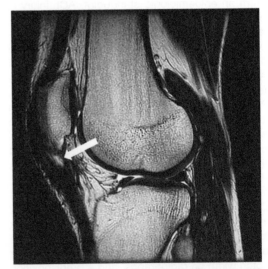

Fig. 20. Jumper's knee and patellar tendinosis in a 29-year-old professional basketball player. Sagittal T2 image illustrates thickening of the proximal patellar tendon. In addition, there is increased signal intensity in the substance of the thickened patellar tendon (*arrow*). The patient subsequently had season-ending surgery to repair the tendinosis.

quadriceps tendon, there are normal striations of signal elevation. With tendinosis signal abnormalities are more pronounced, with a more globular appearance and tendon thickening. Extensor mechanism rupture, including degree of retraction or separation of tendon fibers, is also readily depicted on MR images.[42,43]

The extensor mechanism is also easily evaluated with sonography. Tendinosis manifests as localized tendon thickening and abnormal hypoechogenicity. One study revealed that ultrasonography and MR imaging had similar specificities for the detection of patellar tendinosis, but ultrasonography demonstrated a higher sensitivity for the diagnosis.[44] Tendon rupture is also readily assessed with ultrasonography.[45]

Early patellofemoral arthrosis in basketball players may be asymptomatic.[29] Whether or not symptoms are present, patellofemoral chondromalacia may manifest as cartilage signal alteration, fissuring, or fibrillation (Fig. 21). Focal cartilage defects along patella and/or trochlea may be observed, often with underlying subchondral cysts or bone marrow edema. In all cases of cartilage injury, careful interrogation of the entire knee joint is required to exclude cartilaginous bodies.

PELVIS AND HIP

Although not as frequent as injuries to the ankle and knee, injuries to the pelvis, hip, and upper thigh in basketball players are moderately common. These injuries chiefly involve muscles and tendons with osseous and articular injuries occurring with a significantly lower prevalence.

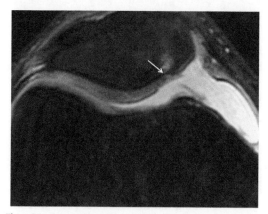

Fig. 21. Asymptomatic chondromalacia patella in a 30-year-old professional basketball player. Axial PD fat-saturated image shows focal chondromalacia and subchondral edema of the right medial patella facet (*arrow*).

In a 16-year longitudinal study of injuries in the NCAA men's basketball program, injuries to the pelvis, hip, and upper leg accounted for approximately 10% of game-related injuries and greater than 11% of injuries sustained during practice. The specific injuries identified were musculotendinous strains and contusions.[5] In the United States High School Sports-Related Injury Surveillance Study conducted between 2005 and 2007, injuries to the hip, thigh, and upper leg comprised 8.2% of injuries in boys and 8.7% in girls.[4] In a review of injuries over 2 consecutive seasons in professional men's and women's basketball teams, hip and groin injuries were relatively infrequent (2.8% and 2.9%, respectively). However, thigh injuries were more prevalent, comprising 11.9% of injuries in women and 6.5% in men.[1]

In the authors' own experience of providing imaging consultation to an NBA men's team for over 2 decades, most injuries occurring about the pelvis, hips, and upper thighs were composed of musculotendinous strains and contusions (Fig. 22), which included adductor and rectus abdominis strains (Fig. 23), hamstring injuries (Fig. 24), and thigh muscle contusions. In contrast to the ankle and foot, where stress injuries were common, hip stress fracture was exceedingly rare. In addition, very few players presented with symptoms of internal derangement at the hip; MR arthrography of the hip was rarely obtained in this population.

UPPER EXTREMITY

Basketball injuries to the upper extremity are far less frequent than those involving the lower extremity. Of upper extremity injuries, those in the hand and arm predominate over injuries to the shoulder or elbow.[19] Upper extremity injuries, overall, accounted for 12% to 13% of injuries sustained at both the high school level and professional levels of play.[4,7]

Excluding stress fractures and nasal bone injuries, the fingers and thumb represent the most likely site of acute fracture in basketball players.[6] The proximal interphalangeal joints (PIP) are the most frequently injured sites. At the PIP joints various injuries are observed, including those involving joint capsule and ligaments, closed tendon injuries, and intra-articular fractures. At the distal interphalangeal joint, injuries to the terminal extensor tendon, flexor profundus tendon injuries, as well as fractures and dislocations have been reported.[19,46] "Dunk lacerations" have also been described in basketball players. These injuries occur secondary to the impact of the player's

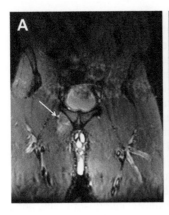
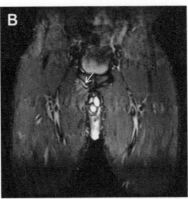

Fig. 22. Groin strain in a 41-year-old professional basketball player. (*A*) Coronal STIR image demonstrates increased signal intensity just distal to the right pubic arch representing a grade I strain in the adductor longus muscle (*arrow*). (*B*) Coronal STIR image shows high signal intensity adjacent to the pubic symphysis (*arrow*), which represents a partial tear of the adductor origin.

hand with sharp edges of the rim or with the flange connecting the rim to the backboard.[47]

At the hand, injuries to the metacarpophalangeal (MCP) joints of the second through fifth rays are observed, as are injuries at the carpometacarpal (CMC) joints of the second through fifth rays. At the ulnar aspect of the hand, dorsal dislocations at the CMC joints may occur. Thumb injuries include fractures at the CMC joint as well as MCP ligament tears (**Fig. 25**).[27]

Suspected fracture and/or dislocation at the hand and wrist are evaluated with conventional radiographs. Complex and intra-articular fractures may benefit from CT with multiplanar image reformation, which is of particular benefit in assessing alignment and fragment position in the setting of CMC fracture/dislocation. Injuries to the joint

capsule, ligaments, and tendons at the hand and wrist are well evaluated by MR imaging or sonography.

Shoulder injuries sustained during basketball are uncommon. In a review of shoulder injuries in high school athletes between 2005 and 2007, the incidence was 0.47 injuries per 10,000 exposures for boys and 0.45 injuries per 10,000 exposures for girls. Injuries were much more commonly sustained during competition than during practice, with most injuries occurring during defending and rebounding (**Fig. 26**).[48] In the NBA, the most

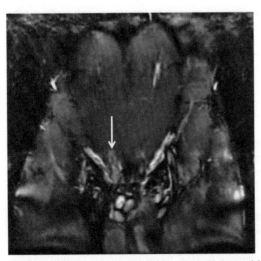

Fig. 23. Rectus abdominis strain in a 32-year-old professional basketball player. Coronal STIR image demonstrates linear areas of increased signal intensity in the distal right rectus abdominis muscle consistent with an abdominal muscle strain (*arrow*).

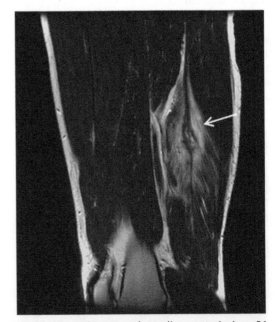

Fig. 24. Hamstring musculotendinous strain in a 31-year-old professional basketball player. Sagittal T2 image of the right femur shows feathery appearance and high signal intensity in the semimembranosus muscle (*arrow*) consistent with grade I musculotendinous strain.

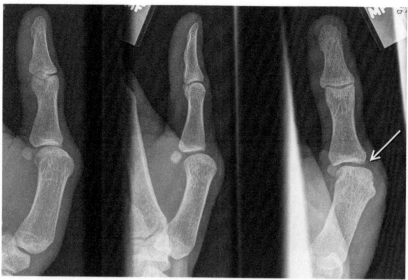

Fig. 25. Radial collateral ligament rupture of the thumb in a 29-year-old professional basketball player. The 3 radiographic views of the left thumb demonstrate ulnar tilt and volar subluxation of the right thumb proximal phalanx in relation to the metacarpal (*arrow*). The patient subsequently underwent surgical repair of the radial collateral ligament of the right thumb MCP joint.

frequently identified shoulder injuries were glenohumeral sprain, acromioclavicular joint sprain (**Fig. 27**), and rotator cuff inflammation.[7]

BACK INJURIES

Back injuries in basketball players are relatively common and account for a substantial proportion of missed games. Despite their relative frequency, a large percentage of these injuries are classified as muscle strains. This classification may account for the low proportion of these injuries that present for imaging evaluation.

Lumbar spine injuries accounted for 6.8% of all injuries sustained by NBA players over a 10-year period but represented 11% of all days missed. Back muscle strain was the most common presentation; disk rupture/herniation was far less prevalent. Cervical spine injuries were significantly less common than lumbar injuries, accounting for 1.3% of injuries overall. Sacral injuries amounted to 0.6% of the total and thoracic spine injuries 0.5% of the total.[7]

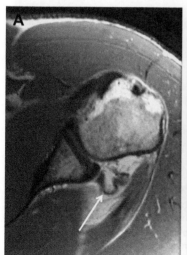
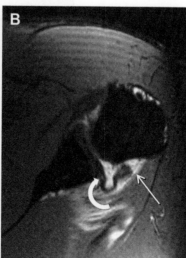

Fig. 26. Posterior shoulder injury in a 21-year-old professional basketball player. (*A*) Axial PD image demonstrates disruption of the posterior shoulder capsule (*arrow*) with edema in the adjacent soft tissues. (*B*) Axial T2* gradient-echo image demonstrates the capsule tear (*arrow*) and edema in the soft tissues secondary to the tear. There is also a posterior labral injury (*curved arrow*). The patient underwent a procedure to repair the posterior capsule and labrum.

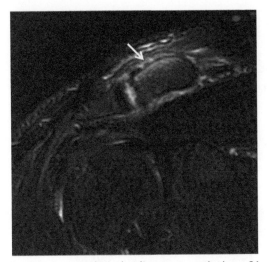

Fig. 27. Acromioclavicular ligament sprain in a 31-year-old professional basketball player. Oblique coronal STIR image of the right shoulder demonstrates mild distal clavicle osseous edema with adjacent superior soft tissue swelling (*arrow*). The patient had symptoms and signs of a grade I acromioclavicular sprain.

Soft tissue injuries, such as muscle strains and contusions, present with localized back pain without radiation to the lower extremities and are treated conservatively with rest and rehabilitation. Symptomatic disk herniations may present with radicular symptoms and are typically evaluated with MR imaging (**Fig. 28**). Radiologists who perform minimally invasive pain management, such as epidural steroid injections, may play an important role in the nonsurgical management of these injuries. Facet syndrome, caused by lumbar facet degenerative changes, may also be managed with fluoroscopically guided facet injection with steroid and anesthetic (**Fig. 29**).[49]

Pars interarticularis defects are an important cause of back pain in young athletes, including basketball players.[49] Pars defects, with or without resultant spondylolisthesis, may be detected on radiographs but are most frequently diagnosed on MR imaging or CT of the lumbar spine (**Fig. 30**). Careful evaluation of the posterior spinal elements, particularly at L5, is critical on cross-sectional imaging studies, even in the absence of spondylolisthesis.

NONORTHOPEDIC INJURIES

Although a detailed discussion of nonorthopedic injuries is beyond the scope of this article, it must be emphasized that these injuries as well as exacerbation of preexisting medical conditions in basketball players are not uncommon. Injuries to the head, face, and neck generally result from a collision with another player. A proportion of these occur during illegal or foul play. Most concussions also result from collision with another player.[4] In the WNBA experience, concussions accounted for 6.5% of all injuries sustained during games and 3.7% of injuries during practices.[6]

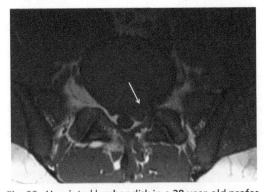

Fig. 28. Herniated lumbar disk in a 28-year-old professional basketball player. Axial T1 image demonstrates a left L5-S1 paracentral disk protrusion, which posteriorly deviates the descending left S1 nerve root sleeve in the lateral recess (*arrow*).

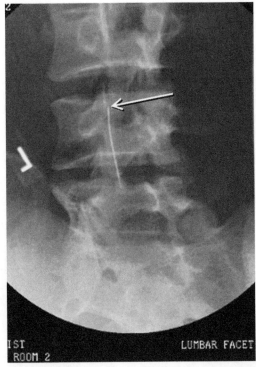

Fig. 29. Facet block in a 31-year-old professional basketball player. Fluoroscopic spot film demonstrates needle placement for a left L3-L4 facet block (*arrow*).

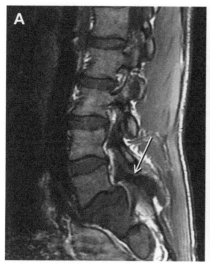
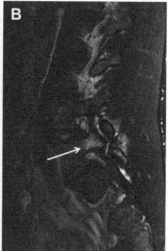

Fig. 30. Spondylolysis and spondylolisthesis L5 in a 23-year-old professional basketball player. (*A*) Sagittal T1 image of the lumbar spine demonstrates right L5-S1 pars interarticularis defect (*arrow*) with grade I spondylolisthesis. (*B*) Sagittal T2 fat-saturated image shows edema around the pars defect as well as fluid in the chronic pars defect with sclerosis of the margins compatible with nonunion (*arrow*).

Concussions were less frequently reported in men's NCAA competition (3.6% of injuries sustained during games)[5] and in NBA competition.[7]

Other basketball injuries to the head and face reported with some frequency include nasal fractures, eye injuries, and dental injuries. Nasal fractures represent 1.5% and 1.7% of injuries in the NBA and NCAA men's competition, respectively.[5,7] Eye injuries range from eyelid lacerations to corneal abrasions to severe orbital fractures and more severe injuries to the globe.[14,50] Oral injuries, particularly to the teeth, have decreased with the increasing use of mouthguards.[14]

Sudden cardiac death in basketball players, although rare, has generated greater interest since the death of Hank Gathers during an NCAA men's game in 1990 and the sudden death of the ex-NBA player Pet Maravich while playing basketball at age 40 years. In most cases, sudden cardiac death in basketball players is caused by a congenital structural cardiac condition, such as hypertrophic cardiomyopathy, Marfan syndrome, or myocarditis.[19,51] Sudden cardiac death in young athletes is often reported in high school or college-age basketball players.[51–53] Prevention of sudden cardiac death requires careful medical screening of prospective players.[19]

SUMMARY

As basketball has increased in popularity among amateur and professional athletes of all ages, there has been an increasing focus on the prevalence and pattern of injuries. Most injuries are orthopedic in nature, and imaging plays an important role in their evaluation and management. MR imaging has supplanted other modalities for the evaluation of soft tissue injuries, including ligament sprain, muscle strain, and occult osseous injuries, including stress fracture.

REFERENCES

1. Zelisko JA, Noble HB, Porter M. A comparison of men's and women's professional basketball injuries. Am J Sports Med 1982;10:297–9.
2. Cumps E, Verhagen E, Meeusen R. Prospective epidemiological study of basketball injuries during one competitive season: ankle sprains and overuse knee injuries. J Sports Sci Med 2007;6: 204–11.
3. Stone WJ, Steingard PM. Year-round conditioning for basketball. Clin Sports Med 1993;12:173–91.
4. Borowski LA, Yard EE, Fields SK, et al. The epidemiology of US high school basketball injuries, 2005-2007. Am J Sports Med 2008;36:2328–35.
5. Dick R, Hertel J, Agel J, et al. Descriptive epidemiology of collegiate men's basketball injuries: National Collegiate Association Injury Surveillance System, 1988-1989 through 2003-2004. J Athl Train 2007;42:194–201.
6. Agel J, Olson DE, Dick R, et al. Descriptive epidemiology of collegiate women's basketball injuries: National Collegiate Association Injury Surveillance System, 1988-1989 through 2003-2004. J Athl Train 2007;42:202–10.
7. Starkey C. Injuries and illnesses in the National Basketball Association: a 10-year perspective. J Athl Train 2000;35:161–7.
8. Deitch JR, Starkey C, Walters SL, et al. Injury risk in professional basketball players: a comparison of Women's National Basketball Association and

National Basketball Association Athletes. Am J Sports Med 2006;34:1077–83.

9. Palmer WE, Kuong SJ, Elmadbouh HM. MR imaging of myotendinous strain. AJR Am J Roentgenol 1999; 173:703–9.

10. Palmer WE, Caslowitz PL, Chew FS. MR arthrography of the shoulder: normal intraarticular structures and common abnormalities. AJR Am J Roentgenol 1995;164:141–6.

11. Kassarjian A, Yoon LS, Belzile E, et al. Triad of MR arthrographic findings in patients with cam-type femoroacetabular impingement. Radiology 2005; 236:588–92.

12. Newman JS. Arthrosonography. Semin Musculoskelet Radiol 1998;2:439–46.

13. Moul JL. Differences in selected predictors of anterior cruciate ligament tears between male and female NCAA division I collegiate basketball players. J Athl Train 1998;33:118–21.

14. Guyette RF. Facial injuries in basketball players. Clin Sports Med 1993;12:247–64.

15. Kofotolis N, Kellis E. Ankle sprain injuries: a 2-year prospective cohort study in female Greek basketball players. J Athl Train 2007;42:388–94.

16. Nelson AJ, Collins CL, Yard EE, et al. Ankle injuries among United States high school athletes, 2005–2006. J Athl Train 2007;42:381–7.

17. Sickles RT, Lombardo JA. The adolescent basketball player. Clin Sports Med 1993;12:207–19.

18. Johnson KA, Teasdell RD. Sprained ankles as they relate to the basketball player. Clin Sports Med 1993;12:363–71.

19. Sonzogni JJ, Gross ML. Assessment and treatment of basketball injuries. Clin Sports Med 1993;12: 221–37.

20. McDermott EP. Basketball injuries of the foot and ankle. Clin Sports Med 1993;12:373–93.

21. Perrich KD, Goodwin DW, Hecht PJ, et al. Ankle ligaments on MRI: appearance of normal and injured ligaments. AJR Am J Roentgenol 2009;193:687–95.

22. O'Loughlin PF, Heyworth BE, Kennedy JG. Current concepts in the diagnosis and treatment of osteochondral lesions of the ankle. Am J Sports Med 2010;38:392–404.

23. Berkowitz MJ, Kim DH. Process and tubercle fractures of the hindfoot. J Am Acad Orthop Surg 2005;13:492–502.

24. Meyer SA, Saltzman CL, Albright JP. Stress fractures of the foot and leg. Clin Sports Med 1993;12:395–413.

25. Kiss ZS, Khan KM, Fuller PJ. Stress fractures of the tarsal navicular bone: CT findings in 55 cases. AJR Am J Roentgenol 1993;160:111–5.

26. Fernandez Fairen M, Guillen J, Busto JM, et al. Fractures of the fifth metatarsal in basketball players. Knee Surg Sports Traumatol Arthrosc 1999;7: 373–7.

27. Major NM. Role of MRI in prevention of metatarsal stress fractures in collegiate basketball players. AJR Am J Roentgenol 2006;186:255–8.

28. Hickey GJ, Fricker PA, McDonald WA. Injuries of young elite female basketball players over a six-year period. Clin J Sport Med 1997;7:252–6.

29. Major NM, Helms CA. MR imaging of the knee: findings in asymptomatic collegiate basketball players. AJR Am J Roentgenol 2002;179:641–4.

30. Kaplan LD, Schurhoff MR, Selesnick H, et al. Magnetic resonance imaging of the knee in asymptomatic professional basketball players. Arthroscopy 2005;21:557–61.

31. Agel J, Arendt EA, Bershadsky B. Anterior cruciate ligament injury in National Collegiate Association Basketball and Soccer: a 13-year review. Am J Sports Med 2005;33:524–31.

32. Prodromos CC, Han Y, Rogowski J, et al. A meta-analysis of the incidence of anterior cruciate ligament tears as a function of gender, sport, and a knee injury-reduction regimen. Arthroscopy 2007;23:1320–5.

33. Trojian TH, Ragle RB. Injuries in women's basketball. Conn Med 2008;72:147–50.

34. Renstrom P, Ljungqvist A, Arendt E, et al. Non-contact ACL injuries in female athletes: an International Olympic Committee current concepts statement. Br J Sports Med 2008;42:394–412.

35. Lombardo S, Sethi PM, Starkey C. Intercondylar notch stenosis is not a risk factor for anterior cruciate ligament tears in professional male basketball players: an 11-year prospective study. Am J Sports Med 2005;33:29–34.

36. Emerson RJ. Basketball knee injuries and the anterior cruciate ligament. Clin Sports Med 1993;12:317–28.

37. Krosshaug T, Nakamae A, Boden BP, et al. Mechanisms of anterior cruciate ligament injury in basketball: video analysis of 39 cases. Am J Sports Med 2007;35:359–67.

38. Busfield BT, Kharrazi FD, Starkey C, et al. Performance outcomes of anterior cruciate ligament reconstruction in the National Basketball Association. Arthroscopy 2009;25:825–30.

39. Moyer RA, Marchetto PA. Injuries of the posterior cruciate ligament. Clin Sports Med 1993;12:307–15.

40. Molnar TJ, Fox JM. Overuse injuries of the knee in basketball. Clin Sports Med 1993;12:349–62.

41. O'Keefe SA, Hogan BA, Eustace SJ, et al. Overuse injuries of the knee. Magn Reson Imaging Clin N Am 2009;17:725–39.

42. Sonin AH, Fitzgerald SW, Bresler ME, et al. MR imaging appearance of the extensor mechanism of the knee: functional anatomy and imaging patterns. Radiographics 1995;15:367–82.

43. Dupuis CS, Westra SJ, Makris J, et al. Injuries and conditions of the extensor mechanism of the pediatric knee. Radiographics 2009;29:877–86.

44. Warden SJ, Kiss ZS, Malara FA, et al. Comparative accuracy of magnetic resonance imaging and ultrasonography in confirming clinically diagnosed patellar tendinopathy. Am J Sports Med 2007;35:427–36.

45. LaRocco BG, Zlupko G, Sierzenski P. Ultrasound diagnosis of quadriceps tendon rupture. J Emerg Med 2008;35:293–5.

46. Wilson RL, McGinty LD. Common hand and wrist injuries in basketball players. Clin Sports Med 1993;265–91.

47. Kirk AA. Dunk lacerations—unusual injuries to the hands in basketball players. JAMA 1979;242:415.

48. Bonza JE, Fields SK, Yard EE, et al. Shoulder injuries among United States high school athletes during the 2005-2006 and 2006-2007 school years. J Athl Train 2009;44:76–83.

49. Herskowitz A, Selenick H. Back injuries in basketball players. Clin Sports Med 1993;12:293–306.

50. Zagelbaum BM, Starkey C, Hersh PS, et al. The National Basketball Association eye injury study. Arch Ophthalmol 1995;113:749–52.

51. Maron BJ, Gohman TE, Aeppli D. Prevalence of sudden cardiac death during competitive sports activities in Minnesota high school athletes. J Am Coll Cardiol 1998;32:1881–4.

52. Drezner JA, Rogers KJ. Sudden cardiac arrest in intercollegiate athletes: detailed analysis and outcomes of resuscitation in nine cases. Heart Rhythm 2006;3:755–9.

53. Subasic K. Athletes at sudden risk for cardiac death. J Sch Nurs 2010;26:18–25.

Skiing and Snowboarding Injuries: A Review with a Focus on Mechanism of Injury

Luke H. Deady, MD[a,b],*, David Salonen, MD[a]

KEYWORDS

- Skiing • Snowboarding • Imaging • Mechanism of injury

Snow skiing in one form or another has been pursued for many years and may date back as long as 5000 years when hunters and fishermen used animal tusks to traverse snow. Competitive skiing started in Norway in 1767, and within 100 years, it was a well-established pastime in Scandinavian countries.[1] It was the 1932 Winter Olympics at Lake Placid that saw a rapid rise in the popularity of skiing.[2] Today skiing is a sport enjoyed by approximately 200 million people worldwide. With an injury rate at around 3 per 1000 skier days, it is certainly a risky sport,[3] and with modern equipment allowing participants to push into higher speeds and more challenging terrain, there has been an evolution in the types and frequency of injuries being seen. The advent of modern boot and binding technology has also seen a shift in injury patterns, with a significant reduction in the number of ankle injuries at the expense of the knee and proximal tibia.[4]

By comparison, snowboarding is a young sport, which has evolved rapidly during the last 30 to 40 years, with the first modern style boards being patented in the early 1970s. The year 1980 marked the year of the first world snowboard competition,[5] with snowboarding being featured in the Winter Olympics for the first time at Nagano in 1998. There has been a huge increase in the popularity of snowboarding recently, with an estimated 80% of children who participate in snow sports having ridden a snowboard by the age of 12 years.[6]

The upper extremity is injured nearly twice as often in snowboarding than skiing, with approximately 50% of injuries involving this region,[7–9] and fractures occur more than twice as frequently as in Alpine skiers.[10] Wrist injuries, particularly fractures, are the most common snowboarding injuries.[7–9] Fracture of the lateral process of the talus, which was previously a rare injury, is now a well-recognized injury pattern in the snowboarder. Knee injuries in snowboarders are usually less severe, with one series reporting a complete ligament rupture in only 2 of 62 reported knee injuries.[10]

SKIING INJURIES
Knee Injuries

With the advent of modern ski boots and binding systems that have been designed to reduce the incidence of ankle injury and lower leg fractures, there has subsequently been an increase in the number of significant knee injuries occurring in Alpine skiers.[1] Since the early 1980s, the number of severe anterior cruciate ligament (ACL)

[a] Division of Musculoskeletal Radiology, Department of Medical Imaging, University of Toronto University Health Network, Toronto Western Hospital, 3MC422, 399 Bathurst Street, Toronto, ON M5T 2S8, Canada
[b] Department of Medical Imaging, Royal Prince Alfred Hospital, Missendon Road, Camperdown, NSW 2050, Australia
* Corresponding author. Department of Medical Imaging, Royal Prince Alfred Hospital, Missendon Road, Camperdown, NSW 2050, Australia.
E-mail address: lukedeady@hotmail.com

Radiol Clin N Am 48 (2010) 1113–1124
doi:10.1016/j.rcl.2010.07.005

disruptions has increased at an alarming rate, with the trend continuing.[11,12]

Injuries to the knee account for one-third of all injuries in adult skiers,[13,14] whereas the rate in children and adolescents is half this number.[14]

Most investigators agree that injury to the medial collateral ligament (MCL) is the commonest knee injury in skiers, accounting for 20% to 25% of all injuries[15]; however, MCL injuries are usually grade I or grade II sprains generally treated nonoperatively. Others believe that a complete rupture of the ACL is the commonest knee injury in adult skiers,[14] and these injuries are often complete ruptures (**Fig. 1**). ACL injury rates in Alpine skiers are amongst the highest in sport,[16] and as seen in other sports, injury rates are significantly higher in female skiers. One study has shown the rate of ACL disruption in women to be double the disruption rate in men[17] and this has been attributed to relative quadriceps weakness, narrower intercondylar notch dimensions, increased joint laxity, and hormonal influences.[18,19]

Because ACL injuries often lead to ongoing instability and the development of secondary osteoarthritis (OA), they are among the most clinically significant injuries to the knee.

Mechanisms of injury

Several common mechanisms are seen in skiers, which differ from the usual mechanisms seen.

Valgus-external rotation This mechanism is the classic mechanism whereby the skier catches the inside edge of the front of the ski, resulting in external rotation of the tibia. As the skiers' momentum continues forward, the lower leg is abducted and externally rotated with a valgus force being exerted on the knee.[20] The leverage created by the length of the ski significantly magnifies the torque acting on the knee. This mechanism usually results in an injury to the MCL; however, in 20% of cases the ACL is also torn.[16,21]

Boot-induced anterior drawer This mechanism occurs when landing a jump, with the center of gravity too far back, known as "being in the back seat".[4] The tail of the ski lands first, levering the tibia anteriorly via force transmitted through the top of the boot and creating an anterior drawer effect, which usually results in an isolated ACL disruption.

Flexion-internal rotation (the phantom foot injury mechanism) The off-balance skier sits with the weight back on the skis and catches an inside edge on the snow, resulting in sudden internal rotation of the knee that continues to flex. The back of the ski provides the torque required to rupture the ACL. This mechanism is believed to be the commonest cause of ACL injury at present.[22]

Other proposed mechanisms include hyperextension injuries and also forceful quadriceps contraction as the skiers try to shift their weight forward after being off balance at the back of the ski. Aggressive quadriceps contraction with the knee in slight flexion can produce significant anterior translation of the tibia and resultant ACL injury.[23]

Reports of the incidence of meniscal tears in association with ACL tears in skiers range from 23% to 55%,[24–26] which is less than the figures reported generally in athletes with ACL tears, which range from 62% to 65%.[26–29] Lateral meniscal

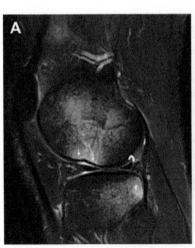
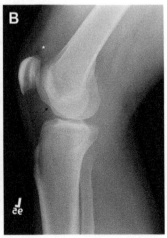

Fig. 1. (*A*) Sagittal fast spin echo (FSE) fat-suppressed T2-weighted image. Left knee demonstrating T2 hyperintense edema within the lateral femoral condyle with a subchondral fracture (*white arrows*) as well as edema within the posterolateral tibial plateau (*white asterisk*) with an effusion secondary to an acute ACL disruption with a pivot-shift pattern of bone marrow edema in a 26–year-old female skier. Note the associated vertical tear through the posterior horn of the lateral meniscus (*curved white arrow*). This type of meniscal tear is often associated with ACL disruptions. (*B*) Same patient as in **Fig.** 1A: there is deepening of the sulcus terminalis (*black arrow*), a plain film finding that is highly associated with an ACL tear. Note also a small effusion within the suprapatellar pouch (*white asterisk*).

tears associated with ACL and MCL tears are more common, with one study reporting a 43% incidence of a torn lateral meniscus versus a 13% incidence of medial meniscal tears.[30] Another group reported a 9 times higher incidence of ACL/MCL/lateral meniscal tears versus ACL/MCL/medial meniscal tears.[25]

Injuries to the lateral collateral ligament (LCL) are relatively uncommon, with 1 investigator reporting a 3% association between LCL injuries and ACL tears.[24] Posterior cruciate ligament (PCL) and knee dislocations are also rarely reported but dislocations are important to recognize. Knee dislocation is a significant injury, and MR imaging demonstrating multiligamentous disruption is often needed to assist in making the diagnosis because it often spontaneously reduces shortly after the injury (**Fig. 2**). A patient with a dislocation may demonstrate evidence of multiligamentous disruption without definite evidence of a dislocation.[31] The popliteal artery and common peroneal nerve are prone to injury in this setting of knee dislocation, and therefore, the possibility of vascular and neural injuries should be considered.

Imaging

MCL injuries are assessed well clinically. MR imaging has been shown to correlate well with the clinical assessment of MCL injury.[32] The advantage of MR imaging is that it allows

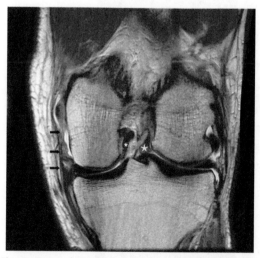

Fig. 2. Coronal FSE PD left knee in a 20-year-old male skier with left knee dislocation. Extensive thickening and complete discontinuity of medial collateral ligament compatible with a complete disruption of both deep and superficial fibers (*black arrows*). Note marked signal abnormality within the ACL (*yellow asterisk*) and PCL (*white asterisk*). Complete tears of both these ligaments were confirmed on sagittal imaging.

assessment of associated ligamentous, cartilaginous, and meniscal injuries.

MR imaging is accurate in the diagnosis of complete disruption of the ACL, with a sensitivity of 87%[33] to 94%[34] and specificity of 91%[33] to 94%,[34] although there is some reduction in accuracy when diagnosing partial tears. Using all 3 imaging planes and looking for abnormal signal intensity, orientation, caliber, and fiber discontinuity is useful in determining whether a partial tear is present.[15] Close scrutiny of the posterolateral bundle near the femoral attachment is required as this is a common place for a partial tear.[35] Complete ACL tears in skiers most commonly involve the proximal 1/3.[35] The presence of bone marrow edema indicates that a tear is at least a high-grade partial if not complete tear, although this does not hold true in the child and adolescent population in whom ligamentous avulsions and ligamentous laxity may also result in bone marrow edema.

Fractures of the Lower Leg

With the advent of modern stiff ski boots, the incidence of ankle ligamentous injuries and fractures has declined significantly since the early 1970s, with the reduction in injury rates being reported as high as 92%.[36] Much improved binding release systems have also seen a significant reduction in cases of spiral tibial fractures; however, poorly adjusted bindings remain a significant problem. One group found that 95% of all bindings tested had at least 1 fault, and 50% of bindings have release settings at least 20% above the recommended standards. When a group of skiers were compared with a group in whom the bindings had been adjusted properly, the nonadjusted group suffered 4 times the incidence of binding-related injuries.[37]

Paralleling the rise in numbers of ligamentous injuries, there has also been a rise in the number of tibial plateau fractures. This rise probably reflects the same phenomenon, resulting in a rise in the number of ACL injuries, namely increased forces being transmitted to the knee.[3] Valgus-type loads on the knee typically result in fractures of the anterolateral tibial plateau, which may or may not be associated with a disruption of the MCL.[3] Tensile ligamentous injuries are more common, however, than the compressive type forces, resulting in fractures of the tibial plateau or femoral condyles.

Fractures of the tibial shaft are a result of failure of the ski binding to release with bending at the cuff of the boot that generates sufficient torque to result in bony failure. This fracture pattern has been named the boot top fracture because of the leverage created at the top of the stiff ski boot cuff.

Imaging

Plain films usually suffice in assessment of tibial fractures. Computed tomography (CT) does add valuable information particularly in characterizing the intra-articular extent of tibial plateau fractures.

Thumb Injuries

Injury to the ulnar collateral ligament (UCL) of the thumb was first described by Campbell[38] as an occupational hazard in Scottish gamekeepers who injured the UCL in the process of killing wounded rabbits, hence the term "gamekeepers' thumb." Now it is also referred to as "skiers' thumb" because of the high prevalence of this injury in Alpine skiers.[39] Today, a skiing fall is the commonest cause of an acute UCL injury,[40] and thumb injuries are the commonest injuries sustained in skiing.[3,41]

Injuries to the UCL and adductor aponeurosis lead to weakness of pinch and grasp strength, with chronic instability leading to the development of secondary OA.[42–45]

Mechanism of injury

Injuries occur during falls, with the pole maintained in the hand, resulting in forced abduction and extension at the metacarpophalangeal (MCP) joint.[3,39–41,46–49] A significant component of the injury may also result from the fact that skiers fall past the thumb as their continued downhill momentum pushes them down the slope, resulting in a severe valgus load at the MCP joint of the thumb, thus resulting in injury to the UCL.[3] The leverage provided by the pole results in considerable forces acting across the MCP joint, and consequently a high number of Stener lesions are encountered. In a Stener lesion, the distal ruptured end of the UCL is displaced and the ulnar expansion of the dorsal aponeurosis is interposed between the ligament and the site of its attachment to the proximal phalanx,[46] which often results in a painful, palpable lump at the site of the "balled-up" ligament.

Some investigators suggest that the use of pole straps increases the risk of thumb injuries and as such, postulate that the number of injuries can be reduced by skiing without using the straps.[41,50]

Imaging

Plain radiographs are the first-line investigation in the assessment of injury to the thumb. Observed fracture rates are in the range of 23.3% to 27.5% (Fig. 3).[41] If no fracture is identified, clinical assessment of ligamentous injury then guides the need for further imaging. Pain and swelling as well as the concern of exacerbating injury can

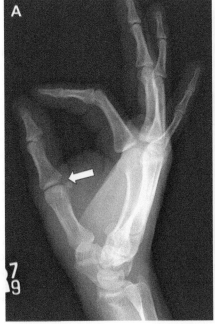
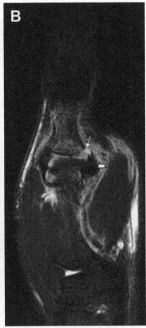

Fig. 3. (A) An avulsion fracture with proximal displacement at the distal attachment of the ulnar collateral ligament of the thumb (*white arrow*). (B) Same patient as in Fig. 3A. Coronal FSE fat-suppressed T2-weighted image demonstrates avulsion of distal UCL attachment (*thin white arrow*) with the balled-up hypointense retracted ligament (*thick white arrow*). Extensive surrounding soft tissue edema is also seen.

make physical examination challenging, and therefore, imaging where the integrity of the ligament can be visualized is helpful in determining best management.

MR imaging is able to characterize tears of the UCL complex. The intact ligament is seen as a taut hypointense band running along the ulnar margin of the MCP joint deep to the adductor aponeurosis. A partial tear is diagnosed when there is signal hyperintensity traversing the ligament or a complete tear when there is total discontinuity of the ligament. A Stener lesion is seen as a retracted balled-up UCL lying superficial to the adductor aponeurosis referred to as a "yoyo" on a string, with the ligament representing the yoyo and the intact aponeurosis representing the string. Coronal T2 fast spin echo sequences are the most useful for assessing ligamentous integrity (Fig. 4).[51]

MR imaging has been shown to be accurate in discerning between displaced and nondisplaced UCL tears in cadaveric specimens with sensitivity and specificity of 100% and 94%, respectively.[52] Noncadaveric studies have reported sensitivity and specificity of 90% to 100% and 87% to 100%, respectively.[53,54] Chronic UCL injuries are accurately assessed with MR imaging; however,

the differentiation between Stener and non-Stener type injuries is more difficult in the chronic setting because of adjacent scar tissue.[51]

Ultrasound is also an effective method of assessing the UCL and has the advantage of allowing dynamic assessment and is less time consuming than MR imaging. The positive predictive value of ultrasound for detecting ruptures of the UCL has been shown to be 94% versus 80% for clinical examination in the hands of specialist hand surgeons.[55]

Shoulder Injuries in Skiers and Snowboarders

Following thumb injuries, shoulder injuries are the second commonest injury to the upper limb in skiing, with instances reported as 4% to 11% of all ski injuries,[41,56,57] and 22% to 41% of upper extremity injuries.[56] The rate of shoulder injuries during Alpine skiing is in the range of 0.2 to 0.5 injuries per 1000 skier days. Shoulder injuries account for 8% to 16% of all injuries and 20% to 34% of upper extremity injuries in snowboarders.[56]

The commonest shoulder injuries are rotator cuff tears, anterior dislocations of the glenohumeral joint, acromioclavicular joint injuries, and clavicular fractures. Less common injuries include

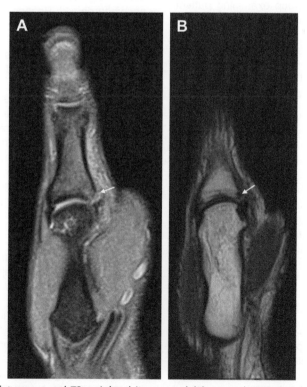

Fig. 4. (A) Coronal FSE fat-suppressed T2-weighted image and (B) coronal FSE PD right thumb demonstrating a complete tear of the UCL at the distal attachment with slight retraction (white arrow).

greater tuberosity fractures, trapezius strains, proximal humeral fractures, biceps strains, glenoid fractures, scapula fractures, humeral head fractures, sternoclavicular separations, and acromial fractures.[56]

Mechanism of injury

Falls are the commonest method of injury with either a direct blow, axial loading from an outstretched arm, or eccentric muscle contraction associated with shoulder abduction during a fall.[56] Pole planting during skiing and aerial maneuvers during snowboarding are also common causes. Anterior dislocations usually occur during a fall, with the shoulder abducted and excessively externally rotated.

The most common mechanism of injury to the acromioclavicular (AC) joint during skiing or snowboarding is a direct fall on the acromion.[56]

Clavicular fractures result from downward forces acting on the shoulder as in AC joint injuries or from a direct blow to the clavicle; the majority of fractures tend to involve the middle third.

Proximal humeral fractures tend to occur from a fall on an outstretched hand with axial loading along the shaft of the humerus.

Rotator cuff tears generally occur during resisted abduction occurring during a fall and can be seen in association with glenohumeral joint dislocations. One group examining patients older than 40 years with first anterior shoulder dislocations occurring during skiing found a 35% associated incidence of rotator cuff tear with a 40% incidence when there was a greater tuberosity fracture and 100% with neurologic deficits involving primarily the axillary nerve (**Fig. 5**).[58]

Imaging

Plain radiographs are the initial imaging modality of choice. These should ideally include an axillary view, and postreduction views in the case of glenohumeral dislocation should assess for the presence of Hill-Sachs and Bankart fractures. Additional Garth or Stryker view may be helpful to assess for Bankart fractures.

MR imaging is the imaging modality of choice in assessing injuries to the rotator cuff and labrocapsular injury (**Fig. 6**).

SNOWBOARDING INJURIES
Lateral Process of Talar Fractures

Fractures of the lateral process of the talus (LPT) were considered rare injuries before the increase in popularity of snowboarding, with the few reported cases in the literature occurring usually as a result of motor vehicle accidents or falls

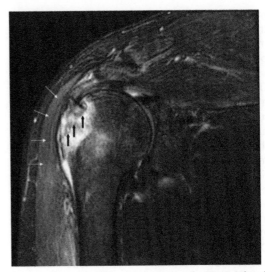

Fig. 5. Coronal FSE fat-suppressed T2-weighted image. Right shoulder demonstrates a fracture of the greater tuberosity (*black arrows*). Note the mild edema within the deltoid muscle (*white arrows*) secondary to traction on axillary nerve at the time of glenohumeral joint dislocation.

from a height[59] and only accounted for 0.86% of ankle fractures.[60] These fractures are being seen with increasing frequency in snowboarders, accounting for 32% of ankle fractures seen in snowboarders.[61] Recognition of this fracture is important because they can masquerade as an anterolateral ankle ligamentous sprain. Also one needs a high index of suspicion because of the fact that they are often difficult to diagnose on plain radiographs. These fractures are often in close proximity to articular surfaces, and intra-articular extension to the ankle joint, the posterior subtalar joint or both is common. Misdiagnosis as a ligamentous sprain may result in inappropriate management and complications, such as nonunion, malunion, or ankle and subtalar joint OA, which can lead to significant morbidity in a young and active patient population.[15,60,62,63]

Mechanism of injury

It is well documented that fractures of the LPT are the result of high-energy injuries.[64]

There is some controversy as to the exact mechanism of injury. It is generally agreed that significant axial loading is involved. Many investigators believe that in addition dorsiflexion and inversion are important components to this type of injury.[10,59,61,65]

Other investigators have demonstrated that a component of external rotation is critical in producing the fracture.[64] This component results

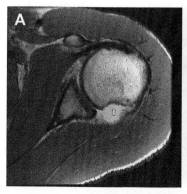 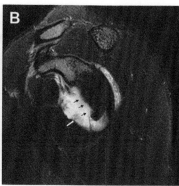

Fig. 6. (A) Left shoulder of a 33-year-old skier with history of dislocation after a fall. Axial FSE PD shows a large Hill-Sachs defect in the posterosuperior humeral head (*white arrow*). (B) Same patient as in Fig. 6A. Sagittal FSE T2 with fat suppression demonstrates an anterior glenoid bony defect consistent with a Bankart fracture (*black arrows*) There is an associated effusion with reactive synovitis (*white arrow*).

in disrupted talocalcaneal congruency, concentrating stress on the LPT.[60,64,65]

Imaging

LPT fractures are difficult to diagnose on plain ankle radiographs because of bony complexity and overlap on standard projections, with as many as 40% to 50% undetected on initial radiographs.[64,66] In addition to standard ankle views, 1 investigator believes that the best radiographic view is the ankle anteroposterior (AP) view with 45° of internal rotation and 30° of plantarflexion,[67] whereas another found an AP view with 20° of internal rotation and neutral plantarflexion to be most helpful.[60] However, the clinician needs to have a low threshold for proceeding to cross-sectional imaging in the snowboarder with antero-lateral pain due to the commonly plain film occult nature of these fractures and also due to the inability of plain films to define the full extent and degree of displacement of these fractures. CT with direct coronal imaging or fine coronal reconstructions is the imaging modality of choice as MR imaging may not be able to distinguish a small cortical avulsion type injury from an adjacent ligamentous injury (Fig. 7).

BOOT-RELATED SOFT TISSUE INJURIES IN SKIERS AND SNOWBOARDERS
Malleolar and Adventitial Bursae

Bursae are fluid containing sacs found throughout the body in regions where tissues are mobile and subject to forces of friction. These bursae reduce friction and allow movement at tissue interfaces. Adventitious bursae develop in areas of the body that are subject to repeated trauma and friction, such as the malleoli in the skier or snowboarder. Bursae do not normally occur at the ankle, and these newly developed bursae are suboptimal in acting as protective structures.[68] They are characterized by thicker fibrous walls and are more prone to becoming inflamed.[68] Chronic irritation of

existing adventitious bursa from an ill-fitting boot may lead to the development of a painful, inflamed mass.

Imaging

Plain radiographs may demonstrate soft tissue swelling localized over the bony promontories of the malleoli. No bone abnormalities are seen.

Bursae are well demonstrated with ultrasound and MR imaging showing fluid containing, lobulated, and septated lesions with varying levels of complexity to the contents.

Pseudotumor of the Lower Leg and Ankle

Chronic irritation of the soft tissue of the lower leg may result in inflammatory reactions in the subcutaneous tissues that are not associated with the formation of adventitial bursae. These tend to occur more in the supramalleolar region and more commonly laterally.[15] The presumed cause is subcutaneous fat compression and shearing between the boot, fibula, and the peroneal muscle group.[69] Chronic repetitive injury is thought to result in localized fat necrosis, with inflammation and fibrosis resulting in a mass-like appearance.

Imaging

MR imaging typically demonstrates loss of T1 hyperintense fat signal, which appears more isointense to muscle and hyperintense on T2-weighted imaging as well as enhancement after intravenous administration of gadolinium. There may be evidence of bone stress in the distal fibula, which typically occurs slightly more proximally to the soft tissue abnormality.[69]

ELBOW, FOREARM, AND WRIST INJURIES

The most common site of upper limb injuries in snowboarders is the wrist. One study of 7430 snowboarding-related injuries found 3645 upper limb injuries of which the most common site of injury was the wrist, accounting for 21.6% of all

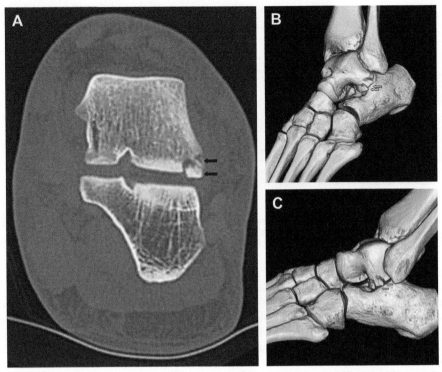

Fig. 7. (*A*) Coronal CT reconstruction on the left talus. Twenty-five-year-old snowboarder with anterolateral ankle pain following hyperdorsiflexion injury demonstrating a fracture through the lateral process of the talus (*black arrows*). (*B*) Same patient as in **Fig.** 7A. 3-dimensional (3D) volume-rendered reconstruction again demonstrates the fracture of the lateral process of the talus (*white arrows*). (*C*) Same patient as in **Fig.** 7A and 7B. 3D volume-rendered reconstruction. The fracture is clearly seen to extend to involve the posterior subtalar facet (*white arrows*).

snowboarding injuries.[70] Wrist injuries accounted for 44% of all upper extremity injuries, with 78% of wrist injuries being fractures. Wrist fractures, except for scaphoid fractures, occurred predominantly in beginners, accounting for 34% of all injuries in the beginner group. Upper limb injuries are more common with backward falls toward the heelside of the board.

Intermediate to advanced snowboarders tended to have higher-energy injuries, resulting in more scaphoid fractures and more severe distal radial fractures than the beginner group. Lunate or perilunate fractures and dislocations are also reported in the expert group, which are a result of a backward fall following an aerial maneuver (**Fig. 8**).

Elbow and forearm injuries are relatively less common, accounting for approximately 8% and 5% of upper extremity injuries, respectively. These injuries are, however, more common in the Alpine skiing population. UCL injuries of the thumb are rarely seen, accounting for approximately 2% of upper extremity injuries.[70] Monteggia and Galeazzi injury patterns are infrequently reported.[70]

Mechanism of Injury

The vast majority of all wrist injuries are a result of a fall. Backward falls result in twice as many fractures as forward falls. It has been reported that snowboarders who wear protective wrist guards are half as likely to sustain wrist injuries as those who did not.

Imaging

Plain radiographs are usually adequate in the diagnosis of distal radial fractures. However, scaphoid fractures are occult in approximately 16% of cases.[71] One study using MR imaging in 195 patients suspected of having scaphoid fractures clinically, but with normal radiographs, demonstrated occult fractures in almost 40%, with 19% of these being scaphoid fractures.[72] Given the risks of nonunion and avascular necrosis complicating approximately 5% to 12% of these fractures,[73,74] MR imaging should be considered in the presence of normal radiographs as this would also avoid over treating the unfractured scaphoid.[75]

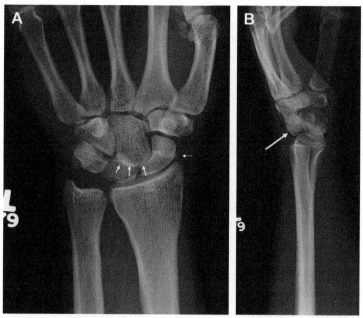

Fig. 8. Transcaphoid perilunate dislocation of the left wrist in a 27-year-old snowboarder. (*A*) There is a transverse fracture through scaphoid waist seen on the PA view (*white arrow*) with overlap of the capitate with respect to the lunate and scaphoid (*yellow arrows*). (*B*) The lateral view confirms the dorsal perilunate dislocation (*white arrow*).

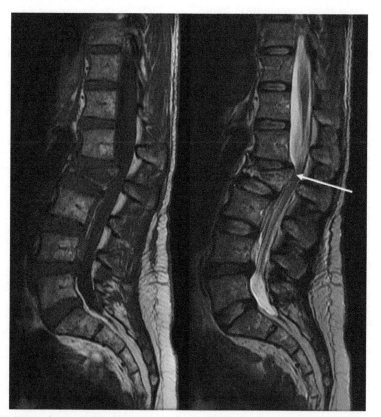

Fig. 9. Sagittal FSE T1- and T2-weighted images through the lumbar spine demonstrating an anterior wedge compression fracture at the L2 level with marked loss of vertebral body height resulting in a focal kyphotic deformity with resultant narrowing of the vertebral canal and crowding of nerve roots (*white arrow*).

Similar results have been noted in the elbow. MR imaging detected occult fractures and soft tissue injuries in 47% to 100% and 16% to 24% of patients with traumatic elbow joint effusions, respectively.[76,77]

SPINAL INJURIES IN SKIERS AND SNOWBOARDERS

Spinal injuries are amongst the most severe and debilitating injuries occurring in sporting activities. These injuries are seen 4 times more commonly in snowboarders than in skiers, with the incidence reported at 0.01 per 1000 skier days versus 0.04 per 1000 snowboarder days.[78] This difference reflects the higher incidence of aerial maneuvers in snowboarding.

Mechanism of Injury

Jumping is seen as the cause in 77% of snowboarding injuries versus 20% of skiing injuries. Although this is a significant difference, jumping is a more intrinsic element in snowboarding,[78] with snowboarders embarking on more frequent aerial maneuvers with increasing skill levels and experience. Burst fractures are the most common patterns, followed by anterior compression fracture. The thoracolumbar junction is the commonest site of injury, with fractures of T12 and L1 accounting for 50% in skiers and 35% in snowboarders. Cervical injuries are most frequently seen in the lower neck, mainly involving C6 and C7.[78,79]

Multisystem injuries occur in one-third of patients, with injuries at the thoracolumbar level more likely to be associated with torso and extremity trauma than those with cervical injuries.[79]

Imaging

Plain films are often the initial imaging modality used in assessing for spinal injury. However, a significant number of spinal injuries may be occult particularly in the presence of degenerative disease. The clinician should have a low threshold for using more advanced imaging techniques, with CT for assessing for bony injury and MR imaging for assessing for disc, ligamentous, and spinal cord injury as well as surrounding soft tissue pathology such as a hematoma (**Fig. 9**).

SUMMARY

Alpine skiing and snowboarding are very popular winter pastimes with ever increasing participation rates. The equipment used in these sports results in large forces acting across specific joints, resulting in unique patterns of injury. Knee injuries are commonly seen in skiers because of large torques occurring at the knee due to the length of the ski, with boots providing relative ankle protection. Ski poles are heavily implicated in UCL injuries of the thumb. LPT fractures are being seen with increasing frequency in snowboarders. Because of the high speed and energy of these sports, upper limb fractures and dislocations are not uncommon. Spinal injuries are also seen particularly in association with aerial maneuvers.

REFERENCES

1. Ascherl R, Schlemmer H, Lechuer F, et al. A ten year survey of skiing injuries. In: Hauser W, Karlsson J, Magi M, editors. Ski trauma and ski safety IV. Munich (German): TUEV Publication; 1982. p. 153–63.
2. Johnson RJ. Skiing and snowboarding injuries: when schussing is a pain. Postgrad Med 1990;88:36–51.
3. Hunter RE. Skiing injuries. Am J Sports Med 1999;27(3):381–8.
4. Rossi MJ, Lubowitz JH, Guttmann D. The skier's knee. Arthroscopy 2003;19(1):75–84.
5. Pino EC, Colville MR. Snowboard injuries. Am J Sports Med 1989;17(6):778–81.
6. Meyers C. On the edge: new riders on the olympic stage. Ski Magazine 1996;25:25.
7. Davidson TM, Laliotis AT. Snowboarding injuries: a four-year study with comparison with alpine ski injuries. West J Med 1996;164:231–7.
8. Chow TK, Corbett SW, Farstad DJ. Spectrum of injuries from snowboarding. J Trauma 1996;41:321–5.
9. Sutherland AG, Holmes JD, Myers S. Differing injury patterns in snowboarding and alpine skiing. Injury 1996;27:423–5.
10. Blandin C, Gidings P, Robinson M. Australian snowboard injury data base study. Am J Sports Med 1993;21:701–4.
11. Johnson RJ, Pope MH. Epidemiology and prevention of skiing injuries. Ann Chir Gynaecol 1991;80:110–5.
12. Natri A, Jarvinen M, Kannus P, et al. Changing injury pattern of acute anterior cruciate ligament tears treated at Tampere University Hospital in the 1980s. Scand J Med Sci Sports 1995;5:100–4.
13. Warme W, Feagin J, King P, et al. Ski injury statistics, 1982 – 1993, Jackson Hole Ski Resort. Am J Sports Med 1995;23(5):597–600.
14. Diebert M, Aronsson D, Johnson R, et al. Skiing injuries in children, adolescents, and adults. J Bone Joint Surg Am 1998;80:25–32.

15. Boutin RD, Fritz RC. MRI of snow skiing and snowboarding injuries. Semin Muscoskel Radiol 2005;9(4):360–78.

16. Ettlinger C, Johnson R, Shealy J. A method to help reduce the risk of serious knee sprains incurred in alpine skiing. Am J Sports Med 1995;23:531–7.

17. Greenwald R, France E, Rosenberg T. Significant gender difference in alpine skiing injuries. Philadelphia: American society of testing and materials; 1996.

18. Gray J, Taunton J, McKenzie D, et al. A survey of injuries to the anterior Cruciate ligament of the knee in female basketball players. Int J Sports Med 1985;6:314–6.

19. Arendt E, Dick R. Knee injury patterns among men and women in collegiate basketball and soccer. Am J Sports Med 1995;24:694–701.

20. Jarvinen M, Natri A, Laurila S, et al. Mechanisms of anterior cruciate rupture in skiing. Knee Surg Sports Traumatol, Arthroscopy 1994;2:224–8.

21. Johnson RJ. Prevention of cruciate ligament injuries. In: Feagin JA Jr, editor. The crucial ligaments. New York: Churchill Livingstone; 1988. p. 349–56.

22. Natri A, Beynnon BD, Ettlinger CF, et al. Alpine ski bindings and injuries. Current findings. Sports Med 1999;28(1):35–48.

23. DeMorat G, Weinhold P, Blackburn T, et al. Aggressive quadriceps loading can induce noncontact anterior cruciate ligament injury. Am J Sports Med 2004;32(2):477–83.

24. Cimino P. The incidence of meniscal tears associated with acute anterior cruciate ligament disruption secondary to snow skiing accidents. Arthroscopy 1994;10:198–200.

25. Duncan J, Hunter R, Purnell M, et al. Meniscal injuries associated with acute anterior cruciate ligament tears in alpine skiers. Am J Sports Med 1995;23:170–2.

26. Paletta G, Levine D, O'Brien S, et al. Patterns of meniscal injury associated with acute anterior cruciate ligament injury in skiers. Am J Sports Med 1992;20:542–7.

27. Clancy W, Ray M, Folton D. Acute tears of the anterior cruciate ligament. Surgical versus conservative treatment. J Bone Joint Surg Am 1988;70:1483–8.

28. DeHaven K. Diagnosis of acute knee injuries with haemarthrosis. Am J Sports Med 1980;8:9–14.

29. Noyes F, Bassett R, Grood E, et al. Arthroscopy in acute traumatic haemarthrosis of the knee: Incidence of anterior cruciate ligament tears and other injuries. J Bone Joint Surg Am 1980;62:687–95.

30. Barber F. Snow skiing combined anterior cruciate ligament/medial collateral ligament disruptions. Arthroscopy 1994;10:85–9.

31. Walls RM, Rosen P. Traumatic dislocation of the knee. J Emerg Med 1984;1:527–31.

32. Mirowitz SA, Shu HH. MR imaging evaluation of knee collateral ligaments and related injuries: comparison of T1-weighted, T2-weighted, and far-saturated T2-weighted sequences — correlation with clinical findings. J Magn Reson Imaging 1994;4(4):725–32.

33. Jackson JL, O'Malley PG, Kroenke K. Evaluation of acute knee pain in primary care. Ann Intern Med 2003;139:575–88.

34. Solomen DH, Simel DL, Bates DW, et al. The rational clinical examination. Does this patient have a torn meniscus or ligament of the knee? Value of the physical examination. JAMA 2001;286:1610–20.

35. Ho CP, Marks PH, Steadman JR. MR imaging of knee anterior cruciate ligament and associated injuries in skiers. Magn Reson Imaging Clin N Am 1999;7:117–30.

36. Johnson RJ, Ettlinger CF, Shealy JE. Skier injury trends — 1972 to 1994. In: Johnson RJ, Mote CD Jr, Ekeland A, editors. Skiing trauma and safety, vol. 11. ASTM STP 1289. Philadelphia: American Society for Testing and Materials; 1997. p. 37–48.

37. Hauser W. Experimental prospective skiing injury study. In: Johnson RJ, Mote CD Jr, Binet MH, editors. Skiing trauma and safety: seventh international symposium. ASTM STP 1022. Philadelphia: American Society for Testing and Materials; 1989. p. 18–24.

38. Campbell CS. Gamekeeper's thumb. J Bone Joint Surg Br 1955;37(B):148–9.

39. Miller RJ. Dislocation and fracture dislocations of the metacarpophalangeal joint of the thumb. Hand Clin 1988;4:45–65.

40. Harper MT, Chandnani VP, Spaeth J, et al. Gamekeeper thumb: diagnosis of ulnar collateral ligament injury using magnetic resonance imaging, magnetic resonance arthrography and stress radiography. J Magn Reson Imaging 1996;6(2):322–8.

41. Carr D, Johnson RJ, Pope MH. Upper extremity injuries in skiing. Am J Sports Med 1981;9(6):378–83.

42. Palmer AK, Louis DS. Assessing ulnar instability of the metacarpophalangeal joint of the thumb. J Hand Surg 1978;3(A):542–6.

43. Nevaiser RJ, Wilson JN, Lievano A. Rupture of the ulnar collateral ligament of the thumb (Gamekeeper's thumb) correction by dynamic repair. J Bone Joint Surg Br 1971;53(A):1357–64.

44. Aldred AJ. Rupture of the collateral ligament of the metacarpophalangeal joint of the thumb. J Bone Joint Surg Br 1955;37(B):443–5.

45. Smith RJ. Post-traumatic instability of the metacarpophalangeal joint of the thumb. J Bone Joint Surg Br 1977;59(A):14–21.

46. Stener B. Displacement of the ruptured ulnar collateral ligament of the metacarpophalangeal joint of the thumb. J Bone Joint Surg Br 1962;44(B):86979.

47. Coonrad RW, Goldner JL. A study of the pathological findings and treatment in soft-tissue injury of

the thumb metacarpophalangeal joint. J Bone Joint Surg Br 1968;50(A):439–51.

48. Bowers WH, Hurst LC. Gamekeeper's thumb. J Bone Joint Surg Br 1977;59(A):519–24.

49. Resnick D, Danzig LA. Arthrographic evaluation of injuries of the first metacarpophalangeal joint: gamekeeper's thumb. Am J Roentgenol 1976;126:1046–52.

50. Fricker R, Hintermann B. Skier's thumb. Treatment, prevention and recommendations. Sports Med 1995;19:73–9.

51. Lohman M, Vasenius J, Kivisaari A, et al. MR imaging of chronic rupture of the ulnar collateral ligament of the thumb. Acta Radiol 2001;42:10–4.

52. Spaeth HJ, Abrabs RA, Bock GW, et al. Gamekeeper's thumb: differentiation of non-displaced and displaced tears of the UCL with MRI. Radiology 1993;188:553–6.

53. Plancher KD, Ho CP, Cofield SS, et al. Role of MR imaging in the management of "skiers thumb" injuries. Magn Reson Imaging Clin N Am 1999;7:73–84.

54. Hergan K, Mittler C, Oser W. Ulnar collateral ligament: differentiation of displaced and nondisplaced tears with US and MR imaging. Radiology 1995;194:65–71.

55. Jones MH, England SJ, Muwanga CL, et al. The use of ultrasound in the diagnosis of injuries of the ulnar collateral ligament of the thumb. J Hand Surg Br 2000;25(1):29–32.

56. Kocher MS, Dupre MM, Feagin JA Jr. Shoulder injuries from alpine skiing and snowboarding. Aetiology, treatment and prevention. Sports Med 1998; 25(3):201–11.

57. Kocher MS, Feagin JA Jr. Shoulder injuries during alpine skiing. Am J Sports Med 1996;24:665–9.

58. Penvy T, Hunter RE, Freeman JR. Primary traumatic anterior shoulder dislocation in patients 40 years of age and older. Arthroscopy 1998;14:289–94.

59. Hawkins LG. Fracture of the lateral process of the Talus: a review of thirteen cases. J Bone Joint Surg Br 1965;47(A):1170–5.

60. Mukherjee SK, Pringle RM, Baxter AD. Fracture of the lateral process of the Talus: a report of 13 cases. J Bone Joint Surg Br 1974;56(B):263–73.

61. Kirkpatrick DP, Hunter RE, James PC, et al. The snowboarder's foot and ankle. Am J Sports Med 1998;26:271–7.

62. Heckman JD, McLean MR. Fractures of the lateral process of the talus. Clin Orthop 1985;199:108–13.

63. Mills HJ, Horne G. Fractures of the lateral process of the talus. Aust NZ J Surg 1987;57:643–6.

64. Boon AJ, Smith J, Zobitz ME, et al. Snowboarder's talus fracture: mechanism of injury. Am J Sports Med 2001;29(3):333–8.

65. Fjeldborg O. Fracture of the lateral process of the talus, supination-dorsal flexion fracture. Acta Orthop Scand 1968;39:407–12.

66. Ebraheim NA, Skie MC, Podeszwa DA, et al. Evaluation of process fractures of the talus using computed tomography. J Orthop Trauma 1994;8:332–7.

67. Dimon JH. Isolated displaced fractures of the posterior facet of the talus. J Bone Joint Surg Br 1961;43(A):275–81.

68. Brown TD, Varney TE, Micheli LJ. Malleolar bursitis in figure skaters. Indications for operative and nonoperative treatment. Am J Sports Med 2000;28(1):109–11.

69. Anderson SE, Weber M, Steinbach LS, et al. Shoe rim and shoe buckle pseudotumour of the ankle in elite and professional figure skaters and snowboarders: MR imaging findings. Skeletal Radiol 2004;33:325–9.

70. Idzikowski JR, Janes PC, Abbott PJ. Upper extremity snowboarding injuries. Ten-year results from the Colorado snowboard injury survey. Am J Sports Med 2000;28(6):825–32.

71. Hunter J, Escobedo E, Wilson A, et al. MR imaging of clinically suspected scaphoid fractures. Am J Roentgenol 1997;168:1287–93.

72. Brydie A, Raby N. Early MRI in the management of clinical scaphoid fracture. Br J Radiol 2003;76:296–300.

73. Leslie IJ, Dickson RA. The fractured carpal scaphoid. Natural history and factors influencing outcome. J Bone Joint Surg Br 1981;63(B):225–30.

74. Dias JJ, Brenkel IJ, Finlay DB. Patterns of union in fractures of the waist of the scaphoid. J Bone Joint Surg Br 1989;71:307–10.

75. Barton N. Twenty questions about scaphoid fractures. J Hand Surg Br 1992;17:289–310.

76. Major N, Crawford S. Elbow effusions in trauma in adults and children: is there an occult fracture? Am J Roentgenol 2002;178:413–8.

77. Burns P, Hunt J, King C, et al. MR imaging of acute trauma of the elbow. Am J Roentgenol 2002;179:1076–7.

78. Tarazi F, Dvorak MF, Wing PC. Spinal injuries in skiers and snowboarders. Am J Sports Med 1999;27(2):177–80.

79. Prall JA, Winston KR, Brennan R. Spine and spinal cord injuries in downhill skiers. J Trauma 1995;39(6):1115–8.

Imaging of Triathlon Injuries

Michael J. Tuite, MD

KEYWORDS

- Triathlon • Swimming • Running • Cycling
- Magnetic resonance imaging

The modern triathlon is a race in which athletes swim, cycle, and run in succession, and their overall time includes the transition time between each sport. Triathlons have become a popular athletic event both in the United States and worldwide. In the United States there are about 300,000 athletes performing triathlons every year, with more than 1000 races, including approximately 15 Ironman-length events per year.[1,2]

Triathlon races can be variable in length, ranging from a "sprint triathlon," to the longer Olympic length, to Ironman, and to even ultradistance. These races became popular after the original Hawaii Ironman Triathlon was established to combine into a single race the Waikiki 2.4-mile "Roughwater swim," a 112-mile bike race around Oahu, and a 26.2-mile marathon. However, the most popular triathlons are the shorter sprint triathlons, which usually involve a 750-m swim, a 20-km cycling course, and a 5-km run. Although termed a "sprint," this race is really an endurance event, which requires training and stamina.

INJURY OVERVIEW

The modern triathlon was devised by runners who were cross-training in swimming and cycling to provide a variety to their workouts and to reduce overuse injuries due to running.[2] When the first triathlons began, many believed that training in the 3 disciplines would mean fewer injuries than in athletes who train in a single sport. In fact, overuse injuries among triathletes are more common than injuries in single-sport athletes.[1,3–5] This higher incidence is thought to be for 2 reasons. First, triathletes train for more hours on average than single-sport athletes, averaging 10 to 14 hours of training per week.[6,7] As discussed in this article, the 3 disciplines can contribute to some of the same overuse injuries. Second, triathletes sometimes have poorer technique or equipment than dedicated single-sport athletes, which has been shown to predispose them to more overuse injuries.[1,2] An example is the distance runner who decides to train for an Ironman triathlon but has a poorly fitted bike and develops patellar tendinosis.

There are several medical issues that can occur in people either training for or racing in a triathlon (Box 1). In this article, the main focus is on those musculoskeletal injuries that may require medical imaging.

About 90% of actively training triathletes will have an acute or overuse injury over the course of the year.[3,8,9] An injury is typically defined as a musculoskeletal symptom that causes an unplanned stop in training or failure to complete a race, or leads the individual to seek medical care.[1,2] Acute injuries in triathletes include, for instance, an acromioclavicular (AC) joint separation from falling off a bike. Overuse injuries have an insidious onset and are much more common in triathletes, representing 75% to 80% of injuries.[1,2,6] Overuse injuries usually occur during training, but 15% to 25% of injuries either present during a race or are exacerbated during the race to a point that it forces the athlete to discontinue.[1,2,6]

The most common site of injury in a triathlete is the knee, accounting for over a quarter of all injuries.[1,2,6,10] Foot, ankle, lumbar spine, and shoulder injuries are also common (Table 1). Although overlap exists, the 3 different sports tend to be associated with somewhat distinct injuries. Running has the highest triathlete injury

Musculoskeletal Division, Department of Radiology, University of Wisconsin Medical School, UW Health, E3/311, 600 Highland Avenue, Madison, WI 53792, USA
E-mail address: mjtuite@wisc.edu

Radiol Clin N Am 48 (2010) 1125–1135
doi:10.1016/j.rcl.2010.07.008

radiologic.theclinics.com

Box 1
Examples of injuries and illnesses in triathletes
Nonmusculoskeletal
Dehydration
Hyperthermia
Blisters
Abrasions
Muscle cramps
Female athletic triad (anorexia, amenorrhea, osteoporosis)
Musculoskeletal, nonimaged
Short-duration low back pain
Muscle strains
Ulnar neuropathy (cyclist's palsy)
Musculoskeletal, imaged
Rotator cuff impingement
Stress fractures
Tendinosis
Plantar fasciitis
Radiculopathy
Osteitis pubis
Meniscal tear
Iliotibial band syndrome

rate and swimming the lowest (**Fig. 1**), although most of the training hours are typically spent cycling.[1,2,11]

In this article, the imaging appearance of injuries in triathletes commonly seen with each of the 3 sports is discussed. The authors highlight those injuries that are associated with more than one of

the disciplines, which often lead to the triathlete seeking medical care because they significantly affect their training regimen. This article also discusses injuries that tend to occur with one sport but are then exacerbated by training in the other disciplines.

SWIMMING

Acute injuries are rare during swim training or during the swim leg of a triathlon.[1,2,6,8] One of the most serious concerns is drowning, because triathletes often train and compete in open water where the underwater visibility is poor.[12] Acute musculoskeletal injuries from shark attacks have also been described in triathletes training in the ocean (http://www.msnbc.msn.com/id/24313314/).

Overuse injuries from swimming are less common than injuries from cycling and running, accounting for only 5% to 10% of injuries in triathletes.[1,2,13] Most clinical complaints are of shoulder tendinitis and impingement pain.[1,2,14] The swimming motion involves repetitive extremes of abduction, flexion, and extension, and "swimmer's shoulder" is common in competitive swimmers. Swimmer's shoulder refers to a combination of rotator cuff tendinosis/impingement and laxity from stretched anterior glenohumeral ligaments.[15] Shoulder impingement pain in triathletes can be exacerbated during cycling when using aerobars, in which the cyclist leans forward and rests the elbows on a pad to maintain an aerodynamic position. This position causes the humeral head to compress against the supraspinatus tendon and subacromial bursa, and may aggravate impingement symptoms.

In one of the few imaging articles on triathletes, shoulder magnetic resonance (MR) imaging findings of triathletes at the Hawaii Ironman Race were assessed.[14] These investigators performed MR imaging scans on athletes with shoulder symptoms and found rotator cuff tendinopathy in 50%, AC joint marrow edema in 62%, and partial

Table 1	
Site and percentage of injuries in triathletes	
Site	**Percentage of All Injuries (%)**
Foot	10–15
Ankle	10–15
Lower leg	5–10
Knee	25–30
Thigh	5–10
Hip/groin	5–10
Shoulder	10–15
Lumbar spine	10–15
Cervical spine	5
Other	5

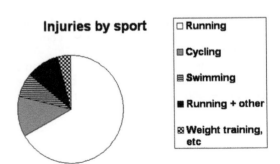

Fig. 1. Percentage of injuries in triathletes that occur from the 3 sports.

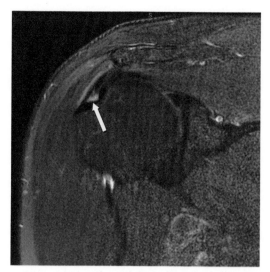

Fig. 2. A 39-year-old man with shoulder pain when swimming and lifting weights. Oblique coronal fat-suppressed T2-weighted MR image shows increased signal within the supraspinatus tendon (*arrow*) consistent with rotator cuff tendinopathy. The finding is common in symptomatic and asymptomatic triathletes.

thickness rotator cuff tears in 19%. From MR imaging, tendinopathy was defined as abnormal signal intensity on short echo-time (TE) images without a defect in the tendon on fluid-sensitive sequences (Fig. 2). Partial-thickness rotator cuff tears were defined as high-signal defects in the tendon on T2-weighted images (Fig. 3). In this study, 29% of asymptomatic triathletes also had rotator cuff tendinopathy, 71% had AC marrow edema, and 29% had partial-thickness rotator cuff tears on MR imaging (Fig. 4). It is difficult to know if these MR imaging abnormalities are actually the cause of shoulder symptoms or if many triathletes ignore minor shoulder pain.

CYCLING

Cycling injuries are relatively uncommon, considering the number of hours triathletes spend on the bike, but they are more common than swimming injuries and represent 10% to 20% of injuries.[1,2,6] Acute injuries during cycling are mainly falls from a bike, with about one-third of triathletes experiencing a fall each year. The most common time to fall is during a race, occurring in 1 out of every 250 competitors. This incidence is probably a result of the higher speeds during the race, and cycling more aggressively down hills and around turns.

Although most falls result only in abrasions and contusions, more serious injuries such as head trauma can also occur. The most common musculoskeletal injury after a fall is to the shoulder, mainly clavicle fractures and dislocations of the AC or glenohumeral joint (Fig. 5).[1,2,6] Serious triathletes become accustomed to training despite pain, so even grade 1 AC separations can progress to chronic injuries if they are not rested, leading to posttraumatic osteolysis (Fig. 6).

The most common site for overuse injuries during cycling is at the knee. Knee injuries are more common if a bike is not properly fitted, such as with a seat positioned too low or too far forward for the size of the rider.[2] The major overuse injuries around the knee are patellar tendinosis, patellofemoral stress syndrome, and ITBS, all 3 of which can also occur from running.[16] Patellar tendinosis is the most common cause of anterior knee pain during cycling, and results from the

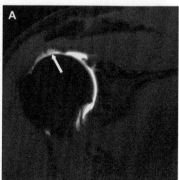
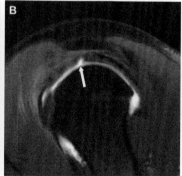

Fig. 3. A 38-year-old man with shoulder pain while training for a triathlon. (*A*) Oblique coronal fat-suppressed T1-weighted MR arthrogram image shows contrast extending into the articular surface of the supraspinatus tendon (*arrow*). (*B*) Oblique sagittal fat-suppressed T1-weighted MR arthrogram image confirms the articular surface partial thickness rotator cuff tear (*arrow*). Impingement and rotator cuff pain is usually worse during swimming but can be exacerbated while cycling when leaning onto aerobars.

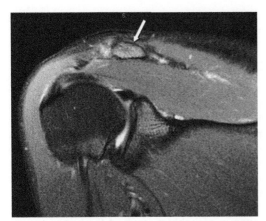

Fig. 4. A 38-year-old woman with shoulder tendinitis from swimming. Oblique coronal fat-suppressed T2-weighted MR image shows increased marrow signal in the distal clavicle (*arrow*), a common finding even in asymptomatic triathletes.

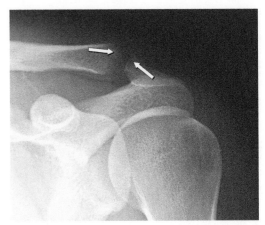

Fig. 6. A 34-year-old man with persistent shoulder pain 2 months after a fall from his bike. Anteroposterior radiograph shows resorption of subchondral bone adjacent to the AC joint (*arrows*) consistent with posttraumatic osteolysis. The patient had continued swim training for an Ironman triathlon despite the continued discomfort after the fall.

high extension forces during the down stroke while pedaling.[17] Patellar tendinosis tends to occur at the ends of the tendon near the enthesis, either proximally or distally (**Fig. 7**). On MR imaging, tendinosis appears as a high signal on T2-weighted images, while on ultrasonography (US) it appears

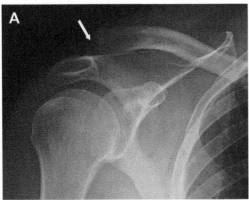

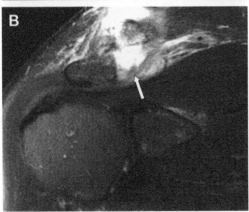

Fig. 5. A 53-year-old man who fell from his bike while training for a triathlon. (*A*) Anteroposterior radiograph shows elevation of the distal clavicle with widening of the AC joint (*arrow*). (*B*) Oblique coronal fat-suppressed T2-weighted MR image shows edema and hemorrhage at the AC separation (*arrow*).

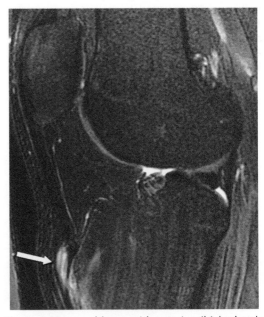

Fig. 7. A 22-year-old man with anterior tibial tubercle pain while cycling and running. Sagittal fat-suppressed T2-weighted image shows high signal in the distal patellar tendon (*arrow*), indicating patellar tendinopathy.

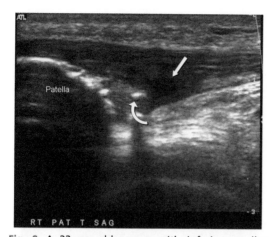

Fig. 8. A 23-year-old person with inferior patellar pain when cycling and running. Longitudinal US image shows swelling and hypoechoic changes (*arrow*) in the proximal patellar tendon, with a small calcification (*curved arrow*). This observation is consistent with superior patellar tendinopathy or "jumper's knee."

as a hypoechoic region within the tendon, usually with increased Doppler flow (**Fig. 8**).

Patellofemoral stress syndrome, or "biker's knee," is seen more often in female triathletes and results from the repetitive loading of the patellofemoral joint.[1,2,18] The higher incidence in women is mainly because of the greater Q angle and resultant lateral displacement forces on the patella. Patients may have abnormal patellar tracking on physical examination tests, such as a positive "J" sign, which refers to the lateral deviation of the patella at full knee extension. Imaging in patients with patellofemoral stress syndrome is usually limited to radiography, including an axial or "sunrise" view of the knee. Although most triathletes with patellofemoral stress syndrome have normal radiographs, some can have patella alta, lateral subluxation, or a shallow trochlear groove. Treatment usually consists of vastus medialis strengthening and an orthotic sleeve, but adjustments to the bicycle seat height or interpedal width may also be helpful.

ITBS is also seen in cyclists and is caused by the friction of the iliotibial band tendon across the lateral femoral condyle with the knee in 10° to 30° of flexion. Although less common than in runners, ITBS occurs in cyclists because of the high number of repetitions of the knee in the "impingement zone" near the bottom of the stroke cycle. ITBS is exacerbated when the seat is too high or too far back.[19] ITBS manifests as a T2 high signal between the iliotibial band and the lateral femoral condyle on MR images, as an obliteration of the fat distal to the vastus lateralis, and occasionally as an adventitial bursa (**Fig. 9**).[20] Although all 3 of these overuse knee injuries can present while cycling, they are often exacerbated by running.

Overuse injuries at the ankle can also result from cycling. The most common ankle injury is Achilles tendinosis, which makes up about 5% of injuries in triathletes.[1,2,6] Achilles tendinosis from cycling results from the repetitive plantar flexion against resistance during the down stroke and, in general, is more common in older athletes.[21] Achilles tendinosis in triathletes is thought to be exacerbated by having to cycle immediately after the foot has been held in plantar flexion for several hours during the swim portion of the race.

Achilles tendinosis is divided into 2 main types: hypoxic and mucoid. The hypoxic type involves focal thickening of the Achilles tendon, which appears as a low signal on T1- and T2-weighted sequences and has relatively normal echogenicity

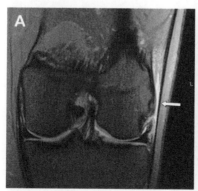
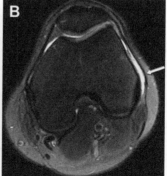

Fig. 9. A 36-year-old woman with lateral knee pain when cycling and running. (*A*) Coronal fat-suppressed intermediate-weighted image shows high signal between the iliotibial band (ITB) and the lateral femoral epicondyle (*arrow*). (*B*) Axial fat-suppressed T2-weighted image confirms the adventitial bursa deep to the ITB (*arrow*) consistent with ITB friction syndrome. ITBS can result from running on a laterally sloped surface.

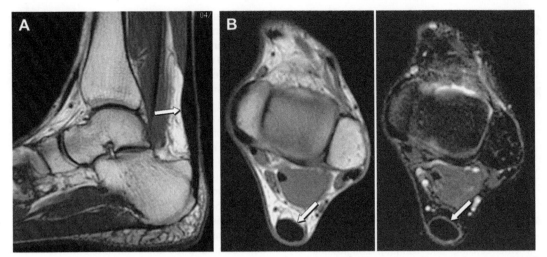

Fig. 10. A 49-year-old man with a lump in the Achilles tendon. (*A*) Sagittal T1-weighted image shows focal thickening of the Achilles tendon (*arrow*). (*B*) Axial proton-density (*left*) and fat-suppressed T2-weighted (*right*) images show low signal in the thickened tendon (*arrow*) consistent with hypoxic tendinopathy.

on US (**Fig. 10**). The hypoxic type usually presents with a painless lump in the tendon, and there is little risk of progressing to tendon rupture. The other type of tendinosis is the mucoid type, which appears on T2-weighted MR images as a thin linear high signal within the tendon and on US as similar linear anechoic areas (**Fig. 11**). The focal thickening of the tendon in the mucoid type is usually painful, and there is increased risk of progressing to a tear, so triathletes with this condition may have to modify their workout. Raising the seat height to reduce the amount of ankle dorsiflexion and the stretch on the ligament can help relieve symptoms.

Pain in the low back or neck is also common during cycling in triathletes. O'Toole and colleagues[8] surveyed Hawaii Ironman Triathlon competitors and found that 78% had experienced back or neck overuse injuries in the year before the race. Lumbar pain during cycling is thought to result partly from holding the trunk in an aerodynamic flexed position for an extended period. The pain is typically of a muscular or ligamentous origin because in three-fourths of triathletes the pain resolves in a few weeks.[11] However, 25% of those with back pain have either radiculopathy or pain for longer than 3 months. Although there is little literature on imaging regarding the prevalence of structural abnormalities in this population, back pain for longer than 3 months is suggestive of an abnormality such as disk or facet disease or unrecognized spondylolysis. Low back pain can be exacerbated when running and, if severe enough, may limit training in both disciplines.

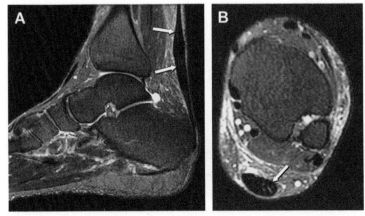

Fig. 11. A 63-year-old man with a painful lump in the Achilles tendon. (*A*) Sagittal fat-suppressed T2-weighted image shows focal thickening and high-signal striations within the Achilles tendon. (*B*) Axial fat-suppressed T2-weighted image confirms the mucoid tendinopathy (*arrow*) of the Achilles tendon.

Neck pain is common in single-sport cyclists and therefore, not surprisingly, is also seen in triathletes. Neck pain is less common than low back pain, seen in about 45% of triathletes at some time during their competitive years.[11] Neck pain and cervical disk disease from cycling is probably caused by maintaining hyperlordosis of the neck while riding in the aerodynamic position with the trunk low and the head looking forward. Similar to low back pain, radiculopathy or neck pain for longer than 3 months suggests a structural abnormality such as a cervical disk disease, and 10% to 20% of triathletes with neck pain have pain for this duration and therefore may undergo imaging (**Fig. 12**).

RUNNING

The running stage of a triathlon is considered to be the most important leg of the race.[2] Most triathletes are former distance runners, and the run time is the best predictor of the overall triathlon success.[22] The running portion is also the most common stage in the race during which an athlete is forced to drop out from an overuse injury. In addition, it is the final stage of the triathlon, and therefore competitors experience the most fatigue and muscle tightness. Running is also associated with most injuries during training, accounting for two-thirds to three-fourths of all skipped workouts.

Knee injuries account for more than one-third of all running injuries in triathletes.[1,2,6] Many of the knee injuries from running are the same as those seen while cycling, including patellofemoral stress syndrome, ITBS, and patellar tendinosis. Patello-femoral stress syndrome, called biker's knee when seen in cyclists, is also called runner's knee and is usually worse when running on hills. ITBS tends to be aggravated by running on a laterally sloped surface, such as a steeply crowned road. Patellar tendinosis appears to be associated with a rapid increase in mileage, especially if running on a hard surface. Patellofemoral stress syndrome and ITBS are more common in female distance runners, while patellar tendinosis is more common in men.[23] When severe, knee injuries may limit training in both running and cycling.

Meniscal tears in triathletes almost exclusively occur as a result of their run training. These tears are usually overuse tears from the repetitive impaction forces across the meniscus, and are more common in older triathletes who have started to develop myxoid change within the meniscus.[24] Meniscal tears are most common in the posterior

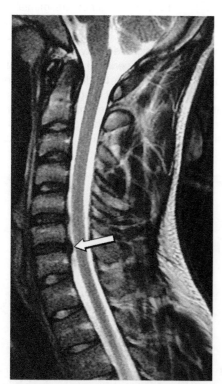

Fig. 12. A 22-year-old man with neck pain radiating into the upper extremity, especially when riding his racing road bike. Sagittal T2-weighted image shows a disk protrusion at C6-C7 (*arrow*). There is a smaller C5-C6 disk bulge.

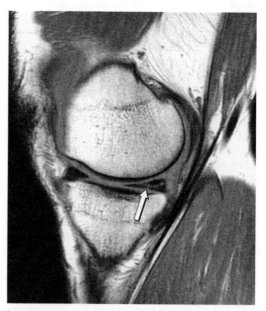

Fig. 13. A 45-year-old man with knee pain when running. Sagittal proton-density–weighted image shows a tear in the posterior horn of the medial meniscus (*arrow*). Meniscal tears are more common in older triathletes.

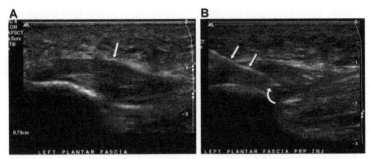

Fig. 14. A 23-year-old person with heel pain when running. (*A*) Longitudinal US image shows a 7.9-mm thick, heterogeneous, hypoechoic plantar aponeurosis (*arrow*) that was tender to palpation with the ultrasound probe, consistent with plantar fasciitis. (*B*) Longitudinal US image during injection of platelet-rich plasma (PRP) shows the needle (*arrows*) and the hyperechoic PRP within the tendon (*curved arrow*).

horn of the medial meniscus and appear as an increased signal unequivocally extending to an articular surface on a short TE sequence and on at least 2 images (**Fig. 13**).

Foot and ankle injuries are also most common during running, and account for 15% to 25% of running injuries in triathletes.[1,2,6] Foot pain can also develop during a race and may be due to worsening of a preexisting metatarsalgia or metatarsal stress reaction. Ankle pain from Achilles tendinopathy can occur while running in addition to cycling, and is more common in older triathletes.

Plantar fasciitis accounts for half of all running foot and ankle injuries.[1,2,6,23] Plantar fasciitis is a tendinopathy or partial tearing of the medial plantar aponeurosis, and is usually an overuse stretch injury.[25,26] The MR imaging findings are T2 high signals within and around a thickened medial plantar aponeurosis. US is also useful in evaluating for plantar fasciitis and demonstrates thickening of the aponeurosis greater than 5 mm, occasionally with increased Doppler flow around the ligament (**Fig. 14**). Plantar fasciitis is treated initially with padded heel cups and stretching exercises, such as rolling the foot across a cold soda can. Refractory cases may benefit from injection, including injection of platelet-rich plasma (PRP).[27] Quality running shoes are also important to prevent or allow healing of plantar fasciitis.[28]

Another common injury of the foot during distance running is metatarsalgia. Metatarsalgia is a clinical term for pain near the metatarsal heads and includes conditions such as tendinitis, metatarsal-phalangeal joint synovitis or capsulitis, and Morton neuroma. Some investigators also include metatarsal stress reaction and sesamoiditis.[1,2] Actual stress fractures of the metatarsals can also be seen in triathletes,[29] although some studies have reported that they are less common than tibial and femoral stress fractures in distance runners.[23,30] The second and third metatarsals are

the most vulnerable to stress injuries, and treatment usually consists of wearing a stiff shoe until the symptoms subside. Stress reaction appears on MR images as T2 high signal within the bone marrow without a cortical abnormality, while stress fractures also have a focal cortical abnormality (**Fig. 15**).[30]

Lower leg (calf/tibia/fibula) injuries are also common during run training in triathletes, accounting for about 10% of triathlete injuries.[1,2,13] The 2 main injuries are medial tibial stress syndrome (shin splints) and stress fractures.[31] Shin splints are thought to be a part of a continuum of overuse injury to the tibia and may be caused by periostitis, stress reaction, and/or repetitive traction tendinopathy by the tibialis posterior muscle. MR images may be normal in triathletes with mild shin splints or can show T2 high-signal periosteal reaction along the tibia at the site of pain (**Fig. 16**). Tibial stress fractures

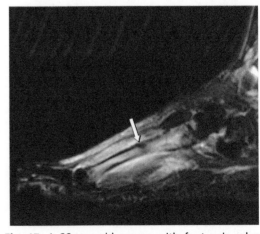

Fig. 15. A 28-year-old person with foot pain when running. There is a metatarsal stress fracture (*arrow*) with surrounding marrow edema on a fat-suppressed T2-weighted image.

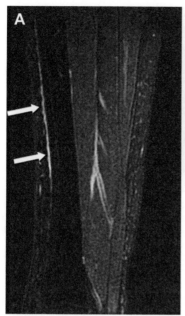
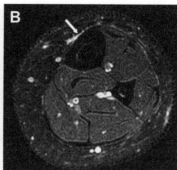

Fig. 16. A 26-year-old person with pain when running. (*A*) Sagittal short-tau inversion recovery image shows periosteal edema along the anterior tibia (*arrows*). (*B*) Axial fat-suppressed T2-weighted image confirms the high signal adjacent to the anteromedial tibia (*arrows*). Periosteal edema without marrow or cortical involvement is consistent with medial tibial stress syndrome or shin splints.

can be difficult to distinguish clinically from medial tibial stress syndrome, so MR imaging is very helpful in making the diagnosis. On MR imaging, stress fractures demonstrate a cortical abnormality between an area of periostitis and T2 high signal within the marrow (Fig. 17).

Another appearance of the tibial stress injury is cortical resorption cavities, typically in the anterior "keel" of the tibia.[32] These cavities appear on computed tomography as linear longitudinal regions of nonmineralized tissue within the cortex. On MR imaging, these linear resorption cavities are high signal on T2-weighted images. Resorption cavities may be an isolated finding on MR images or may be associated with other more typical stress injury findings.

Upper leg, hip, and groin injuries account for 10% to 20% of injuries in triathletes and usually result from run training.[1,2,13] Stress fractures of the proximal femur are always a concern in triathletes with hip pain, and typically occur along the medial concave portion of the femur in the region of the lesser trochanter. Thigh pain in triathletes can result from overuse injuries of the hamstrings, typically tendinopathy at the hamstring origin.[13] These injuries appear on MR images as T2 high signal in the proximal tendon, and can be treated with an image-guided injection of anesthetic and corticosteroid or PRP (Fig. 18). Gluteus medius pain from distance running is more common in

women.[23] Finally, triathletes can develop groin pain due to osteitis pubis. Osteitis pubis results from the repetitive vertical shear forces across the pubic symphysis that occurs with the alternating foot strike during distance running (Fig. 19).

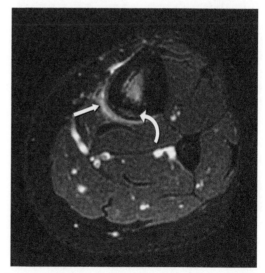

Fig. 17. A 24-year-old person with lower leg pain when running. Axial fat-suppressed T2-weighted image shows periostitis (*arrow*), marrow edema, and abnormal signal within the tibial cortex (*curved arrow*), indicating a stress fracture.

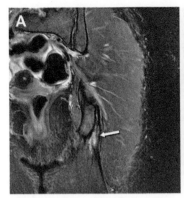
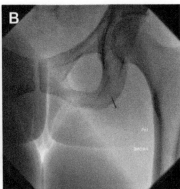

Fig. 18. A 45-year-old woman who competes in Ironman and ultradistance triathlons. (*A*) Coronal fat-suppressed T2-weighted image shows increased signal in the proximal hamstring tendons (*arrow*). (*B*) Anteroposterior fluoroscopic image shows a needle placed into the abnormal area of tendon for injection of anesthetic and corticosteroid. Two weeks after the injection, this woman set a course record in the Hawaii Ultraman World Championship triathlon.

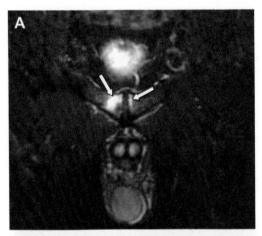
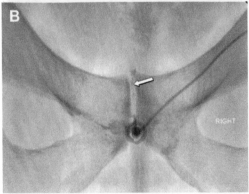

Fig. 19. A 47-year-old man with groin pain while training for a triathlon. (*A*) Coronal short-tau inversion recovery image shows edema around the pubic symphysis (*arrow*) consistent with osteitis pubis. (*B*) Anteroposterior fluoroscopic image during an injection of anesthetic and corticosteroid shows the needle in the pubic symphysis with contrast in the joint (*arrow*). This man went on to finish an Ironman triathlon race several months later.

SUMMARY

Injuries in triathletes are common and are mostly overuse injuries. Rotator cuff tendinitis is the most common complaint from swimming, but the incidence of tendinopathy and rotator cuff tears on MR imaging is comparable in triathletes without and with shoulder pain. Cycling injuries are mainly to the knee, including patellar tendinosis, ITBS, and patellofemoral stress syndrome, and to the cervical and lumbar spine. Running is associated with most injuries in triathletes, during both training and the event, causing the person to discontinue a triathlon. In addition to knee injuries from running, foot and ankle, lower leg, and hip injuries are also seen. Some injuries in triathletes may be mainly symptomatic during 1 of the 3 sports but are also exacerbated by one or both of the other disciplines.

REFERENCES

1. Burns J, Keenan AM, Redmond AC. Factors associated with triathlon-related overuse injuries. J Orthop Sports Phys Ther 2003;33:177–84.
2. Strock GA, Cottrell ER, Lohman JM. Triathlon. Phys Med Rehabil Clin N Am 2006;17:553–64.
3. Levy CM, Kolin E, Berson BM. The effect of cross training on injury incidence, duration and severity (part 2). Sports Med Clin Forum 1986;3:1–8.
4. Gosling CM, Gabbe BJ, Forbes AB. Triathlon related musculoskeletal injuries: the status of injury prevention knowledge. J Sci Med Sport 2007;11: 396–406.
5. Cipriani DJ, Swartz JD, Hodgson CM. Triathlon and the multisport athlete. J Orthop Sports Phys Ther 1998;27:42–50.

6. Collins K, Wagner M, Peterson K, et al. Overuse injuries in triathletes: a study of the 1986 Seafair Triathlon. Am J Sports Med 1989;17:675–80.

7. Shaw T, Howat P, Trainor M, et al. Training patterns and sports injuries in triathletes. J Sci Med Sport 2004;7:446–50.

8. O'Toole ML, Hiller WD, Smith RA, et al. Overuse injuries in ultraendurance triathletes. Am J Sports Med 1989;17:514–8.

9. Egermann M, Brocai D, Lill CA, et al. Analysis of injuries in long-distance triathletes. Int J Sports Med 2003;24:271–6.

10. Wilk BR, Fisher KL, Rangelli D. The incidence of musculoskeletal injuries in an amateur triathlete racing club. J Orthop Sports Phys Ther 1995;22:108–12.

11. Villavicencio AT, Burneikiene S, Hernandez TD, et al. Back and neck pain in triathletes. Neurosurg Focus 2006;21:E7.

12. Dallam GM, Jonas S, Miller TK. Medical considerations in triathlon competition: recommendations for triathlon organisers, competitors and coaches. Sports Med 2005;35:143–61.

13. Korkia PJ, Tunstall-Pedoe DS, Maffulli N. An epidemiological investigation of training and injury patterns in British triathletes. Br J Sports Med 1994;28:191–6.

14. Reuter RM, Hiller WDB, Ainge GR, et al. Ironman triathletes: MRI assessment of the shoulder. Skeletal Radiol 2008;37:737–41.

15. Rupp S, Berninger K, Hopf T. Shoulder problems in high level swimmers—impingement, anterior instability, muscular imbalance? Int J Sports Med 1995;16:556–62.

16. Clements K, Yates B, Curran M. The prevalence of chronic knee injury in triathletes. Br J Sports Med 1999;33:214–6.

17. Bailey MP, Maillardet FJ, Messenger N. Kinematics of cycling in relation to anterior knee pain and patellar tendinitis. J Sports Sci 2003;21:649–57.

18. Mellion MB. Common cycling injuries. Management and prevention. Sports Med 1991;11:52–70.

19. Farrell KC, Reisinger KD, Tillman MD. Force and repetition in cycling: possible implications for iliotibial band friction syndrome. Knee 2003;10:103–9.

20. Muhle C, Ahn JM, Yeh L, et al. Iliotibial band friction syndrome: MR imaging findings in 16 patients and MR arthrographic study of six cadaveric knees. Radiology 1999;212:103–10.

21. Cohen GC. Cycling injuries. Can Fam Physician 1993;39:628–32.

22. Vleck VE, Burgi A, Bentley DJ. The consequences of swim, cycle, and run performance on overall result in elite Olympic distance triathlon. Int J Sports Med 2006;27:43–8.

23. Taunton JE, Ryan MB, Clement DB, et al. A retrospective case-control analysis of 2002 running injuries. Br J Sports Med 2002;36:95–101.

24. Shellock FG, Hiller WD, Ainge GR, et al. Knees of Ironman triathletes: magnetic resonance imaging assessment of older (>35 years old) competitors. J Magn Reson Imaging 2003;17:122–30.

25. Theodorou DJ, Theodorou SJ, Farooki S, et al. Disorders of the plantar aponeurosis: a spectrum of MR imaging findings. AJR Am J Roentgenol 2001;176:97–104.

26. Theodorou DJ, Theodorou SJ, Kakitsubata Y, et al. Plantar fasciitis and fascial rupture: MR imaging findings in 26 patients supplemented with anatomic data in cadavers. Radiographics 2000;20 (Spec No):S181–97.

27. Sampson S, Gerhardt M, Mandelbaum B. Platelet rich plasma injection grafts for musculoskeletal injuries: a review. Curr Rev Musculoskelet Med 2008;1:165–74.

28. Wilk BR, Fisher KL, Gutierrez W. Defective running shoes as a contributing factor in plantar fasciitis in a triathlete. J Orthop Sports Phys Ther 2000;30:21–8 [discussion: 29–31].

29. Sell S, Konermann W. [Triathlon—continuous stress on muscles, tendons and bones?]. Sportverletz Sportschaden 1988;2:112–4 [in German].

30. Fredericson M, Jennings F, Beaulieu C, et al. Stress fractures in athletes. Top Magn Reson Imaging 2006;17:309–25.

31. Clement DB, Ammann W, Taunton JE, et al. Exercise-induced stress injuries to the femur. Int J Sports Med 1993;14:347–52.

32. Gaeta M, Minutoli F, Vinci S, et al. High-resolution CT grading of tibial stress reactions in distance runners. AJR Am J Roentgenol 2006;187:789–93.

Overhead Throwing Injuries of the Shoulder and Elbow

Mark W. Anderson, MD*, Bennett A. Alford, MD

KEYWORDS

- Magnetic resonance imaging • Throwing • Injury
- Shoulder • Elbow

Injuries to the shoulder and elbow are common in athletes involved in sporting activities that require overhead motion of the arm such as baseball, volleyball, tennis, and some track and field events.[1–3] Baseball pitchers are most often affected, both before and after skeletal maturation. The purpose of this article is to review the biomechanics of throwing, how the throwing motion is related to specific injuries in the shoulder and elbow, and the magnetic resonance (MR) imaging appearances of the most common injuries.

THE BIOMECHANICS OF THROWING

The throwing motion provides a prototype for evaluating the effects of overhead athletic activities on the upper extremity. As a pitch is thrown, energy is transferred from the lower extremities via a kinetic chain through the trunk to the upper extremity, ultimately resulting in ball release from the fingers. This familiar motion is classically divided into 6 stages: windup, early cocking, late cocking, acceleration, deceleration, and follow-through.[1,4] The most significant forces act on the shoulder and elbow during the late cocking and acceleration phases.

As the arm is abducted and externally rotated, anterior translational force of the humeral head on the glenoid can reach up to one-half body weight,[5] and is resisted by static stabilizers that include the glenoid labrum, glenohumeral ligaments, and anterior joint capsule. Dynamic stabilization is provided by the rotator cuff and other muscles of the shoulder girdle and chest wall.[6,7] Of note, the long head of the biceps tendon also plays a role in stabilizing the humeral head, and has been shown to be a more important stabilizer of the humerus than the rotator cuff in patients with underlying anterior instability.[7]

During the acceleration phase, humeral torque reaches levels that are typically higher than the torsional strength of the humerus, as determined in cadaver studies.[8] The arm is decelerated after ball release by contraction of the posterior shoulder musculature resulting in distraction forces at the joint equal to body weight.[5,9]

Tremendous valgus forces also occur at the elbow during these same phases of throwing and result in tensile stresses on the medial collateral ligament, the common flexor tendon, and the ulnar nerve. Compressive forces occur along the radial aspect of the joint, and shear forces are generated across the posteromedial aspect of the joint, primarily affecting the ulnohumeral articulation.[3]

THROWING INJURIES: RISK FACTORS AND FINDINGS IN ASYMPTOMATIC PATIENTS

Adolescent throwers are especially vulnerable to shoulder and elbow injuries. Young throwers who develop symptoms tend to throw more pitches, throw at higher velocities, and continue to throw despite arm pain and fatigue. Symptomatic individuals also tend to be taller and heavier, and

Department of Radiology, Division of Musculoskeletal Imaging, University of Virginia Health Sciences Center, 1218 Lee Street, Charlottesville, VA 22908, USA
* Corresponding author.
E-mail address: mwa3a@virginia.edu

Radiol Clin N Am 48 (2010) 1137–1154
doi:10.1016/j.rcl.2010.07.002

poor pitching mechanics likely play a role as well.[10–12]

Many findings are present in both symptomatic and asymptomatic throwers, suggesting that some of these may represent adaptive changes to repetitive forces. In a group of asymptomatic skeletally immature throwers, 55% were found to have widening of the proximal humeral physis on radiographs compared with 62% of those in a symptomatic group.[13] Similarly, approximately half of adolescent throwers with radiographic evidence of fragmentation and/or separation of the medial epicondylar apophysis at the elbow were asymptomatic.[14]

Mature throwers also demonstrate a high incidence of asymptomatic abnormalities in the shoulder and elbow. Seventy-nine percent of asymptomatic elite throwers were found to have abnormalities of the glenoid labrum, and 40% had partial- or full-thickness rotator cuff tears.[15,16] In another group of asymptomatic throwers, chronic ulnar collateral ligament injury was observed in 87%, and 81% were shown to have osteochondral abnormalities in the posteromedial elbow.[17]

THE THROWER'S SHOULDER: MR IMAGING TECHNIQUE
Standard MR Imaging

The patient is scanned in the supine position with the arm at the side using a surface coil. The upper arm should be externally rotated such that the bicipital groove is positioned directly anteriorly (at 12 o'clock on an axial image) (**Fig. 1**). Images are obtained in the axial, oblique coronal, and oblique sagittal planes with the oblique sequences oriented relative to the plane of the supraspinatus muscle.

For a standard MR imaging examination of the shoulder, T1-weighted (T1W) and/or proton density sequences as well as T2-weighted (T2W) sequences are typically obtained. Proton density and T2W images are usually acquired using a fat-saturation technique. Gradient echo (T2*W) images are useful for labral evaluation. The exact choice of scanning parameters will vary according to the MR system employed and the operator's preferences.

MR Arthrography

The injection of a dilute gadolinium solution (1:200 dilution in sterile saline), distends the joint, which results in improved visualization of intra-articular structures. Much has been written about the advantages of MR arthrography compared with standard MR imaging of the shoulder, including its specific benefits in overhead athletes with suspected internal derangement. Numerous studies have demonstrated its superior sensitivity and specificity for diagnosing the most common abnormalities in overhead athletes including superior labral anterior to posterior (SLAP) lesions and other types of labral tears, as well as partial-thickness undersurface tears of the rotator cuff tendons.[18–20]

The ABER position (abduction, external rotation) has been advocated as a useful adjunct to MR arthrography in the overhead athlete related to its ability to better demonstrate undersurface cuff tears, and because anterior stabilizing structures are placed under tension with the arm in this position (**Fig. 2**).[21–27]

SPECIFIC INJURIES: SHOULDER

Injuries to the shoulder often involve more than one structure because of the complex forces generated during the throwing motion. Each entity is addressed individually here, and any commonly associated injuries are mentioned in that section as well.

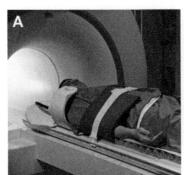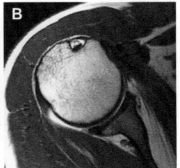

Fig. 1. Shoulder MR technique: standard position. (*A*) The patient is positioned with the arm at the side and externally rotated so that the biceps tendon is positioned anteriorly (12 o'clock) on an axial image (*B*).

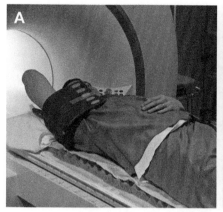
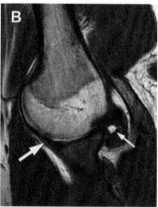

Fig. 2. Shoulder MR technique: ABER position. (*A*) The patient's hand is placed behind the head so that the arm is abducted and externally rotated. (*B*) An oblique axial T1W image with the arm in this position shows the undersurface of the supraspinatus tendon (*small arrow*) as well as the anterior labrum and capsule under tension (*large arrow*).

Rotator Cuff

Internal impingement

Mechanism of injury Internal impingement refers to impaction of the greater tuberosity of the humerus against the posterosuperior aspect of the glenoid as the arm is abducted and externally rotated. A portion of the rotator cuff (the posterior fibers of the supraspinatus and anterior fibers of the infraspinatus tendons) may be entrapped between the bones, often along with the postero-superior aspect of the labrum.[4,7,28] This contact is seen in normal, asymptomatic throwers, but can become symptomatic and produce a constellation of typical injuries.[28]

Internal impingement has been thought to be secondary to microinstability that results from chronic stretching of the anterior capsular structures during the throwing motion.[28] Tightening of the posterior capsular tissues, also known as glenohumeral internal rotation deficit (GIRD), has also been implicated as a possible cause.[29,30] This tightening leads to a loss of internal rotation and a posterosuperior shift of the axis of rotation of the humeral head on the glenoid, thereby worsening the osseous and soft tissue impingement.

Associated injuries include superficial undersurface tears of the posterior cuff tendons, fraying or tears of the posterior superior labrum, and subchondral cysts and/or sclerosis in the greater tuberosity or posterosuperior glenoid.

MR imaging The superficial undersurface cuff tears are often extremely subtle on MR images.[31] MR arthrography has been shown to be more sensitive the conventional MR imaging for detecting partial tears of the cuff.[19,20] Scanning of these patients in the ABER position has also been recommended because it results in better separation of the cuff tendons from the humeral head, allowing for improved visualization of these undersurface tears.[20,32] Findings commonly associated with these undersurface cuff tears include abnormalities of the posterior superior labrum and subchondral cystic foci in the greater tuberosity or superior glenoid (**Fig. 3**). The presence of one or more of these findings in an overhead athlete should suggest the diagnosis of internal impingement.[33]

External impingement

Mechanism of injury Impingement of the supraspinatus tendon at the level of the coracoacromial arch ("outlet" of the shoulder) may be secondary to spurring along the anterior acromion or distal clavicle, a "hook-like" acromion, lateral downsloping of the acromion, or a thickened coracoacromial ligament. This type of impingement is the most common cause of cuff pathology in older patients, and whereas it may occur in older overhead athletes, it is rare in young throwers.[7,20,34] The spectrum of cuff pathology ranges from tendinopathy to partial- or full-thickness tears.

MR imaging Anatomic features that may lead to the development of impingement symptoms, including acromioclavicular joint spurring and abnormal acromial morphology, are best demonstrated on oblique sagittal and oblique coronal images. Supraspinatus tendinopathy manifests as thickening of the tendon with diffuse, heterogeneous intrasubstance signal intensity on T1W and T2W images. A partial-thickness tear is diagnosed when focal, fluid-equivalent signal intensity is identified along the articular or bursal surface of the tendon (**Fig. 4**). Fluid-equivalent signal intensity confined to the substance of the tendon indicates an interstitial tear. A full-thickness tear

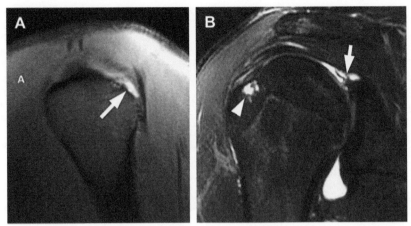

Fig. 3. Internal impingement. (*A*) Sagittal fat-saturated T1W image (MR arthrogram) demonstrates a focal under-surface tear of the infraspinatus tendon (*arrow*). A, anterior. (*B*) Oblique coronal fat-saturated T2W image reveals irregularity and tearing of the posterior superior labrum (*arrow*). Note also the cystic foci in the greater tuberosity (*arrowhead*).

demonstrates fluid (or contrast) extending across the tendon, and it is important to assess the dimensions of the tear, the degree of tendon retraction, and any associated atrophy within the muscles involved (see **Fig. 4**).

Tensile failure ("rim rent"/"PASTA" tears)
Mechanism of injury During the deceleration phase of the throwing motion, the muscles of the rotator cuff contract to slow the arm, and in so doing, place the cuff tendons under tension. These tensile forces can result in superficial undersurface tears involving the distal supraspinatus or infraspinatus tendons.[5,35,36] These lesions are known as "rim rent" or "PASTA" (partial articular surface tendon avulsion) tears.[37]

MR imaging Foci of fluid-equivalent signal intensity are noted on T2W images along the articular surfaces of the distal supraspinatus and/or infraspinatus tendons near their insertions.[36–38] In some cases, retracted fibers are identified along the undersurface of the tendon just proximal to the tear (**Fig. 5**). However, these can be very difficult to detect, especially if the arm is internally rotated.[36] MR arthrography and scanning in the ABER position have been advocated for improved detection.[32]

Subscapularis tendon/biceps tendon
Mechanism of injury Injuries of the subscapularis tendon are much less common than those involving the supraspinatus and infraspinatus tendons. Impingement of the undersurface of the

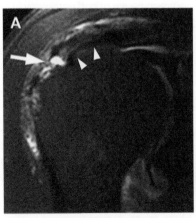
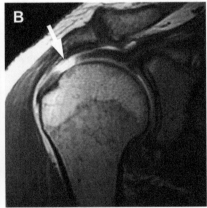

Fig. 4. External impingement. (*A*) Oblique coronal T2W image shows focal, fluid-intensity signal in the distal supraspinatus tendon with disruption of its bursal surface (*arrow*) consistent with a partial-thickness bursal surface tear. Note that the articular surface is intact (*arrowheads*). (*B*) Oblique coronal T1W image (MR arthrogram) demonstrates a full-thickness tear of the supraspinatus tendon (*arrow*) with gadolinium extending into the subacromial/subdeltoid bursa.

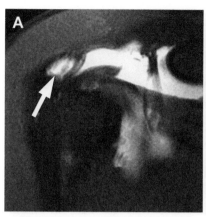 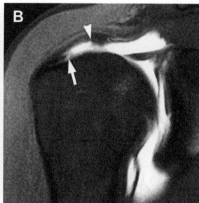

Fig. 5. Rim-rent/"PASTA" lesions. (*A*) Oblique coronal fat-saturated T1W image (MR arthrogram) shows partial-thickness undersurface tearing of the far anterior fibers of the supraspinatus tendon near its insertion (*arrow*). (*B*) Oblique coronal fat-saturated T1W image (MR arthrogram) in a different patient displays partial-thickness undersurface tearing of the distal supraspinatus tendon (*arrow*) with retraction of the torn fibers (*arrowhead*).

subscapularis tendon against the anterior superior glenoid with flexion and internal rotation of the arm has been suggested as a cause of undersurface tears of the tendon in overhead athletes.[39] Partial disruption of the distal fibers of the subscapularis allows for subluxation or dislocation of the long head of the biceps tendon from the bicipital groove, and may be a source of anterior symptoms.[40] The long head of the biceps tendon is also subjected to stretching and traction forces, especially in the setting of anterior instability. Pathology of the biceps tendon ranges from tendinopathy to partial or complete tears.

MR imaging The subscapularis tendon is best evaluated on axial images as it courses anterior to the joint to insert on the lesser tuberosity. Tears of the distal subscapularis tendon may be quite subtle and only noticed because of associated medial subluxation of the biceps tendon (**Fig. 6**).

The vertical portion of the biceps tendon lies within the bicipital groove and is easiest to assess on axial images. The horizontal portion of the tendon courses over the humeral head and is more difficult to evaluate, especially on nonarthrographic studies; it is best evaluated in the oblique sagittal and oblique coronal planes. Accurate assessment of the tendon is especially challenging where it curves to enter the bicipital groove, because it is not orthogonal to the standard imaging planes and is susceptible to magic angle artifact at that site. Careful analysis of the few slices that cover that portion of the tendon should be performed in all 3 planes.

Biceps pathology can range from tendinopathy (enlarged tendon, displaying heterogeneous signal intensity) to partial or complete tears (**Fig. 7**). Focal pathology of the tendon at a level just proximal to

the upper bicipital groove, described as a "groove entrance" lesion, is especially difficult to detect because of the curving morphology of the tendon at that site (see **Fig. 7**).[41]

Labrum

SLAP tear
Mechanism of injury Injuries to the superior labrum at the biceps-labral anchor (superior labrum anterior to posterior—SLAP—tears) are common in

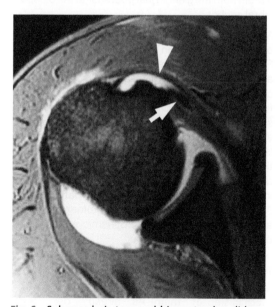

Fig. 6. Subscapularis tear and biceps tendon dislocation. Axial fat-saturated T1W image (MR arthrogram) reveals a partial tear of the distal subscapularis tendon (*arrowhead*) that is more apparent because of the medial dislocation of the long head of the biceps tendon into its substance (*arrow*).

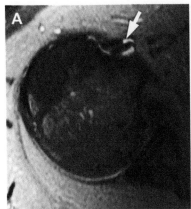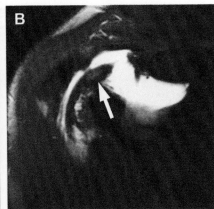

Fig. 7. Biceps tendon injuries. (*A*) A longitudinal split tear of the long head of the biceps tendon is evident on this axial fat-saturated T1W image (*arrow*). (*B*) Oblique coronal T2W image (MR arthrogram) in a different patient reveals slight thickening and focal signal abnormality in the biceps tendon just proximal to the bicipital groove (*arrow*) compatible with focal tendinopathy. The tendon appeared normal proximal and distal to this point.

throwers. Chronic traction on the long head of the biceps tendon, primarily during the deceleration phase, has been implicated as a causative factor.[9] SLAP tears in throwers may also result from a "peel-back" phenomenon in which the tendon assumes a more vertical and posterior orientation with abduction and external rotation of the arm. Simultaneous twisting of the tendon at its labral attachment acts to separate the posterior superior labrum from the glenoid just posterior to the biceps/labral anchor.[9,42]

MR imaging Injuries of the superior labrum are best demonstrated in the oblique coronal plane. Fluid or contrast, extending between the labrum and superior glenoid, is diagnostic; however, it can be impossible to distinguish a true SLAP tear from a normal sublabral sulcus that occurs in that same region (**Fig. 8**).[43,44] Helpful MR findings that support the diagnosis of a true SLAP tear include lateral extension of abnormal signal intensity into the substance of the labrum, irregularity of the labral margin, and extension of the signal into the proximal biceps tendon.[45,46] Scanning the patient in the ABER position has also been recommended in an attempt to provide a quasi-dynamic assessment of the biceps-labral anchor.[47]

Posterior superior labrum (internal impingement)
Mechanism of injury As already described, impingement of the greater tuberosity of the humerus against the posterior superior glenoid is common in throwers, and may become symptomatic. In addition to the superficial fraying and tears noted along the undersurface of the infraspinatus tendon, labral degeneration and tearing along the

posterosuperior glenoid is also a common associated finding.[31] Other pathologic features include subchondral cysts in the posterior portion of the greater tuberosity, chondral abnormalities involving the humeral head, and subchondral cysts or sclerosis in the posterosuperior glenoid.[33]

MR imaging The posterior superior labrum is best assessed on oblique coronal and axial images. An oblique axial scanning plane may provide additional diagnostic information because of the orientation of the labrum at this level. MR arthrography has also been advocated as being more sensitive for detecting labral pathology.[20]

The labral findings in internal impingement may consist only of subtle fraying and irregularity of the posterosuperior labrum (**Fig. 9**). Even so, the labral findings may be easier to identify with MR imaging than the superficial undersurface tears along the posterior cuff tendons. Subcortical marrow edema and cysts in the greater tuberosity or posterosuperior glenoid are also helpful secondary signs, and are most conspicuous on fat-saturated T2W images owing to their high signal intensity.[33] Subchondral sclerosis, when present, is best identified on T1W images because its low signal intensity contrasts sharply with the high signal intensity of the adjacent marrow fat.

Anterior/posterior labral pathology
Mechanism of injury The anterior labrum and glenohumeral ligaments are placed under tension when the arm is abducted and externally rotated during the late cocking phase of the throwing motion. Over time the accumulation of microdamage in these structures may result in anterior instability.[7] Similarly, when the forward momentum of

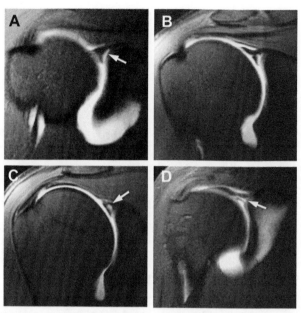

Fig. 8. SLAP tear. (*A*) Oblique coronal fat-saturated T1W image (MR arthrogram) demonstrates a normal sublabral sulcus along the superior labrum (*arrow*). (*B*) Oblique coronal fat-saturated T1W image (MR arthrogram) in a different patient shows a similar appearing sulcus at the level of the biceps-labral anchor, however the image immediately posterior to this level (*C*) demonstrates lateral extension of contrast into the substance of the labrum compatible with a SLAP tear (*arrow*). (*D*) Oblique coronal fat-saturated T1W image (MR arthrogram) in a third patient displays extension of a superior labral tear into the proximal biceps tendon (*arrow*).

the arm is rapidly slowed during the deceleration phase by both dynamic posterior muscle contraction and static posterior labrocapsular structures, associated stretching of the posterior soft tissue

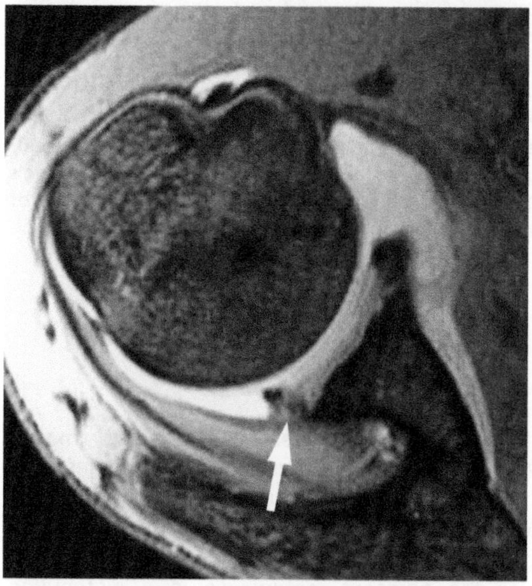

Fig. 9. Internal impingement: posterosuperior labrum. Axial fat-saturated T1W image (MR arthrogram) in a 12-year-old baseball pitcher reveals heterogeneous signal abnormality and irregularity of the posterior superior portion of the labrum (*arrow*).

restraints over time may result in posterior instability.[9] Although frank labral avulsions are rare in throwers, other forms of anterior and/or posterior labral pathology may result.

MR imaging The anterior and posterior portions of the labrum are best evaluated on axial images. As with labral pathology at other sites, MR findings of a labral tear include abnormal signal within the labrum or interposed between the labrum and glenoid (**Fig. 10**). The morphology of the labrum can be variable, so labral "irregularity" is less specific. With posterior instability, the posterior joint recesses may appear capacious, but because that is a very subjective determination, a more specific finding is that of posterior capsular stripping along the posterior margin of the glenoid. In that region, the normal capsule attaches consistently along the base of the labrum at its junction with the osseous glenoid (**Fig. 11**). Assessment of anterior capsular stripping is much more difficult because of extreme variability of the normal capsular attachments along the anterior glenoid.

Little leaguer's shoulder: epiphysiolysis
Mechanism of injury In a skeletally immature athlete, the physis is the "weak link" in the muscle-tendon-bone complex. Repetitive stresses of throwing may lead to the development of a stress reaction along the proximal humeral physis

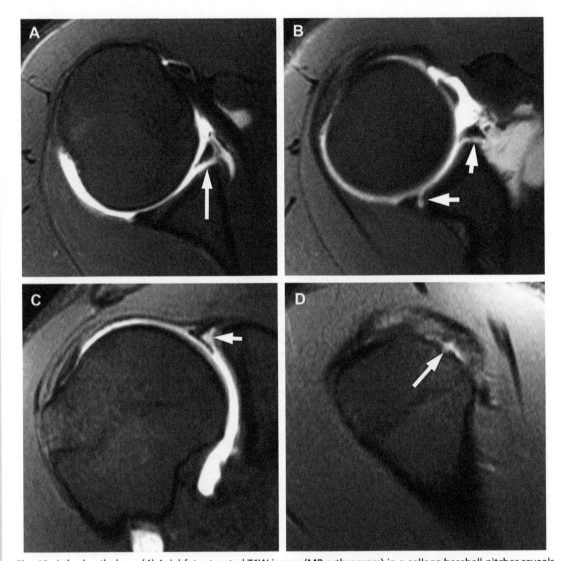

Fig. 10. Labral pathology. (*A*) Axial fat-saturated T1W image (MR arthrogram) in a college baseball pitcher reveals a tear of the anterior inferior portion of the labrum (*arrow*). Axial scans at more superior levels (*B, C*) show extension of the tear superiorly into the posterior superior quadrant to involve approximately 270° of the labrum (*arrows*). (*D*) Oblique sagittal fat-saturated T1W image also revealed an undersurface tear of the infraspinatus tendon (*arrow*) consistent with internal impingement.

(epiphysiolysis) and may be a source of activity-related shoulder pain in this age group.[48] These stresses result in an ingrowth of cartilage from the physis into the adjacent metaphysis, which may appear as widening of the lucent physis on radiographs. As with other throwing injuries, physeal widening may be seen in young asymptomatic throwers.[48]

MR imaging The signal intensity of the physis varies depending on the pulse sequence used.

In general, it will appear dark on T1W images and bright on fat-saturated T2W images and many gradient echo sequences. The most notable MR finding in patients. with little leaguer's shoulder is extension of physeal signal intensity into the adjacent metaphysis in a distribution similar to what is seen on radiographs (**Fig. 12**).[49,50] Early physeal injury is more easily identified with MR imaging, partly because of its tomographic nature but also because associated

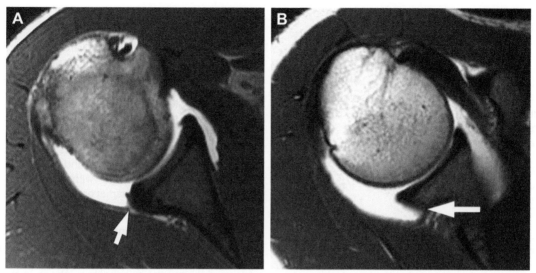

Fig. 11. Posterior instability. (*A*) Axial T1W image (MR arthrogram) shows normal posterior capsular insertion at the base of the labrum (*arrow*). (*B*) Axial T1W image (MR arthrogram) in a different patient reveals posterior capsular stripping related to posterior instability (*arrow*).

marrow edema often provides improved conspicuity in the early stages of injury.

THE THROWER'S ELBOW: MR IMAGING TECHNIQUE
Standard MR Imaging

The patient is scanned in a supine position using a surface coil, with the elbow at the side. If necessary, the patient can lie prone with the elbow positioned above the head, nearer to the center of the bore of the magnet. Images are obtained in axial, coronal, and sagittal planes. Coronal images are proscribed parallel to a line connecting the humeral epicondyles on an axial image. Sagittal images are oriented perpendicular to that axis. T1W and/or proton density sequences and T2W sequences are typically obtained. Proton density and T2W images are usually acquired with a fat-saturation technique. The use of

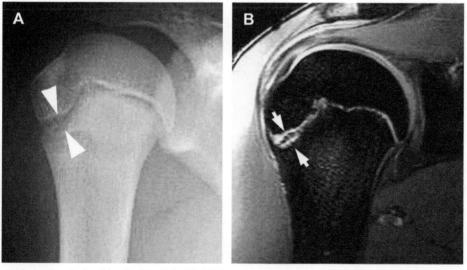

Fig. 12. Little leaguer's shoulder (epiphysiolysis). (*A*) Frontal radiograph of the right shoulder in this adolescent pitcher demonstrates widening of the proximal humeral physis along its lateral aspect (*arrowheads*). This was asymmetrically prominent compared with his asymptomatic left shoulder. (*B*) Oblique coronal gradient echo T2*W image shows high signal intensity cartilage extending into the adjacent metaphysis (*arrows*).

high-resolution scanning parameters is mandatory for obtaining maximal diagnostic information.[51]

MR Arthrography

Injection of a dilute gadolinium solution (1:200 dilution in sterile saline) results in excellent joint distention and has been shown to be especially helpful in depicting subtle partial-thickness tears of the ulnar collateral ligament, evaluating the stability of osteochondral lesions of the capitellum, and demonstrating intra-articular loose bodies.[52]

SPECIFIC INJURIES: ELBOW

As mentioned earlier, during the late cocking and acceleration phases of the throwing motion, a tremendous valgus force occurs at the elbow. The resulting distractive forces along the medial aspect of the joint place medial-sided structures such as the ulnar collateral ligament, common flexor tendon, and ulnar nerve under tensile stresses.[53] The radiocapitellar joint is subjected to compressive forces, and the posteromedial joint, in particular the humeral-olecranon articulation, experiences shear forces. Based on these biomechanical factors, a constellation of injuries is common in the thrower's elbow, referred to as the "valgus overload syndrome."[53,54]

Medial Structures

Ulnar collateral ligament

Mechanism of injury The ulnar collateral ligament (UCL) is composed of 3 bands: anterior, posterior, and transverse/oblique.[54] The anterior band is the primary restraint against valgus force at the elbow during the throwing motion while the posterior band plays a much less significant role. The transverse band plays no significant part in stabilizing the elbow.[54,55] Repetitive valgus stresses during throwing can cause the anterior band of the UCL to accumulate microdamage within its fibers, leading to stretching and partial or complete tears of the ligament.[55]

MR imaging The normal anterior band of the UCL is best seen on coronal and axial MR images as a low signal structure extending from the undersurface of the medial epicondyle to attach to the medial margin of the coronoid process of the ulna at the sublime tubercle. Its humeral attachment is relatively broad, and often demonstrates slightly heterogeneous signal intensity compared with the more distal fibers that taper toward their ulnar attachment (**Fig. 13**). The anterior band is well demonstrated in cross section on axial images, where the posterior band is also seen as a thin low signal structure forming the floor of the adjacent cubital tunnel.

Following ligamentous sprain, the anterior band appears somewhat thickened, typically with adjacent edema.

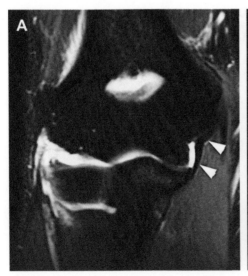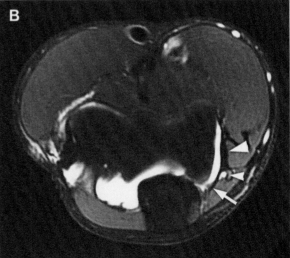

Fig. 13. Normal ulnar collateral ligament. (*A*) Coronal fat-saturated T2W image (MR arthrogram) demonstrates the anterior band of the ulnar collateral ligament (*arrowheads*). (*B*) Axial fat-saturated T2W image (MR arthrogram) displays the ulnar collateral ligament in cross section with the larger anterior band (*large arrowhead*) lying anterior to the posterior band (*arrow*). Note its proximity to the ulnar nerve (*small arrowhead*).

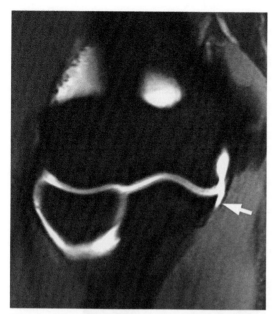

Fig. 14. Ulnar collateral ligament: partial tear. Coronal fat-saturated T1W image (MR arthrogram) reveals a small partial tear of the UCL at its distal attachment to the sublime tubercle forming a "T" sign (*arrow*).

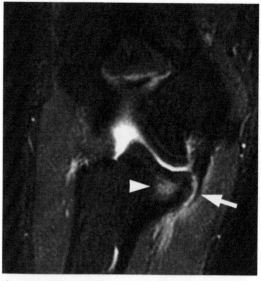

Fig. 16. Ulnar collateral ligament: complete tear. Coronal fat-saturated T2W image (MR arthrogram) demonstrates thickening of the anterior band of the UCL, which is completely torn at its ulnar attachment (*arrow*). Note also the marrow edema in the coronoid (*arrowhead*) and adjacent soft tissues.

Partial tears may involve any portion of the ligament, and result in some degree of fiber disruption. An often subtle lesion involves partial stripping of the distal fibers at their ulnar attachment, producing the "T" sign on routine or, more commonly, arthrographic MR images (**Fig. 14**).[56–59] This may be difficult to differentiate

from a reported normal variation of mild separation of the fibers from the sublime tubercle,[60] and the distinction is usually based on the degree of separation of the ligament from the bone and the amount of fluid or contrast undercutting the ligament at that site. The normally heterogeneous signal within its proximal fibers may be difficult to

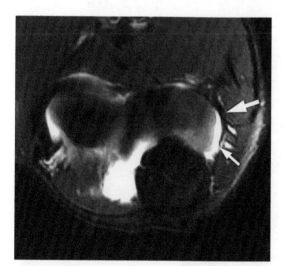

Fig. 15. Ulnar collateral ligament: partial tear (posterior band). Axial fat-saturated T2W image (MR arthrogram) in this college baseball player presenting with medial elbow pain reveals disruption of the posterior band of the UCL (*small arrow*). Note the intact anterior band (*large arrow*).

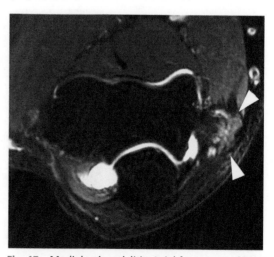

Fig. 17. Medial epicondylitis. Axial fat-saturated T2W image (MR arthrogram) reveals abnormally increased signal in a markedly thickened common flexor tendon at its origin on the medial epicondyle (*arrowheads*) compatible with medial epicondylitis.

distinguish from a partial tear at its humeral attachment. A partial tear of the posterior bundle is much less common, but may clinically mimic an anterior bundle injury. Such a tear is best demonstrated on axial images (Fig. 15).

Complete tears of the UCL demonstrate full-thickness disruption of the ligament, often with associated edema, hemorrhage, and/or extravasation of fluid or contrast into the adjacent soft tissues (Fig. 16).[61]

Avulsion fracture of the sublime tubercle also occurs in throwers, and though it may be identified on radiographs, MR imaging is helpful for demonstrating radiographically occult fractures.[62]

Common flexor tendon (flexor-pronator mass)
Mechanism of injury As the UCL fails, adjacent structures are affected, including the common flexor tendon, a dynamic stabilizer of the medial aspect of the elbow.[3,63] Progressive injury causes tendinopathy and tears of the tendon at its medial epicondylar origin, producing clinical symptoms of medial "epicondylitis." Differentiation from UCL pathology is difficult clinically and MR imaging is often helpful.

MR imaging The normal common flexor tendon demonstrates homogeneously low signal intensity on all MR imaging pulse sequences and is best evaluated in the coronal and axial planes.

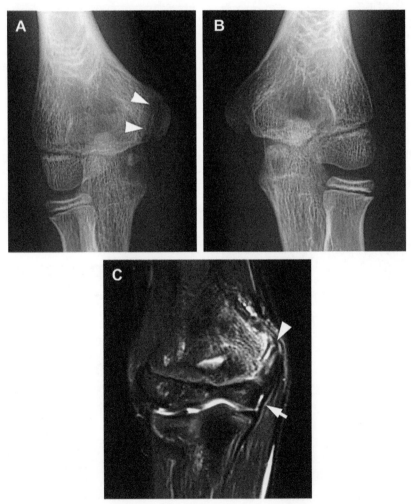

Fig. 18. Little leaguer's elbow (medial apophysitis/epiphysiolysis). (*A*) Frontal view of the left elbow in this young thrower with medial elbow pain shows widening and ill definition of the medial epicondylar apophysis (*arrowhead*) relative to the normal comparison view of the right elbow (*B*). (*C*) A corresponding coronal fat-saturated T2W image shows physeal widening (*arrowhead*) and prominent edema in the adjacent marrow. The UCL is normal (*arrow*).

Injury to the tendon ranges from tendinopathy to a partial or, rarely, a complete tear.[54,63] Tendinopathy is manifest as a thickened, slightly ill-defined proximal tendon that demonstrates intermediate intrasubstance signal intensity, with or without adjacent edema (**Fig. 17**). Focal, fluid-intensity signal within the fibers of the tendon indicate a partial tear. Complete discontinuity of tendon fibers is seen with a tendon rupture.

Medial epicondylar apophysis ("little leaguer's elbow")

Mechanism of injury The elbow is the most frequent site of injury in the skeletally immature thrower.[64] The UCL is usually stronger than the physis of the medial epicondyle in this age group, and tensile forces acting on the medial aspect of the elbow combined with the dynamic pull of the flexor-pronator mass often result in fragmentation or separation of the medial epicondylar apophysis.[65] It is extremely difficult to clinically differentiate between injury to the UCL and the physis in this age group, and imaging often plays an important role in that regard.

MR imaging Widening of the physis on radiographs can be seen in symptomatic as well as asymptomatic throwers (using the opposite elbow is for comparison).[14,65] MR imaging is sensitive for the detection of radiographically occult injuries because it can demonstrate subtle widening of the physis and edema-like signal intensity within the adjacent marrow, which is often readily apparent on fat-saturated T2 or inversion recovery images relative to the dark background of suppressed marrow fat (**Fig. 18**). Because UCL pathology is also in the differential in a young thrower with medial elbow pain, a further advantage of MR imaging is its ability to provide for simultaneous evaluation of the ligament.

Ulnar nerve

Mechanism of injury There are several causes for ulnar neuritis in a thrower, one of which is increasing traction on the nerve within the cubital tunnel as the UCL fails.[54] Impingement from adjacent posteromedial osteophytes is another cause, discussed in a subsequent section.

MR imaging The normal ulnar nerve is best evaluated on axial images as it courses through the cubital tunnel. On T2W images the individual fascicles of the nerve are often discernible and should be of uniform size. With ulnar neuritis, the nerve is typically enlarged and demonstrates bright fascicles, often of varying sizes (**Fig. 19**).

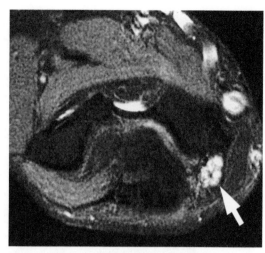

Fig. 19. Ulnar neuritis. Axial fat-saturated T2W image at the level of the cubital tunnel demonstrates an enlarged ulnar nerve containing high signal fascicles of varying sizes (*arrow*), compatible with ulnar neuritis.

Lateral Structures

Radiocapitellar joint

Mechanism of injury As the medial sided stabilizers fail, the valgus forces occurring during the late cocking and acceleration phases result in increasing compressive forces along the lateral aspect of the elbow. Over time, these forces can lead to the development of a focal osteochondral injury in the capitellum, typically along its anterolateral aspect.[66,67] These osteochondral lesions (also known as osteochondritis dissecans or OCD) are thought to result from a combination of repetitive trauma and a tenuous blood supply to this portion of the bone. A subchondral fragment may develop and ultimately heal, or become unstable and displace into the joint.[68]

MR imaging An osteochondral lesion of the capitellum is diagnosed on MR imaging when focal subchondral signal abnormality is identified, especially when accompanied by a low signal linear margin or a separate fragment beneath the articular surface of the capitellum. Subchondral edema within the capitellum on fat-saturated T2W images is a helpful and often conspicuous secondary finding (**Fig. 20**). It is important to attempt to assess the integrity of the overlying cartilage and whether the fragment appears unstable, and MR arthrography is often helpful on both counts.[66,68–71] The primary MR sign of instability is fluid or contrast extending between the lesion and underlying bone (see **Fig. 20**).[66,67] There is also some evidence that intravenous contrast

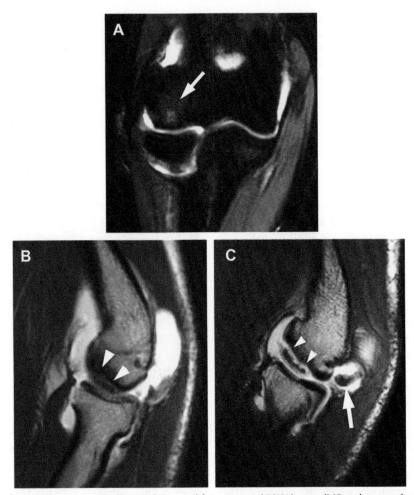

Fig. 20. Osteochondral lesion, capitellum. (*A*) Coronal fat-saturated T2W image (MR arthrogram) reveals marrow edema within the capitellum (*arrow*). (*B*) Sagittal T1W image in the same patient demonstrates a subchondral fragment in the capitellum (*arrowheads*). There is no contrast tracking between the fragment and underlying bone, compatible with a stable fragment. (*C*) Sagittal T1W image from an MR arthrogram in a different patient shows an osteochondral lesion with an unstable fragment, as evidenced by contrast extending between the fragment and capitellum (*arrowheads*). Note also a loose body within the posterior joint recess.

may be of use in determining whether a fragment is viable.[65]

Posteromedial Structures

Olecranon

Mechanism of injury As the medial stabilizers of the elbow fail under repetitive valgus stress, shear forces increase across the posterior aspect of the joint. The olecranon tends to impact against the posteromedial trochlea and olecranon fossa of the humerus, producing chondral loss and posteromedial osteophytes.[53] Of note, these posteromedial osteophytes are the most common indication for surgery in professional baseball players.[72] An olecranon stress fracture may rarely occur.

MR imaging Posteromedial elbow pathology is best evaluated in the axial plane. Focal cartilage loss may be identified along the ulnar or humeral articular surfaces, and associated subchondral edema on fat-saturated T2W images is a helpful secondary sign (**Fig. 21**). Periarticular osteophytes along the posteromedial joint line may be more easily detected on T1W images. These osteophytes can also impinge on the adjacent ulnar nerve.

Trochlear osteochondral lesion

Mechanism of injury Osteochondral lesions of the trochlea are much less common than those involving the capitellum. These lesions are most

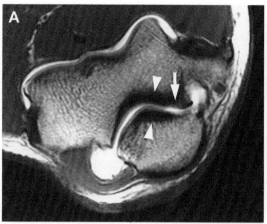 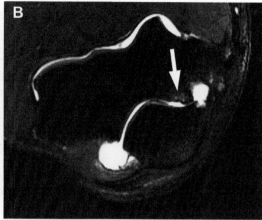

Fig. 21. Posteromedial impingement. (*A*) Axial T1W image (MR arthrogram) in a pitcher shows subchondral sclerosis along the medial ulnotrochlear joint (*arrowheads*) as well as a small trochlear cartilage defect (*arrow*) that is better seen in a corresponding fat-saturated T2W image (*B*).

commonly seen in young throwers and may involve either the posteromedial or posterolateral margins of the trochlea.[73] Posteromedial trochlear lesions are likely related to repetitive shear forces and ulnotrochlear abutment related to UCL insufficiency. The etiology of lesions along the lateral trochlear surface is uncertain, but they probably result from repetitive hyperextension of the elbow, resulting in compromise of the tenuous trochlear blood supply at that site.[73,74]

MR imaging As with capitellar lesions, focal subchondral signal abnormality, cystic change, and/or fragmentation are present and are typically most conspicuous on fat-saturated T2W images (**Fig. 22**).[73,74] Extension of fluid-equivalent signal intensity or gadolinium, in the case of an MR arthrogram, beneath a fragment is considered a sign of an unstable fragment. Should the fragment displace in later stages, a focal subchondral defect will be seen.

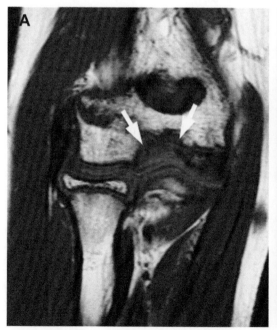 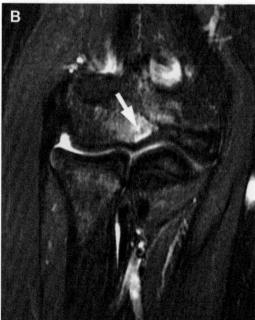

Fig. 22. Osteochondral lesion: trochlea. (*A*) Coronal T1W image in a pediatric thrower shows abnormal, intermediate subchondral signal intensity along the lateral margin of the trochlea (*arrows*). (*B*) Coronal fat-saturated T2W image shows to better advantage a small osteochondral lesion at that site (*arrow*). Note that the overlying articular cartilage is intact.

Table 1
Common injuries in the overhead athlete

SHOULDER: Internal Impingement		ELBOW: Valgus Overload Syndrome	
Structure	Pathology	Structure	Pathology
Posterior supraspinatus Anterior infraspinatus	Undersurface tears	Ulnar collateral ligament	Sprain Partial tear Compete tear
Posterior superior labrum	Fraying and/or tears	Common flexor tendon (flexor-pronator mass)	Tendinopathy Partial tear Complete tear
Superior labrum	SLAP tears	Medial epicondyle apophysis (immature thrower)	Stress reaction Fragmentation Separation
Greater tuberosity Posterior superior glenoid	Subcortical cysts Sclerosis	Ulnar nerve	Neuritis
		Capitellum Ulnohumeral joint	Osteochondral lesion Osteophytes Cartilage loss
		Trochlea (immature thrower)	Osteochondral lesion

SUMMARY

Shoulder and elbow injuries are common in overhead athletes. A thorough understanding of the forces acting on these joints and the anatomic structures involved will lead to improved diagnostic accuracy when interpreting MR imaging studies in these patients. Internal impingement in the shoulder and the valgus overload syndrome in the elbow lead to common injury patterns, summarized in Table 1. By focusing on these structures when interpreting MR examinations in these patients, the chances of detecting these often subtle imaging findings should be markedly improved.

REFERENCES

1. Limpisvasti O, ElAttrache NS, Jobe FW. Understanding shoulder and elbow injuries in baseball. J Am Acad Orthop Surg 2007;15:139–47.
2. Nassab PF, Schickendantz MS. Evaluation and treatment of medial ulnar collateral ligament injuries in the throwing athlete. Sports Med Arthrosc 2006;14:221–31.
3. O'Holleran JD, Altchek DW. The thrower's elbow: arthroscopic treatment of valgus extension overload syndrome. HSS J 2006;2:83–93.
4. Meister K. Injuries to the shoulder in the throwing athlete: part one: biomechanics/pathophysiology/classification of injury. Am J Sports Med 2000;28(2):265–75.
5. Wilk KE, Obma P, Simpson CD II, et al. Shoulder injuries in the overhead athlete. J Orthop Sports Phys Ther 2009;39(2):38–54.
6. Altchek DW, Dines DM. Shoulder injuries in the throwing athlete. J Am Acad Orthop Surg 1995;3:159–65.
7. Park SS, Loebenberg ML, Rokito AS, et al. The shoulder in baseball pitching: biomechanics and related injuries—part 1. Bull Hosp Jt Dis 2002–2003;61(1–2):68–79.
8. Sabick MB, Torry MR, Kim YK, et al. Humeral torque in professional baseball pitchers. Am J Sports Med 2004;32(4):892–8.
9. Park SS, Loebenberg ML, Rokito AS, et al. The shoulder in baseball pitching biomechanics and related injuries—part 2. Bull Hosp Jt Dis 2002–2003;61(1–2):80–8.
10. Olsen SJ II, Fleisig GS, Dun S, et al. Risk factors for shoulder and elbow injuries in adolescent baseball pitchers. Am J Sports Med 2006;34(6):905–12.
11. Davis JT, Limpisvasti O, Fluhme D, et al. The effect of pitching biomechanics on the upper extremity in youth and adolescent baseball pitchers. Am J Sports Med 2009;37(8):1484–91.
12. Sciascia A, Kibler WB. The pediatric overhead athlete: what is the real problem? Clin J Sport Med 2006;16(6):471–7.
13. Mair SD, Uhl TL, Robbe RG, et al. Physical changes and range-of-motion differences in the dominant shoulders of skeletally immature baseball players. J Shoulder Elbow Surg 2004;13:487–91.

14. Hang DW, Chao CM, Hang Y. A clinical and roentgenographic study of little league elbow. Am J Sports Med 2004;32(1):79–84.

15. Miniaci A, Mascia AT, Salonen DC, et al. Magnetic resonance imaging of the shoulder in asymptomatic professional baseball pitchers. Am J Sports Med 2002;30(1):66–73.

16. Connor PM, Banks DM, Tyson AB, et al. Magnetic resonance imaging of the asymptomatic shoulder of overhead athletes: a 5-year follow-up study. Am J Sports Med 2003;31(5):724–7.

17. Kooima CL, Anderson K, Craig JV, et al. Evidence of subclinical medial collateral ligament injury and posteromedial impingement in professional baseball players. Am J Sports Med 2004;32(7):1602–6.

18. Magee T. 3-T MRI of the shoulder: is MR arthrography necessary? AJR Am J Roentgenol 2009;192:86–92.

19. Magee T, Williams D, Mani N. Shoulder MR arthrography: which patient group benefits most? AJR Am J Roentgenol 2004;183:969–74.

20. Tuite MJ. MR imaging of sports injuries to the rotator cuff. Magn Reson Imaging Clin N Am 2003;11: 207–19.

21. Tirman PFJ, Bost FW, Steinbach LS, et al. MR arthrographic depiction of tears of the rotator cuff: benefit of abduction and external rotation or the arm. Radiology 1994;192:851–6.

22. Cvitanic O, Tirman PF, Feller JF, et al. Using abduction and external rotation of the shoulder to increase the sensitivity of MR arthrography in revealing tears of the anterior glenoid labrum. AJR Am J Roentgenol 1997;169:837–44.

23. Choi J-A, Suh SI, Kim BH, et al. Comparison between conventional MR arthrography and abduction and external rotation MR arthrography in revealing tears of the antero-inferior glenoid labrum. Korean J Radiol 2001;2:216–21.

24. Cochet H, Coudere S, Pele E, et al. Rotator cuff tears: should abduction and external rotation (ABER) positioning be preformed before image acquisition? A CT arthrography study. Eur Radiol 2010;20:1234–41.

25. Jung JY, Jee WH, Chun HJ, et al. Magnetic resonance arthrography including ABER view in diagnosing partial-thickness tears of the rotator cuff: accuracy, and inter- and intra-observer agreements. Acta Radiol 2010;2:194–201.

26. Ito Y, Sakai T, Tomo H, et al. Computerized assessment of Bankart lesions under tension with magnetic resonance arthrography. J Shoulder Elbow Surg 2005;14(3):247–51.

27. Roger B, Skaf A, Hooper AW, et al. Imaging findings in the dominant shoulder of throwing athletes: comparison of radiography, arthrography, CT arthrography, and MR arthrography with arthroscopic correlation. AJR Am J Roentgenol 1999;172: 1371–80.

28. Heyworth BE, Williams RJ III. Internal impingement of the shoulder. Am J Sports Med 2009;37(5): 1024–37.

29. Burkhart SS, Morgan CD, Kibler WB. The disabled throwing shoulder: spectrum of pathology. Part 1, pathoanatomy and biomechanics. Arthroscopy 2003;19:404–20.

30. Myers JB, Laudner KG, Pasquale MR, et al. Glenohumeral range of motion deficits and posterior shoulder tightness in throwers with pathologic internal impingement. Am J Sports Med 2006;34(3):385–91.

31. Kaplan LD, McMahon PJ, Towers J, et al. Internal impingement: findings on magnetic resonance imaging and arthroscopic evaluation. Arthroscopy 2004;20(7):701–4.

32. Tirman PFJ, Bost FW, Garvin GJ, et al. Posterosuperior glenoid impingement of the shoulder: findings at MR imaging and MR arthrography with arthroscopic correlation. Radiology 1994;193:431–6.

33. Giaroli EL, Major NM, Higgins LD. MRI of internal impingement of the shoulder. AJR Am J Roentgenol 2005;185:925–9.

34. Ouellette H, Labis J, Bredella M, et al. Spectrum of shoulder injuries in the baseball pitcher. Skeletal Radiol 2008;37:491–8.

35. McConville OR, Iannotti JP. Partial-thickness tears of the rotator cuff: evaluation and management. J Am Acad Orthop Surg 1999;7:32–43.

36. Vinson EN, Helms CA, Higgins LD. Rim-rent tear of the rotator cuff: a common and easily overlooked partial tear. AJR Am J Roentgenol 2007;189:943–6.

37. Tuite MJ, Turnbull JR, Orwin JF. Anterior versus posterior, and rim-rent rotator cuff tears: prevalence and MR sensitivity. Skeletal Radiol 1998;27:237–43.

38. Ostlere S, Marmery H. Imaging the shoulder. Imaging 2007;19:191–200.

39. Gerber C, Sebesta A. Impingement of the deep surface of the subscapularis tendon and the reflection pulley on the anterosuperior glenoid rim: a preliminary report. J Shoulder Elbow Surg 2000; 9:483–90.

40. Braun S, Kokmeyer D, Millett PJ. Shoulder injuries in the throwing athlete. J Bone Joint Surg Am 2009;91: 966–78.

41. Gaskin CM, Anderson MW, Choudhri A, et al. Focal partial tears of the long head of the biceps brachii tendon at the entrance to the bicipital groove: MR imaging findings, surgical correlation, and clinical significance. Skeletal Radiol 2009;38:959–65.

42. Bedi A, Allen A. Superior labral lesions anterior to posterior evaluation and arthroscopic management. Clin Sports Med 2008;27:607–30.

43. Waldt S, Metz S, Burkart A, et al. Variants of the superior labrum and labro-bicipital complex: a comparative study of shoulder specimens using MR arthrography, multi-slice CT arthrography and anatomical dissection. Eur Radiol 2006;16:451–8.

44. Tuite MJ, Rutkowski A, Enright T, et al. Width of high signal and extension posterior to biceps tendon as signs of superior labrum anterior to posterior tears on MRI and MR arthrography. AJR Am J Roentgenol 2005;185:1422–8.

45. Jin W, Ryu KN, Kwon SH, et al. MR arthrography in the differential diagnosis of type ii superior labral anteroposterior lesion and sublabral recess. AJR Am J Roentgenol 2006;187:887–93.

46. Tuite MJ, Cirillo RL, DeSmet AA, et al. Superior labrum anterior posterior (slap) tears: evaluation of three MR signs on t2-weighted images. Radiology 2000;215:841–5.

47. Borrero CG, Casagranda BU, Towers JD, et al. Magnetic resonance appearance of posterosuperior labral peel back during humeral abduction and external rotation. Skeletal Radiol 2010;39:19–26.

48. Osbahr DC, Kim HJ, Dugas JR. Little league shoulder. Pediatrics 2010;22:35–40.

49. Obembe OO, Gaskin CM, Taffoni MJ, et al. Little leaguer's shoulder (proximal humeral epiphysiolysis): MRI findings in four boys. Pediatr Radiol 2007;37:885–9.

50. Hatem SF, Recht MP, Profitt B. MRI of little leaguer's shoulder. Skeletal Radiol 2006;35:103–6.

51. Carrino JA, Morrison WB, Zou KH, et al. Noncontrast MR imaging and MR arthrography of the ulnar collateral ligament of the elbow: prospective evaluation of two-dimensional pulse sequences for detection of complete tears. Skeletal Radiol 2001;30:625–32.

52. Ouellett H, Bredella M, Labis J, et al. MR imaging of the elbow in baseball pitchers. Skeletal Radiol 2008;37:115–21.

53. Cain EL Jr, Dugas JR, Wold RS, et al. Elbow injuries in throwing athletes: a current concepts review. Am J Sports Med 2003;31(4):621–35.

54. Chen FS, Rokito AS, Jobe FW. Medial elbow problems in the overhead-throwing athlete. J Am Acad Orthop Surg 2001;9:99–113.

55. Lynch JR, Waitayawinyu T, Hanel DP, et al. Medial collateral ligament injury in the overhand throwing athlete. J Hand Surg Am 2008;33:430–7.

56. Timmerman LA, Andrews JR. Undersurface tear of the ulnar collateral ligament in baseball players. A newly recognized lesion. Am J Sports Med 1994;22(1):33–6.

57. Schwartz ML, Al-Zahrani S, Morwessel RM, et al. Ulnar collateral ligament injury in the throwing athlete: evaluation with saline-enhanced MR arthrography. Radiology 1995;197:297–9.

58. Timmerman LA, Schwartz ML, Andrews JR. Preoperative evaluation of the ulnar collateral ligament by magnetic resonance imaging and computed tomography arthrography: evaluation in 25 baseball players with surgical confirmation. Am J Sports Med 1994;22(1):26–31.

59. Nakanishi K, Masatomi T, Ochi T, et al. MR arthrography of elbow: evaluation of the ulnar collateral ligament of elbow. Skeletal Radiol 1996;25(7):629–34.

60. Munshi M, Pretterklieber ML, Chung CB, et al. Anterior bundle of ulnar collateral ligament: evaluation of anatomic relationships by using MR imaging, MR arthrography, and gross anatomic and histologic analysis. Radiology 2004;231:797–803.

61. Mirowitz SA, London SL. Ulnar collateral ligament injury in baseball pitchers: MR imaging evaluation. Radiology 1992;185:573–6.

62. Salvo JP, Rizio L III, Zvijac JE, et al. Avulsion fracture of the ulnar subline tubercle in overhead throwing athletes. Am J Sports Med 2002;30(3):426–31.

63. Walz DM, Newman JS, Konin GP, et al. Epicondylitis: pathogenesis, imaging, and treatment. Radiographics 2010;30:167–84.

64. Magra M, Caine D, Maffulli N. A review of epidemiology of paediatric elbow injuries in sports. Sports Med 2007;37(8):717–35.

65. Klingele KE, Kocher MS. Little league elbow valgus overload injury in the paediatric athlete. Sports Med 2002;32(15):1005–15.

66. Baker CL III, Romeo AA, Baker CL Jr. Osteochondritis dissecans of the capitellum. Am J Sports Med 2009;20(10):1–12.

67. Kijowski R, Tuite M, Sanford M. Magnetic resonance imaging of the elbow. Part 1: normal anatomy, imaging technique, and osseous abnormalities. Skeletal Radiol 2004;33:685–97.

68. Takahara M, Mura N, Sasaki J, et al. Classification, treatment, and outcome of osteochondritis dissecans of the humeral capitellum. J Bone Joint Surg Am 2007;89:1205–14.

69. Janarv PM, Hesser U, Hirsch G. Osteochondral lesions in the radiocapitellar joint radiographic, MRI, and arthroscopic findings in 13. J Pediatr Orthop 1997;17(3):311–4.

70. Kijowski R, DeSmet AA. MRI findings of osteochondritis dissecans of the capitellum with surgical correlation. AJR Am J Roentgenol 2005;185:1453–9.

71. Peiss J, Adam G, Casser R, et al. Gadopentetate-dimeglumine-enhanced MR imaging of osteonecrosis and osteochondritis dissecans of the elbow: initial experience. Skeletal Radiol 1995;24:17–20.

72. Andrews JR, Timmerman LA. Outcome of elbow surgery in professional baseball players. Am J Sports Med 1995;23(4):407–13.

73. Marshall KW, Marshall DL, Busch MT, et al. Osteochondral lesions of the humeral trochlea in the young athlete. Skeletal Radiol 2009;38:479–91.

74. Pruthi S, Parnell SE, Thapa MM. Pseudointercondylar notch sign: manifestation of osteochondritis dissecans of the trochlea. Pediatr Radiol 2009;39:180–3.

Hip Injuries in Athletes

Donna G. Blankenbaker, MD*, Arthur A. De Smet, MD

KEYWORDS

• Hip • Injury • Labrum • Cartilage • Tendon • Muscle
• Apophyseal injury

Hip pain is a common complaint in the active athletic population with a variety of possible causes. The differential diagnosis of hip pain is extensive, and affected athletes may have acute or chronic symptoms of widely ranging intensity, location, and duration. Clinical findings are highly variable, and the numerous regional anatomic structures make the clinical evaluation difficult. The demand for improved diagnosis of hip conditions has led to several advanced imaging techniques, including magnetic resonance (MR) imaging, MR arthrography, computed tomographic (CT) arthrography, and sonography. MR imaging is considered the imaging technique of choice for examining injured athletes after initial radiography. Sonography plays a role in the evaluation of other maladies around the hip. This article discusses the normal anatomy of the hip joint and surrounding structures of the hip, including abnormalities of the hip, both commonly and less commonly encountered in the active athletic population.

NORMAL ANATOMY

The hip is the prototypical ball-and-socket joint that allows a wide range of motion in all directions. The osseous components consist of the femoral head and the acetabulum. The acetabulum is oblique to all planes, with mild anteversion and lateral opening in the normal hip. The socket of the acetabulum is deficient centrally, where the cotyloid fossa is filled with fibrofatty tissue and is lined with synovium. The depression of the cotyloid fossa is continuous with the inferiorly positioned acetabular notch. Thus, the articular surface of

the acetabulum is essentially an upside-down horseshoe, which is covered by hyaline cartilage. The femoral head is entirely covered with hyaline cartilage except for the region of the fovea capitis. The fovea is a depression along the central surface of the femoral head. The ligamentum teres femoris arises from this depression and courses inferiorly within the joint to attach medially to the transverse ligament and to several surrounding structures. The ligamentum teres is a conduit for a small branch of the obturator artery, but that branch is often occluded in adults. The primary blood supply for the femoral head passes retrograde up the femoral neck; this blood supply can be disrupted by displaced femoral neck fractures and hip dislocations.

Labrum

The labrum is a fibrocartilaginous structure lining the horseshoe-shaped acetabulum. The labrum is thought to have several important functions, including the containment of the femoral head during acetabular formation and stabilization of the hip by deepening the acetabulum.[1,2] The labrum is generally triangular in cross section[3,4] as it arises from the rim of the acetabulum, although it can have a variable shape at MR imaging.[5] These labral shapes include triangular (most common), round, flat, or absent.[5] The labrum is thinner anteriorly and thicker posteriorly.[3,4,6] The acetabular labrum overlies the hyaline cartilage around the perimeter of the acetabulum.[3,7] The acetabular labrum blends with the transverse ligament at the margins of the acetabular notch, except for a small area where the

Musculoskeletal Division, Department of Radiology, University of Wisconsin School of Medicine and Public Health, 600 Highland Avenue, Madison, WI 53792-3252, USA
* Corresponding author.
E-mail address: dblankenbaker@uwhealth.org

Radiol Clin N Am 48 (2010) 1155–1178
doi:10.1016/j.rcl.2010.07.003
0033-8389/10/$ — see front matter © 2010 Elsevier Inc. All rights reserved.

ligament and labrum join. The appearance of a "cleft" or "sulcus" can often be seen between the labrum and transverse ligament where they join.[8] The labrum is innervated by nerves that play a role in proprioception and pain production.[9] The vascular supply to the labrum is limited, without significant penetration of vessels from the underlying acetabular bone into the labral substance, thus leaving the majority of the labrum avascular with limited potential for an injured labrum to heal.[10,11] The labrum is not designed to withstand significant weight-bearing forces; when subjected to such forces it eventually degenerates and tears.

Capsule

The capsule of the hip joint extends just above the acetabular rim proximally and down to the intertrochanteric ridge distally; the anterior extent of the capsule is more distal than the posterior extent. The capsule attaches to the acetabulum above the base of the labrum in most people, creating a normal perilabral recess between the labrum and the capsule.[3,12] Most of the femoral neck lies within the joint capsule. A series of ligaments helps to reinforce the capsule, including the iliofemoral, ischiofemoral, and pubofemoral ligaments; these are described as thickenings of the joint capsule. Along the middle of the femoral neck, there is a band of thickening of the capsule, called the zona orbicularis.

Iliopsoas

The iliopsoas musculotendinous unit consists of 3 muscles: the psoas major, the psoas minor, and the iliacus. The major action of the psoas and iliacus muscles is to flex the thigh on the pelvis, as well as function as a lateral flexor of the lower vertebral column.[13] The fibers of the iliacus and psoas muscles converge to form the iliopsoas tendon. Anatomic dissections have shown that with the hip in a neutral position, the iliopsoas tendon at the brim of the pelvis lies in a groove between the anterior inferior iliac spine laterally and the iliopectineal eminence medially. The muscular portions of the iliacus and psoas that surround the tendon cover the anterior inferior iliac spine and the iliopectineal eminence.[14,15] The tendon proper remains within the groove even at its far lateral and medial points of excursion. The iliopsoas tendon is closely related to the anterior aspect of the hip joint. The musculotendinous unit is separated from the adjacent bony structures by the iliopsoas bursa. A direct communication exists between the joint capsule and the iliopsoas bursa in 15% of adult individuals.[16,17]

Trochanteric Anatomy

The greater trochanter serves as the main attachment site for the strong abductor tendons. Four facets of the greater trochanter each have a specific tendinous attachment and specific nearby bursa.[18] The anterior facet is located on the anterolateral surface of the trochanter, has an oval appearance, and shares a medial border with the intertrochanteric line. The lateral facet has an inverted triangular shape and the caudal portion representing the palpable part at physical examination. The superoposterior facet forms the most cranial and posterior part of the trochanter, and has an oblique transverse orientation. The posterior facet is the most posterior aspect of the trochanter.

The trochanteric bursa is located immediately posterior to the cortex of the posterior facet of the greater trochanter, the distal lateral part of the gluteus medius tendon (lateral facet), and the proximal part of the vastus lateralis insertion. The subgluteus medius bursa is located deep to the lateral part of the gluteus medius tendon and covers the superior part of the lateral facet. The subgluteus minimus bursa is located beneath the gluteus minimus tendon, medial and superior to its insertion in the area of the anterior facet.

The gluteus medius attachment has been divided into 3 parts.[18] The tendon attaches onto the superoposterior facet (main tendon), the lateral facet from posterior to anterior (lateral portion of the tendon), and the anterior portion of the tendon to the gluteus minimus tendon. The gluteus minimus attachment consists of 2 parts.[18] The main tendon of the gluteus minimus inserts onto the anterior facet of the trochanter on its lateral and inferior aspect. The second part of the tendon inserts in the ventral and superior capsule of the hip joint.

Avulsion injuries in the pelvis primarily occur at 6 sites. The anterior-superior iliac spine is the site of origin of the sartorius tendon and the tensor muscle of the fascia lata. The anterior inferior iliac spine is the site of origin of the straight head of the rectus femoris tendon. The rectus femoris is composed of 2 tendons: one, the anterior or straight head, from the anterior inferior iliac spine; the other, the posterior or short head, from a groove above the brim of the acetabulum.[19] The ischial tuberosity is the site of origin of the hamstring tendons. The iliac crest is the site of attachment of the abdominal musculature and the pubic symphysis, and the inferior pubic ramus is the site of origin of the adductors of the hip, which includes the adductor longus, adductor brevis, and gracilis muscles, and is also the site of distal attachment of the rectus abdominis.

IMAGING TECHNIQUES
Radiography

The imaging workup of hip pain should still almost always begin with radiographs. According to American College of Radiology (ACR) criteria, radiography of a hip should always include an anteroposterior view of the pelvis centered at the level of the hips. Including the other hip in the image provides valuable information regarding symmetry or asymmetry of findings. Imaging the entire pelvis allows one to evaluate for causes of "hip pain" that are outside the hip joint proper. This view should be accompanied by at least one other view of the hip, such as the frog-lateral, cross-table lateral, and false profile views.

Computed Tomography

CT scanning is indispensable in the setting of trauma. The cortical detail is unparalleled, and small intra-articular fragments are readily apparent. Outside of the setting of major trauma, though, CT is seldom used in the evaluation of hip pain. CT arthrography of the hip, although seldom performed, has been shown to accurately define articular cartilage defects in patients with hip dysplasia.[20] The efficacy of CT arthrography in diagnosing labral tears has not been published.

MR Imaging

Hip MR imaging protocols vary from institution to institution, depending on the patient population, the physician's experience, clinical question to be answered, and the MR imaging equipment. There are 2 different types of MR imaging protocols that often are employed depending on the clinical concern for internal derangement (ie, labral tear, cartilage lesion) or nonspecific hip pain (stress fracture, bursitis, muscle or soft tissue injury).

When the differential for a patient's hip pain remains broad, MR imaging is the best imaging technique after initial radiographs. Indications for routine MR imaging include fracture (stress/insufficiency), muscle/tendon injuries, osteonecrosis, pubalgia, and the individual with nonspecific hip pain. MR imaging provides excellent soft tissue contrast, and edema often points the way to pathologic processes on fluid sensitive sequences. MR imaging is very effective at evaluating the regional muscles and tendons as well as the bone marrow.

Whether an MR imaging or MR arthrogram should be the study of choice in the evaluation of the patient with hip pain depends on the referring physician and clinical question to be answered. When the referral comes from primary care physicians, the authors advocate starting with a global assessment to include the entire pelvis and dedicated small-field-of-view imaging of the symptomatic hip. Often the authors have found pathology remote from the hip as the cause of the patient's pain. Therefore, their imaging protocol consists of coronal T1-weighted, coronal T2-weighted fat-suppressed or short-tau inversion recovery (STIR), axial T1-weighted and axial T2-weighted fat-suppressed sequences from just above the iliac crests to below the lesser trochanters with a field of view of 48 cm × 48 cm, at least a 256 × 224 matrix with 5-mm slice thickness. Additional small-field-of-view images are obtained through the symptomatic hip to assess for labral tears, cartilage lesions, or tendinous pathology. The authors obtain coronal T2-weighted fat-suppressed and sagittal proton density fat-suppressed sequences with a field of view of 24 cm through the symptomatic hip.

Alternatively, when the referring physician specializes in musculoskeletal disease and has a specific question with regard to the hip (ie, labral tear, stress fracture), dedicated small-field-of-view imaging of the symptomatic hip can be employed. A comprehensive hip examination would include coronal T1-weighted, coronal T2-weighted fat-suppressed/STIR, axial T1-weighted, axial T2-weighted fat-suppressed, sagittal proton density fat-suppressed, and axial oblique (parallel to the femoral neck) proton density fat-suppressed sequences through the hip with a field of view from 22 cm × 22 cm to 24 cm × 24 cm, at least a 320 × 192 matrix, and 3- to 4-mm slice thickness. Some investigators advocate radial imaging.[21]

MR Arthrography

MR arthrography is an ideal technique for evaluating the internal structures of the hip joint. Indications for MR arthrography include assessment of the acetabular labrum for tears or degeneration, detection of cartilage defects, evaluation of the intrinsic ligaments and hip capsule, evaluation for intra-articular loose bodies, and assessment of the morphologic changes of femoroacetabular impingement. Numerous structural alterations within the joint are visible with joint distention created by the intra-articular administration of contrast. Several anatomic variants and potentially asymptomatic lesions have been described.[4,6,8,22] As arthroscopy of the hip continues to emerge, knowledge about the clinical significance of these structural alterations grows. MR arthrography remains the preferred technique for imaging of the acetabular labrum.

The sensitivity and accuracy of MR arthrography for detection of labral tears and detachments is 90% and 91%, respectively, versus 30% and 36% for conventional MR imaging.[6,7,23] However, Mintz and colleagues[24] found a high accuracy for labral tear detection using optimized noncontrast MR imaging. MR arthrography has been shown to have a sensitivity of 79% and specificity of 77% in the detection of cartilage lesions.[25] Most investigators prefer MR arthrography over conventional MR imaging in the assessment of cartilage lesions, although the study by Mintz and colleagues[24] reported a higher accuracy with conventional MR imaging. In their study, the accuracy for detection of cartilage lesions of the femoral head was 82% to 87% and acetabular cartilage lesion detection was 84% to 88%; however, they graded the cartilage into disease positive (grades 2, 3, and 4) and disease negative (grades 0 and 1), and did not directly compare the exact grade of cartilage lesion detection.

The technique of MR arthrography has been well described.[6,23] A needle is passed into the hip joint, usually under fluoroscopic guidance using an anterior approach. Once the joint is entered, iodinated contrast is injected confirming intra-articular location. Subsequently, a dilute gadolinium solution is injected. There are numerous recipes for the contrast solution. The authors' choice is to combine 5 mL saline, 5 mL iodinated contrast (300 mg/mL, Amersham Health Inc, Princeton, NJ, USA), 5 mL 0.5% ropivacaine HCl (5 mg/mL, Novation, Irving, TX, USA), 5 mL 1% preservative free lidocaine (10 mg/mL, Hospira Inc, Lake Forest, IL, USA), and 0.1 mL (0.2 mmol/L) gadolinium dimeglumine solution (Magnevist; Berlex Laboratories, Wayne, NJ, USA). Recently, several experimental studies have suggested that some local anesthetics may damage articular cartilage, and that 0.5% bupivacaine is toxic to both bovine articular chondrocyte cultures and bovine articular osteochondral tissue.[26,27] Although this is a small risk as only a small amount of diluted anesthetic is injected, most of these patients are young and any chondrolysis would be tragic. The authors therefore have changed their long-acting anesthetic to ropivacaine. This mixture is injected until the joint is distended (approximately 12–15 mL), stopping if the patient feels an uncomfortable fullness or a higher pressure impedes injection. Inclusion of anesthetic in the solution is not mandatory, but provides additional diagnostic information as studies have shown supporting evidence that relief of pain with intra-articular anesthetic confirms that the source of pain is from within the joint.[22,28–30] Pain relief following injection at MR arthrography is important to orthopedic surgeons in considering hip arthroscopy. If no pain relief is achieved, the treating physician must consider that the hip pain may be referred from another site (ie, sacroiliac joint, lumbar spine) and therefore the patient is not a candidate for hip arthroscopy.

A surface phased-array coil should be used to obtain an adequate signal-to-noise ratio. Imaging parameters include a field of view of 16 to 18 cm, at least a 256–320 × 224–256 matrix, and 3.0 to 4.0 mm slice thickness. T1-weighted fast spin echo with fat suppression images are obtained in at least 3 imaging planes. The authors obtain these images in the standard sagittal and coronal imaging planes, with an axial T1 sequence without fat suppression (to assess bone marrow and fatty changes within muscle) and an oblique axial T1-weighted fat-suppressed sequence parallel to the femoral neck. These images allow better evaluation of the anterosuperior portion of the labrum, where most tears occur. Alternatively, some investigators have described using radial imaging for identifying these tears of the labrum.[21] However, a recent study by Yoon and colleagues[31] evaluating the radial sequences with MR arthrography did not find any additional morphologic changes in patients with femoroacetabular impingement. Finally, a coronal T2-weighted fat-suppressed or STIR sequence is included to detect edema, fluid collections, and surrounding soft tissue pathology. A prior study has shown that the axial oblique imaging plane has the highest individual detection rate of labral tears[32] with a greater than 95% detection rate of labral tears achieved with 3 imaging sequences (axial oblique T1-weighted fat-suppressed, sagittal T1-weighted fat-suppressed, and coronal T2-weighted fat-suppressed). Leg traction has been suggested to improve visualization of the femoral head and acetabular cartilage surfaces[33]; however, no studies have been performed to determine if this technique improves the accuracy in detecting cartilage lesions.

Finally, does it matter whether the patients are scanned on the 1.5-T or 3-T magnet? The authors prefer 3-T scans for dedicated hip imaging and MR arthrography if available. For MR arthrography, it is recommended the gadolinium concentration be more dilute at 3-T imaging[34] to optimize contrast. A concentration of 1 to 1.23 mmol Gd/L has been suggested to optimize the signal-to-noise ratio of T1-weighted sequences. Moreover, the addition of iodinated contrast lowers the signal intensity more at 3 T than 1.5 T, and therefore the concentration of iodinated contrast at 3 T should be limited to the least amount possible.

Sonography

As with most joints, the role of sonography in the hip is probably best limited to evaluation of a specific question or two. For instance, ultrasonography is a fine technique for evaluating pathology of individual tendons, but should not be routinely used to survey the entire joint. Especially in small children, sonography is ideal for defining joint effusions and guiding subsequent aspiration.[35] Sonography can also pinpoint suspected bursitis and can demonstrate snapping tendons. It is ideal for performing imaging-guided injections. The labrum can be visualized at the anterior attachment onto the acetabulum with sonography[36]; however, MR arthrography remains the primary imaging technique of choice for evaluation of the acetabular labrum.

HIP PATHOLOGY
Osseous Injuries

MR imaging can be used to diagnose fractures and contusions, and helps to exclude other uncommon osseous pathology in the athletic population, for example, osteonecrosis and transient osteoporosis. Most traumatic fractures of the hip are diagnosed by radiographs, but the diagnosis of nondisplaced fractures may be difficult at radiography and may be missed, especially in the osteoporotic patient. In the traumatic setting following identification of fractures on radiographs, CT is used for fracture assessment and extent as well as for surgical planning.

Stress Fracture

Fatigue-type stress fractures result from repetitive stress on normal bone, resulting in a region of accelerated bone remodeling.[37] At the microscopic level, repetitive overloading leads to increased osteoclastic activity that exceeds the rate of osteoblastic new bone formation; this results in bone weakening, microtrabecular fractures (stress injury), and eventually may lead to a cortical break (stress fracture).[38] These injuries often occur along the medial aspect of the femoral neck, where compressive forces are pronounced, but can also develop along the outer aspect, where tensile forces predominate.[39–41]

The diagnosis of stress injuries can be made based on the clinical history and characteristic radiographic findings of focal periosteal reaction, cortical disruption, and trabecular sclerosis.[41] The subtle, ill-defined area of the affected cortex, the "gray cortex sign," may also be seen during the early stages of stress fractures. However, these fractures are frequently occult on initial radiographs, and MR imaging is the best imaging method for diagnosing stress fractures (**Fig. 1**). On MR imaging, a focal or diffuse, ill-defined

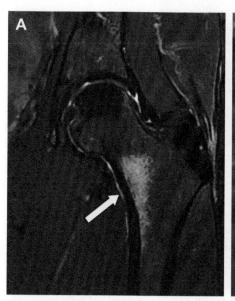
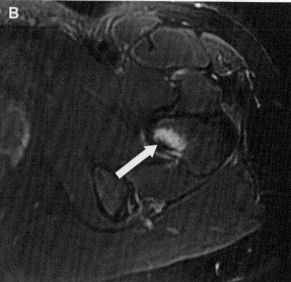

Fig. 1. A 36-year-old woman with left hip pain. She has been recently training for a marathon. (*A*) Coronal T2-weighted fat-suppressed MR image demonstrates periosteal edema (*arrow*), endosteal edema, and increased signal within the medial femoral neck cortex representing a stress fracture. (*B*) Axial T2-weighted fat-suppressed MR image shows a small low-signal intensity line within the endosteal edema (*arrow*).

hypointense area on T1-weighted images that has increased signal on fluid-sensitive sequences is characteristic of stress injury (microtrabecular fracture).[42,43] The identification of periosteal edema, endosteal edema, and high signal within the cortex, even without a fracture line, should suggest the diagnosis of a stress fracture, as the slice thickness may have missed a small fracture line. In addition, an accurate diagnosis of a stress fracture of the hip is important, as many athletes would otherwise be reluctant to reduce their activity so as to protect the hip from a more extensive fracture.

Traumatic Hip Subluxation or Dislocation

The spectrum of traumatic hip malalignment ranges from subluxation to dislocation with or without concomitant injuries (Fig. 2).[44] The diagnosis of a traumatic hip injury is obvious in severe cases of dislocation; however, more subtle traumatic subluxation of the hip can occur with seemingly minimal trauma. The radiologic workup after a presumed traumatic hip injury begins with radiographs. In many cases, this provides a definitive diagnosis. CT imaging is commonly performed to evaluate associated known acetabular fractures, or to look for a subtle nondisplaced fracture of the proximal femur or acetabulum. MR imaging is typically not performed acutely, but to assess for the sequelae of traumatic malalignment such as chondral injuries, labral tears, capsular injuries, and injuries to the surrounding supporting soft tissue

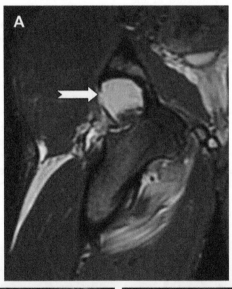

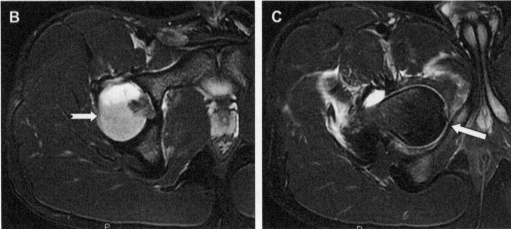

Fig. 2. A 17-year-old football player following acute injury. Coronal (A) T2-weighted fat-suppressed, axial T2-weighted fat-suppressed (B, C) MR images through the right hip demonstrate anterior and inferior dislocation of the femoral head (arrow). A large hemarthrosis fills the acetabulum (notched arrow). There has been tearing of the adductor muscles and ligamentum teres.

structures. Injury patterns depend on the age of the patient and the competency of the surrounding supporting soft tissue structures. In the athlete, a forward fall on the knee with a flexed hip or a blow from behind while down on all 4 limbs can cause a wide range of associated injuries.[44] Traumatic dislocation in the athlete is accompanied by a variety of intra-articular pathologies, the most common being labral, chondral, and intra-articular loose fragments and disruption of the ligamentum teres.[45] One of the complications following hip dislocation is osteonecrosis of the femoral head, which must not be overlooked. MR imaging is useful in the detection of osteonecrosis. However, MR imaging is not an accurate predictor of osteonecrosis in the acute setting following trauma.[46] A repeat MR imaging scan can be performed at 6 weeks to exclude traumatic osteonecrosis.[44] If patients have no evidence of osteonecrosis at 6 to 12 weeks, they may return safely to sports activity.

Apophyseal Avulsion Injuries

Avulsion injuries of the pelvis occur most often in the adolescent athlete, usually resulting in displacement of an unfused apophysis at the site of the tendon attachment due to the inherent weakness at this site.[19,47] The ischial tuberosity is the most common location for apophyseal injury in the pelvis.[19,48] Apophyseal avulsion injuries are usually detected on radiographs, but may require CT, MR imaging, or sonography to identify subtle lesions or to better define the extent of the injury.

Avulsion injuries may be caused by sudden forceful (often eccentric) contraction of the musculotendinous unit during running, jumping, or kicking a ball.[39] In addition, repetitive microtrauma from intensive training can cause biomechanical failure at the physeal plate.[39]

An anteroposterior radiograph of the pelvis should be the first imaging study for patients suspected of having these injuries, because the diagnosis of avulsion injury may be documented without further imaging. Apophyseal avulsions, however, may be radiographically occult if the apophysis is not ossified, so further imaging may be needed for confirmation. Although MR imaging can reveal these injuries, sonography is advantageous because of its faster examination time and decreased cost.[49] MR and CT imaging improves detection of the subtle avulsion injury: CT depicts the amount of displacement and retraction of the apophysis, while MR imaging better defines the extent of adjacent soft tissue injuries and retraction of tendons (**Fig. 3**).[48]

Labrum and Labral Tears

MR appearance of the asymptomatic labrum

There is a wide spectrum of appearances of the acetabular labrum in asymptomatic individuals.[5,50] The shape of the labrum is triangular on conventional MR images in the majority of asymptomatic patients.[1,5,50] The posterior labrum is more commonly triangular in shape than the anterior labrum.[50] The labrum has a tendency to become rounded and irregular with age.[1,5] A previous study by Abe and colleagues[50] showed a triangular labral shape in 96% of patients 10 to 19 years old, but in only 62% of patients older than 50 years. These investigators proposed that the loss of the normal triangular-shaped labrum may be caused by degenerative changes. Abe and colleagues also found that an irregularly shaped labrum was only seen in patients older than 40 years, and an absent labrum only in patients 50 years or older.[50] This irregularity of the labrum, thought to represent degeneration, may be difficult to distinguish from small tears.[50] Other studies have documented an absent labrum on one or more MR images in 10% to 14% of asymptomatic patients.[1,5] Therefore, when the labrum is absent or irregular in a middle-aged or elderly patient it may represent degeneration, but a tear should be considered, especially in symptomatic patients.

The acetabular labrum consists mainly of fibrocartilage tissue, accounting for the single most common appearance on MR of low signal intensity on T1- and T2-weighted images. Several studies have demonstrated a homogeneous low signal intensity labrum in 44% to 56% of asymptomatic individuals.[1,5,23]

About half of asymptomatic individuals have intermediate or high signal intensity within the labrum.[1] A common location for intralabral intermediate signal intensity is at the junction between the labrum and acetabulum.[7] Additional increased intralabral signal is most commonly seen within the superior labrum.[1] This intralabral signal may be linear, globular, or curvilinear, and can involve the capsular or articular surfaces of the labrum, or both.[1,5] Therefore, this appearance may mimic a labral tear on conventional MR imaging images. Degeneration within the fibrocartilage can produce high signal intensity, and may explain some of the labral heterogeneity seen on MR imaging. However, a study in elderly cadavers[7] found a poor correlation between intralabral signal abnormalities and histologic evidence of degeneration. The investigators described this increased intralabral signal as the presence of small intralabral fibrovascular bundles.[7] Another cause for this increased intralabral signal of the acetabular

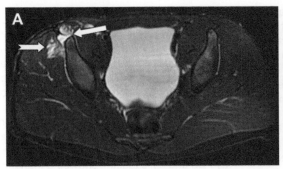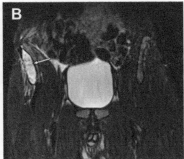

Fig. 3. A 14-year-old boy with right-sided hip pain following hockey injury. Axial T2-weighted fat-suppressed (*A*) and coronal short-tau inversion recovery (*B*) MR images show an acute avulsion injury of the sartorius from the anterior-superior iliac spine (*large arrow*). There is underlying hematoma (*small arrow*). Additional partial avulsion of the origin of the gluteus minimus muscle is also present (*notched arrow*).

labrum on T1-weighted images could be the magic angle effect.[1]

Clinical findings of labral tears

If an active patient has a catching or clicking sensation in the hip after a twisting or slipping injury, a labral tear should be suspected. Labral tears may also occur in the absence of specific recognizable trauma.[10] More commonly the symptom presentation is subtle, characterized by dull activity-induced or positional pain that fails to improve over time. Often patients describe a "deep" discomfort within the anterior groin or occasionally laterally, just proximal to the greater trochanter.[10] Although a clicking mechanical symptom suggests an acetabular-labral tear, other entities such as snapping iliopsoas tendon may give a similar presentation. The physical examination is variable, although pain is often provoked with flexion and internal rotation of the hip.[12,51–53]

Labral tears

Tears of the acetabular labrum have been increasingly recognized as a cause of mechanical hip pain. Labral tears have been reported in patients with hip dysplasia, Legg-Calve-Perthes disease, osteoarthritis, instability, trauma, and femoroacetabular impingement, but may occur in young patients with normal radiographs or no previous injury to the hip.[1,6,53–56] A high percentage of patients with intra-articular hip pain from synovitis, loose bodies, and cartilage defects also have acetabular-labral tears.[6,54] Individuals with even mild degrees of hip dysplasia are at increased

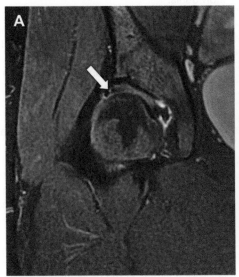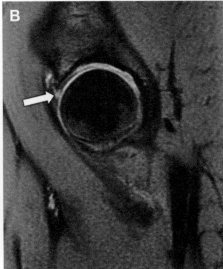

Fig. 4. A 25-year-old woman with hip pain. Clinical concern was stress fracture. Coronal T2-weighted fat-suppressed (*A*) and sagittal proton density (*B*) conventional MR images demonstrate a tear of the anterosuperior labrum confirmed at arthroscopy (*arrows*).

risk for labral tears because decentering of the femoral head generates high loads at the acetabular rim. Certain types of athletic activities, such as gymnastics and dance, may self-select for athletes with greater arcs of hip motion.[57] In these individuals, increased forces on the labrum can result in biomechanical overload and injury.[39]

Athletes are particularly vulnerable to labral tears because their hip joints are exposed to extremes of motion (**Fig. 4**). It is theorized that the forces exerted on the labrum, either periodically or repetitively, are responsible for the injury patterns as seen at arthroscopy.[10] Certain sports such as golf, hockey, or soccer involve frequent external rotation of the hip. It is these repetitive motion sports that may produce an insidious onset of a labral tear. Hyperextension combined with femoral external rotation is the injury pattern most commonly associated with an acute presentation of anterior acetabular-labral pathology, which may result from mild subluxation and sheer injury of the femoral head on the anterior acetabulum.[10] Posterior labral lesions typically occur in an athlete as a result of axial loading of the hip in a flexed position.[10] Tears of the acetabular labrum may result in disabling mechanical symptoms, which limit daily activities as well as participation in athletics.

Labral tears have been diagnosed by conventional arthrography, CT arthrography, conventional MR, and MR arthrography.[7,50,58–61] When labral tears are identified either clinically or radiologically, these tears are now often treated with hip arthroscopy. Early diagnosis and treatment of tears is important because it not only provides pain relief but may prevent the early onset of osteoarthritis.[11,53,59]

Labral abnormalities include partial tears or labral detachments, with detachments more common than tears (**Figs. 5–7**).[12,23,30] The terms labral "tears" and "detachments" are often used interchangeably. Labral tears can be classified according to location, etiology, and morphologic features. The location of tears can be divided into quadrants: anterior, anterior-superior, posterior-superior, or posterior. Tears can also be described by the extent of the tear using a clock face.[62] Tears occur anteriorly in most reported series.[2,11,30,51,54,58] Tears of the posterior-superior labrum have been described in younger patients.[59] Isolated posterior labral tears are also most frequently seen after a posterior hip dislocation or in patients with hip dysplasia (**Fig. 8**).[11]

Labral tears can also be classified with respect to etiology. Tears can be degenerative, dysplastic, traumatic, or idiopathic. Degenerative tears can be seen with long-standing inflammatory arthropathies,

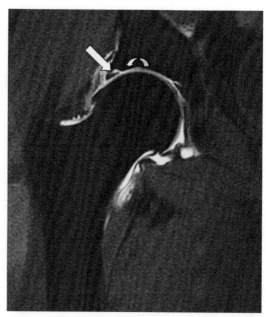

Fig. 5. A 28-year-old male runner with hip pain. Coronal T1-weighted fat-suppressed MR arthrogram image shows a partial-thickness tear of the superior labrum (*arrow*). Notice the acetabular and femoral head cartilage loss (*curved arrow*) and osteophytes at the head-neck junction.

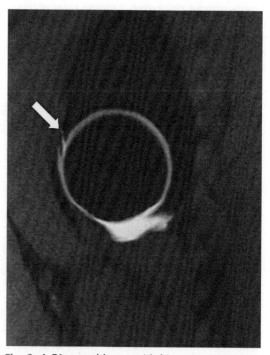

Fig. 6. A 51-year-old man with hip pain. Sagittal T1-weighted fat-suppressed MR arthrogram images demonstrate a full-thickness tear of the superior labrum (*arrow*).

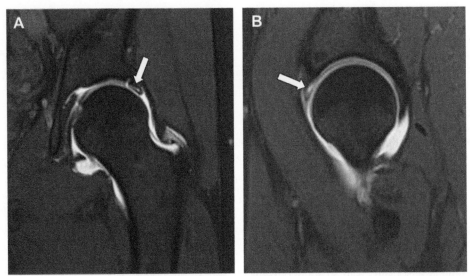

Fig. 7. A 40-year-old woman with hip pain. Coronal (*A*) and sagittal (*B*) T1-weighted fat-suppressed MR arthrogram images show a complex type tear with a vertical and horizontal component (*arrows*).

osteoarthritis, or related to old trauma. Tears associated with hip dysplasia occur most frequently anteriorly but also can occur posteriorly or be diffuse. The anterior labrum in patients with acetabular dysplasia is commonly hypertrophied and torn. Labral tears secondary to trauma are typically isolated to one particular region. Patients who have a labral tear after trauma without dislocation typically have anterior tears. These tears occur in the same region as those seen in athletes or secondary to mild hip dysplasia.[11] Idiopathic tears are those that do not fall into any of the above categories.

Labral tears as seen at arthroscopy have been morphologically classified by Lage and colleagues[2] into radial flap, radial fibrillated, longitudinal peripheral, and unstable tears. It is difficult for MR arthrography to subtype tears into these types. A recent study comparing the Lage classification[2] for hip labral tears did not correlate well with the Czerny MR arthrography classification[23] or an MR arthrography modification of the Lage classification system.[62] Most hip arthroscopists resect or repair the labrum based on other features, and morphologic type usually does not affect surgery.

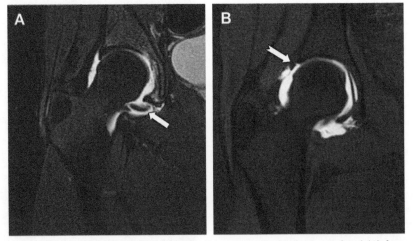

Fig. 8. A 21-year-old woman with history of prior hip dislocation. Coronal T2-weighted (*A*) fat-suppressed and coronal T1-weighted (*B*) fat-suppressed MR arthrogram images show a large intra-articular bony fragment (*arrow*) off the medial femoral head representing sequelae of prior dislocation injury. (*B*) A posterosuperior labral tear is present (*notched arrow*). In the setting of prior posterior dislocation, the posterosuperior labrum should be closely scrutinized for labral lesions.

Therefore, a more useful classification system for labral tears includes the descriptive terms: frayed (irregularity of the free edge of the labral substance seen with degeneration), partial-thickness tear, full-thickness tear, and complex tear.

MR arthrography of labral tears

In the assessment of the labrum at MR arthrography, 4 items should be addressed: (1) what is the morphology, such as triangular, thickened, or distorted/irregular (representing a tear)?; (2) does contrast extend into the labrum (indicating a tear)?; (3) does contrast extend between the labrum and acetabulum indicating labral detachment?; and (4) is there increased signal intensity within the labrum indicating mucoid degeneration but not a tear?

Acetabular-labral tears are recognized on MR arthrography by the presence of contrast material extending into the labrum (see **Fig. 5**).[4,23,63] Detachments are identified by the presence of contrast material interposed at the acetabular-labral junction with or without labral displacement (see **Fig. 6**).[4,23,64] The signal intensity within a tear does not have to be equal to that of gadolinium or fluid to confirm the diagnosis of labral tear.[32] It is important to assess the acetabular labrum on all imaging planes, as a tear may be detected on only one image; however, tears are typically seen on more than one imaging plane and on more than one image.[32]

Secondary findings

Labral lesions may be associated with several abnormalities in the adjacent cartilage, bone, and soft tissues.[39,65] Common associated findings seen in individuals with labral lesions are subchondral bone marrow edema, subchondral cystic change, and cartilage lesions. Within the adjacent soft tissues, paralabral cysts can also be found.

Paralabral cysts have been described in patients with developmental dysplasia of the hip, osteoarthritis, and both acute and remote hip trauma.[66] The cysts are associated with either degeneration or tears of the labrum.[55,65,67] When a labral tear is present, there is an increase in intra-articular pressure secondary to the loss of congruency between the femoral head and the acetabulum.[55] It is this elevated pressure that forces synovial fluid through the labral tear, resulting in a paralabral cyst.[58]

Paralabral cysts are of low to intermediate signal intensity on T1-weighted images and high signal intensity on T2-weighted images (**Fig. 9**). The differential diagnosis of a homogeneous fluid signal intensity mass adjacent to the acetabulum would include a ganglion unrelated to a labral tear, an atypical synovial cyst, neural tumor,[65] and iliopsoas bursitis. Determining the location of the fluid collection in relation to the iliopsoas tendon has been useful in differentiating between iliopsoas bursitis and a paralabral cyst. In the authors' experience, a paralabral cyst frequently is located lateral to the iliopsoas tendon, whereas iliopsoas bursal fluid collections are located medial to the iliopsoas tendon.[65] Another useful sign in determining the cause of the paralabral cyst is to look for a communication of the cyst with a torn acetabular labrum. At MR arthrography,

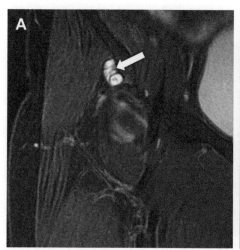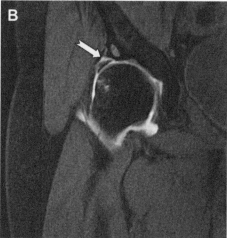

Fig. 9. A 56-year-old active man with hip pain. (*A*) Coronal T2-weighted fat-suppressed MR and coronal (*B*) T1-weighted fat-suppressed MR arthrogram images of the hip show a paralabral cyst anterior to the acetabular labrum (*arrow*). A complex tear is seen involving the anterosuperior labrum (*notched arrow*). Note the subchondral cyst within the superior acetabulum.

high signal intensity contrast filling the paralabral cystic structure on T1-weighted fat-suppressed images adjacent to an abnormal labrum confirms the diagnosis. Occasionally a paralabral cyst can have an unusual low signal appearance on T2-weighted images, which may be due to gelatinous/mucinous material, debris, or proteinaceous products. Recognizing a paralabral cyst is helpful because this observation may confirm an uncertain diagnosis of a labral tear (**Fig. 10**). Care should be taken to recognize a normal variant, the obturator externus bursa. There is a potential communication between the hip joint and obturator bursa, seen in approximately 5.5% of MR arthrograms, which could be misinterpreted as a paralabral cyst.[68]

Pitfalls

One pitfall of MR imaging of the labrum is the normal posterior inferior acetabular sublabral sulcus or groove.[8,69] The posterior inferior location of the sublabral sulcus is helpful, differentiating it from most labral injuries that occur at the anterior or anterior-superior acetabulum.[2,11,30,70] Dinauer and colleagues[8] defined the presence of a posteroinferior sulcus when labral separation from the articular cartilage was clearly observed on at least 2 MR images in the absence of surgical pathology in the same region of the acetabulum; this is a commonly seen finding and should not be misinterpreted as a tear.

The presence of a sublabral sulcus other than in the posteroinferior acetabulum has been raised as a potential pitfall in the diagnosis of labral tears,[4,6] although this topic remains controversial. Several investigators have suggested that a normal sublabral sulcus mimicking a traumatic labral detachment may exist at the anterior-superior acetabulum.[12,22] Byrd[22] described a partial separation of the labrum from the margin of the superior bony acetabulum as a normal variation in patients with acetabular dysplasia.

Two recent studies have evaluated the presence of sublabral sulci at MR imaging and arthroscopy. In the study by Saddik and colleagues,[69] 30 sulci were identified at hip arthroscopy in 25% (27) of 121 patients. Of the 30 sulci found at arthroscopy, 12 were located anterosuperiorly, 14 posteroinferiorly, 2 anteroinferiorly, and 2 posterosuperiorly, indicating that sulci may be seen within any quadrant. In the arthroscopy study by Studler and colleagues,[71] 10 (18%) of 57 patients had sublabral sulci in the anteroinferior part of the acetabulum. Contrast material interposed at the labral base within the anterosuperior portion of the labrum always indicated a labral tear.[71]

It is the authors' experience that there can be a normal sublabral sulcus at the anterior-superior acetabulum at the labral acetabular junction. The differentiating characteristics of a sulcus from a tear are that: (1) contrast should not completely extend through the labrum, (2) smooth borders are seen with a sulcus, whereas irregular borders are seen with tears, and (3) sulci are generally shallow, whereas tears extend deeper within the labrum (**Fig. 11**).[72] The authors do not know exactly how deep a sulcus can extend into the labrum. However, as in the study by Dinauer and colleagues,[8] whenever the authors have noted contrast extending greater than 50% across the anterior-superior labral base at MR arthrography, this finding has surgically correlated with labral injury.[73] Lastly, if there is a high clinical suspicion for labral tear and the patient gets pain relief with

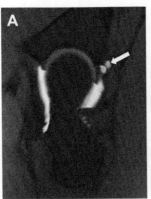 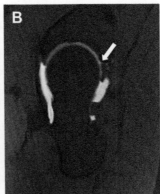 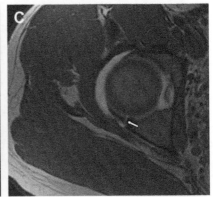

Fig. 10. A 28-year-old male soccer player with chronic hip pain. (*A, B*) Two sequential axial oblique T1-weighted fat-suppressed and axial (*C*) T1-weighted MR arthrogram images demonstrate a small posterior-superior paralabral cyst (*arrow* in *A*). A neck from this cyst can be seen to extend to the labrum (*arrow* in *B*). Axial T1 image help to confirm the posterior labral tear (*arrow* in *C*). Whenever a cyst is identified around the hip, close inspection of the labrum to evaluate for associated labral tear should be made.

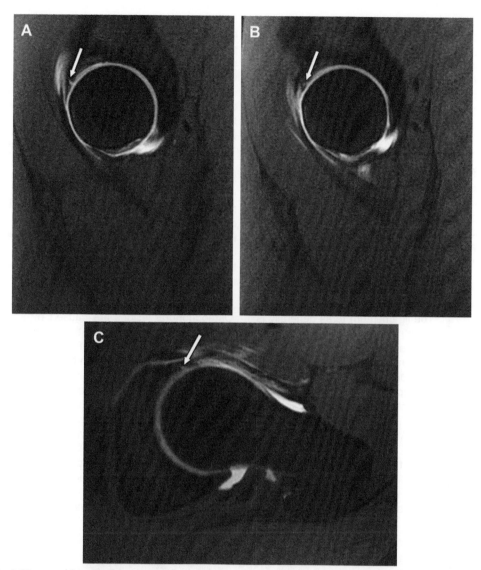

Fig. 11. A 17-year-old male athlete with hip pain. He had symptomatic relief of his hip pain following anesthetic injection. Two sequential sagittal (*A, B*) and axial oblique (*C*) T1-weighted MR arthrogram images of the left hip show high signal at the labral cartilage interface. Initial sagittal image (*A*) could be interpreted as a sulcus; however, this is slightly irregular and deep (*arrow*). The next image (*B*) demonstrates irregularity, distortion, and abnormal morphology of the anterior labrum with subtle high signal within the labral substance indicating a tear (*arrow*). The high signal also extends greater than 50% across the labral base (*arrow* in *C*).

intra-articular injection of anesthetic, and MR arthrography imaging findings are equivocal for labral tear, it may be helpful to point out this pain relief and indicate that this is suspicious for a labral tear rather than a normal sulcus.

Diagnostic difficulties can also result from extra-articular injection or leak of contrast material through the capsular puncture site, which may simulate a tear within the capsule. However, injecting less than 15 mL into the joint decreases

the likelihood of an extracapsular leak.[74] Inadvertent injection of air into the joint could lead to a false-positive diagnosis of intra-articular loose bodies, and depending on the location may cause difficulty in assessing for labral pathology.

Surgical treatment

The management of hip abnormalities has evolved significantly in the past few years with the advancement of arthroscopic techniques, and arthroscopy has been shown to be of benefit in the treatment of labral tears.[53,75] Surgical treatment for labral tears includes either resection or repair of a tear.[11,30,52,53,76,77] Recently a new technique has been described using the ligamentum teres for labral reconstruction.[78]

Ligamentum Teres

Injury of the ligamentum teres has been increasingly recognized at hip arthroscopy and considered as a source of hip pain in athletes.[79] With advances in imaging techniques in assessing intra-articular structures of the hip, ligamentum teres pathology should be evaluated on all hip MR imaging and should be part of the search pattern. Injury of the ligamentum teres is known to occur with dislocation of the joint, but disruption in the absence of a dislocation has also been described.[79,80] The ligamentum teres generally is not thought to contribute to hip joint stability, although this remains uncertain.[81,82] Tear of the ligamentum teres can be a source of persistent hip pain following injury, with the disrupted fibers catching within the hip joint.[79] At arthroscopy, ligamentum teres pathology has been classified as complete ligamentum teres rupture, partial tear, and degeneration.[82] At MR arthrography, the diagnosis of a complete rupture of the ligament is made when no intact ligament can be identified or only wavy incomplete fibers are visualized. A partial tear may be more difficult to diagnose, with irregularity of the fibers or thickening of the ligament (Fig. 12). Treatment consists of limited debridement of the entrapping fibers.[83]

Capsule and Extrinsic Ligaments

With MR imaging, injuries to the extrinsic ligaments may be diagnosed using the criteria commonly used for ligaments elsewhere in the body. The most common injury following traumatic dislocation of the femoral head is injury to the iliofemoral ligament of the hip joint capsule, easily diagnosed at MR imaging.[84] The capsule may also be injured following dislocation or during sports-related activities. The identification of contrast across the capsule (not at the site of puncture during arthrography) indicates a capsular injury (Fig. 13).

Osteochondral Lesions, Chondral Defects, and Intra-Articular Loose Bodies

Osteochondral lesions are caused by impaction injuries that result in laceration of the articular cartilage and microfracture of the underlying subchondral trabeculae.[85] Within the hip joint, osteochondral injuries have been reported most commonly following hip dislocation.[86] The location of osteochondral impaction injury depends on the direction of dislocation. Following anterior dislocation, the site of impaction is typically located along the posterolateral aspect of the femoral head, whereas following posterior dislocation the anterior margin of the femoral head is mostly involved. Patients who have chronic, persistent hip pain following injury, with negative or equivocal

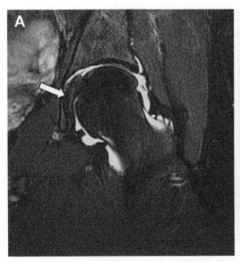 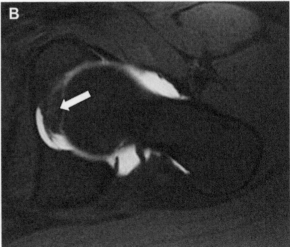

Fig. 12. A 16-year-old runner with hip pain. Coronal (A) T2-weighted fat-suppressed and axial oblique (B) T1-weighted fat-suppressed MR arthrogram images demonstrate a thickened and slightly irregular ligamentum teres (arrows).

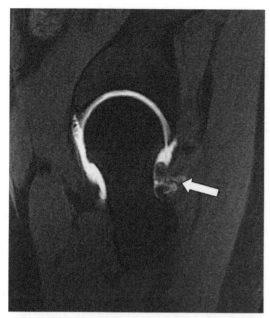

Fig. 13. A 22-year-old football player with hip pain. Axial oblique T1-weighted MR arthrogram image shows contrast extravasation through the posterior capsule (*arrow*) indicating a posterior capsular tear.

radiographic findings, may benefit from evaluation with MR imaging or MR arthrography. When chondral injury is suspected, MR arthrography is preferred.[87]

Cartilage assessment

Normal hyaline cartilage has intermediate to bright signal on MR imaging images, although typically less intense than gadolinium solution.[88] The articular cartilage should be closely scrutinized on all imaging planes. The gadolinium solution outlines the articular margins, defining any cartilage surface irregularities and filling partial- or full-thickness defects (Figs. 14 and 15).[89] With a cartilage flap tear, there is undercutting of the chondral surface with fluid/gadolinium visualized. MR arthrography has been shown to have a sensitivity of 50% to 79%, specificity of 77% to 84%, and accuracy 69% to 78% in detection of cartilage lesions overall.[25] Most investigators prefer MR arthrography over conventional MR images, although the study by Mintz and colleagues[24] reported a similar accuracy for detection of cartilage lesions on conventional nonarthrographic MR images. However, as noted previously, this study did not compare the exact grades of cartilage lesions at MR imaging with those seen at arthroscopy.

Chondral lesions are often noted in association with labral tears. In the study by Fitzgerald,[30] 33% of patients at arthroscopy had alterations of the articular surface of the femoral head associated with a labral tear. A more recent study by McCarthy and colleagues[11] showed a highly significant association between the presence of labral lesions and degeneration of the articular cartilage. Labral and articular lesions are commonly located in the same zone of the acetabulum.[11] In the study by McCarthy and colleagues,[70] they observed a preponderance of chondral lesions involving the anterior labral cartilage junction in their arthrographic and cadaveric series. It is thought that certain repetitive rotational maneuvers preferentially subject the anterior portion of the cartilage near the labral junction to recurrent microtrauma and eventual mechanical attrition. Arthroscopic and anatomic observations support the concept that labral tears and chondral lesions frequently are part of a continuum of degenerative joint disease.[70] As in other joints, the long-term consequences of chondral lesions are a major concern. Symptomatic improvement has been shown from arthroscopic debridement of unstable cartilage flaps, although future advances in cartilage resurfacing procedures may promote long-term overall health of the hip joint.[52]

The detection of a discrete chondral or osteochondral defect should prompt a thorough search for a displaced intra-articular body (Fig. 16). Osteochondral lesions of the femoral head have been described in athletes, and have an MR imaging appearance similar to osteochondral lesions in other locations such as the knee and ankle.[90,91] Intra-articular loose bodies manifest as a low signal intensity filling defect within the fluid-filled joint (Fig. 17). Ossific bodies may be isointense to fat containing bone marrow. Progressive joint space narrowing after traumatic hip subluxation or dislocation, occurring in the months immediately following trauma, may indicate post-traumatic chondrolysis.[92]

Newer MR imaging techniques in cartilage imaging with dGEMRIC and T2 mapping may provide more detailed information regarding early changes within articular cartilage, and may guide surgical intervention.[20,93,94] Additional cartilage sequences performed during MR arthrography may provide increased lesion conspicuity (Fig. 18).[95,96]

Plicae

Synovial plicae are normal anatomic structures that sometimes become symptomatic (Fig. 19). Symptomatic plicae are a well-known cause of knee pain.[97,98] Hip plicae have been described in

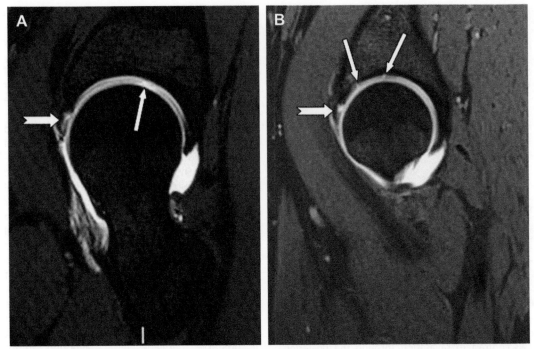

Fig. 14. A 40-year-old woman with hip pain (same patient as **Fig. 7**). (*A*) Axial oblique and sagittal (*B*) T1-weighted fat-suppressed MR arthrogram images demonstrate articular cartilage lesions within the femoral head and 2 focal lesions within the acetabulum (*arrows*). If subchondral cysts or bone marrow edema are present, one should closely evaluate the overlying articular cartilage for lesions.

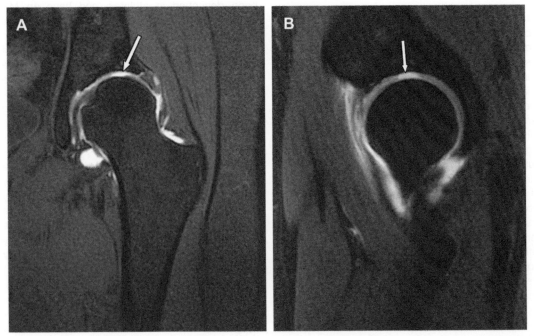

Fig. 15. A 52-year-old active woman with hip pain. Coronal (*A*) and sagittal (*B*) T1-weighted fat-suppressed MR arthrogram images of the left hip demonstrate gadolinium signal intensity filling a cartilage defect within the acetabulum and femoral head (*arrows*).

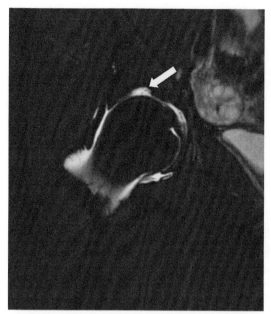

Fig. 16. A 16-year-old girl with recurrent catching, locking, and mechanical symptoms. Coronal T2-weighted fat-suppressed MR image at arthrography shows an osteochondral lesion within the superior acetabulum (*arrow*). There is no surrounding bone marrow edema. Osteochondritis dissecans has been described in the hip, classically within the femoral head.

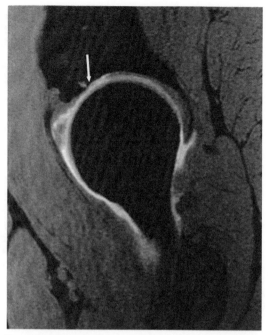

Fig. 18. A 25-year-old man with hip pain. Sagittal Iterative Decomposition of water and fat with Echo Asymmetry and Least-squares estimation Spoiled Gradient Echo (IDEAL-SPGR) image shows a cartilage lesion (*arrow*). This cartilage sequence may increase the conspicuity of cartilage lesions and help to detect shallow defects.

cadavers[99] and in patients undergoing diagnostic hip arthroscopy.[100] Symptomatic hip plicae are now becoming recognized and treated at hip arthroscopy.[100] The normal pectinofoveal fold should be recognized at MR imaging, has been shown to have various appearances and attachment sites, and should not be misinterpreted as a thickened hip plicae.[101]

Femoroacetabular Impingement

Another cause of hip pain is femoroacetabular impingement (FAI). There is some overlap of this entity with labral tears because some tears seen at MR arthrography may be caused by FAI. FAI can result from anatomic abnormalities of the proximal femur and/or acetabulum. FAI occurs with hip flexion, adduction, and internal rotation (described as the "anterior impingement position") in individuals who have subtle predisposing anatomic features.[25,102–104] These anatomic features result in decreased clearance between the anterior acetabular rim and the anterior femur at the head-neck junction. This impingement can lead to labral tears, cartilage lesions, and eventually premature osteoarthritis.

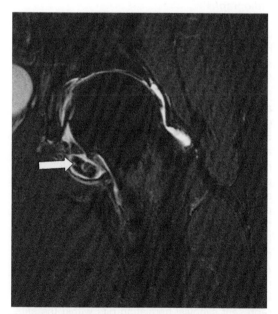

Fig. 17. A 27-year-old man with hip pain. Coronal T2-weighted fat-suppressed MR arthrographic image demonstrates a low signal intensity structure within the hip joint compatible with a loose body (*arrow*). Note the diffuse cartilage loss of the femoral head and acetabulum, abnormal morphology of the labrum, and osteophytes.

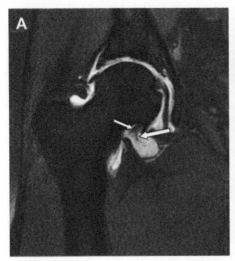
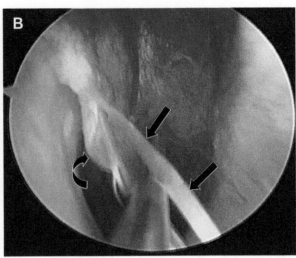

Fig. 19. A 52-year-old man with hip pain. (*A*) Coronal T1-weighted MR arthrogram image demonstrates a mildly thickened plicae (*arrow*) within the medial hip joint space just medial to the normal pectinofoveal fold (*notched arrow*). (*B*) Arthroscopic image depicts the irregular, thickened plicae (*arrows*) adjacent to the pectinofoveal fold (*curved arrow*); this was excised at arthroscopy.

The anatomic abnormalities that lead to FAI and can be divided into 2 main types of impingement: cam and pincer. The most common situation is a mixed cam and pincer pathology, occurring along the anterior femoral neck and the anterior-superior acetabular rim.[56] Cam impingement is due to an abnormal morphology of the anterior femoral head-neck junction, and is typically seen in younger individuals.[102,105,106] The prominence of the femoral head-neck junction can be seen as an overall decreased offset at the femoral head-neck junction. This decreased offset has been termed the "pistol-grip deformity," which describes a flattened head-neck junction seen on standard anteroposterior radiographs of the hip.[107] Pincer impingement is caused by an abnormally retroverted acetabulum contacting a normal femur during hip flexion, and is more common in older women. Retroversion, a cause of pincer impingement, may be seen as a result of trauma, as part of a complex acetabular dysplasia, or in isolation, and is thought to play a role in early-onset degenerative joint disease. This condition can result from decreased acetabular anteversion or coxa profunda. Acquired causes can be acetabular protrusion, or postsurgical prominent antero-superior acetabulum. Another cause can be coxa vara.[108] Both types of FAI are common in athletes presenting with hip pain, loss of range of motion, and disability.[56]

Imaging FAI

The diagnosis of femoroacetabular impingement is based on the patient's distinct clinical history and physical examination. The morphologic abnormalities help confirm the diagnosis and may be identifiable on radiographs, but some cases are apparent only on CT or MR imaging.

Anteroposterior pelvis and frog-leg lateral radiographs

In cam FAI there may be an osseous prominence in the anterosuperior region of the femoral head-neck junction (femoral bump), or the femoral neck may have a pistol-grip deformity.[109] Pincer-type FAI can be visualized as acetabular retroversion, coxa profunda, protrusio acetabuli, and acetabular rim ossification.[110] One radiographic sign of acetabular retroversion that has been described is the crossover sign.[111] In a positive crossover sign, the anterior acetabular rim is projected laterally relative to the same point of the posterior rim in the superolateral aspect of the acetabulum. Another sign seen in pincer-type FAI is when the acetabular fossa or the femoral head lies medial to the ilioischial line, indicating increased acetabular socket depth, as seen with protrusion acetabuli.[111,112] A lucency within the anterosuperior femoral neck may be associated with femoroacetabular impingement.[110] These lucencies are known to represent synovial herniation pits within the subcapital femoral neck. The lucencies are often seen in athletes, and have been thought to represent an abnormal interaction between the iliopsoas tendon and the joint capsule, which produces increased pressure on the anterior portion of the proximal femur.

MR imaging

MR imaging is ideal for evaluation of the anatomic changes of FAI (**Fig. 20**). On MR images an abnormal morphology of the anterior femoral head-neck junction is clearly seen in the cam type of FAI. The abnormal head-neck morphology can be seen on conventional MR images, but MR arthrography is preferred because it also provides better evaluation of the labrum and cartilage. Radial imaging may be helpful is assessing FAI morphology.[113] An alpha angle greater than 55° has been shown to be closely associated with symptomatic cam-type femoroacetabular impingement.[103,106] The alpha angle is used as an objective representation of the prominence of the anterior femoral head-neck junction. The greater the alpha angle, the greater the likelihood for impingement of the anterior/anterosuperior femoral head-neck against the acetabulum. However, the alpha angle measurement is fraught with inconsistencies. A recent study by Lohan and colleagues[114] found that the alpha angle performed poorly and was statistically of no value in suggesting the presence or absence of cam FAI. There is often MR imaging evidence for corresponding impaction damage at the superior portion of the superolateral femoral head-neck junction. One can also often see acetabular-labral damage resulting from this structure being impinged between the acetabulum and the adjacent femoral head-neck region.

Patients with clinical symptoms of FAI have been found to have increased ratios of femoral neck size relative to the femoral head as compared with patients without clinical symptoms.[102] The larger the neck radius in the superior and anterior aspects of the neck, the more likely there is to be impingement, although no absolute measurements are defined.[102]

Treatment of FAI

Arthroscopic treatment of FAI allows athletes to return to sports competition.[56] The treatment of symptomatic cam-type FAI unresponsive to conservative measures is surgical, and consists of excision osteoplasty of the nonspherical portion of the femoral head and neck.[105,106,115] This procedure improves the head-neck offset and increases bony clearance during hip motion. The procedure is often combined with resection of the soft tissue anterior to the hip joint that may also be involved in impingement. For pincer impingement, periacetabular osteotomy or excision of the bony prominence at the anterior acetabular rim is performed to reduce anterior over-coverage.[105] Articular cartilage smoothing and/or debridement near the acetabular rim are also done. A torn or degenerated labrum may need to be excised and/or repaired. If there has been development of an extra-articular bony prominence along the femoral head-neck region, excision osteoplasty may also be performed to increase the femoral neck offset and create a better waist at the head-neck junction.[105,106]

The Snapping Hip

Another cause of hip pain, usually in young individuals, is the snapping hip syndrome, a symptom

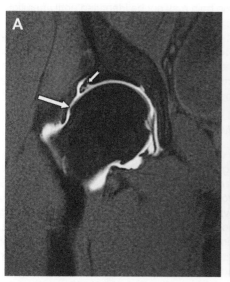
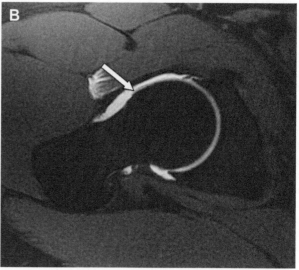

Fig. 20. A 27-year-old man with persistent hip pain. (*A*) Coronal and axial oblique (*B*) T1-weighted MR arthrogram images of the right hip demonstrate loss of the concavity at the femoral head-neck junction and an osseous "bump" (*arrows*) compatible with cam FAI. Note the anterosuperior labral tear (*notched arrow*).

complex characterized by pain and an audible or perceived snapping of the hip during movement of the hip. Symptoms are reproduced during specific movements of the hip but most frequently when the hip moves from a position of flexion-abduction-external rotation (frog-leg position) to the neutral position.[116] Snapping hip has various causes, which have been categorized as external, internal, and intra-articular. Diagnosing the exact cause clinically is sometimes difficult.

The external type of snapping hip is the most common, and occurs as a result of catching of either the posterior iliotibial band (ITB) or the anterior aspect of the gluteus maximus muscle as it moves over the greater trochanter during flexion and extension of the hip joint.[17,116–118] An external snapping hip is typically a clinical diagnosis, so imaging is seldom needed.

Intra-articular causes of a snapping hip include labral tears, loose bodies, synovial osteochondromatosis, synovial folds, and fracture fragments. Hip MR arthrography is commonly used to assess for these intra-articular conditions, and they often require surgery for relief of symptoms.[17,116,117,119–121]

An internal snapping hip is most often related to the iliopsoas tendon, and has been suggested as a more common cause of snapping hip than the extrinsic type.[116] There are 3 proposed mechanisms to explain the snapping: contact between the iliopsoas tendon and the iliopectineal eminence, or at the lesser trochanter ("friction syndrome"),[15,72] and catching between the iliopsoas tendon and its muscle.[122]

Snapping iliopsoas tendon (internal snapping hip)

The normal iliopsoas tendon glides smoothly over the pelvic brim during hip rotation.[15] Sonography has demonstrated a snapping or abnormal jerky movement of the iliopsoas tendon in the snapping hip.[123] Sonography has emerged as the preferred technique for examining the iliopsoas tendon because it allows both static and dynamic evaluation of the soft tissues around the hip joint.[116,119,123] Sonography also provides an accurate method for injection into the iliopsoas bursa. However, because sonography may not allow accurate evaluation of intra-articular pathologic conditions, some combination of radiography, hip arthrography, CT, or MR imaging is still recommended if an intra-articular cause for hip pain is suspected.[123]

Although iliopsoas tendinopathy and bursitis can be seen,[120] sonographic signs of tendinopathy are not a common feature of a snapping iliopsoas tendon.[72,116] When it does occur, iliopsoas bursitis and tendinitis are interrelated in the

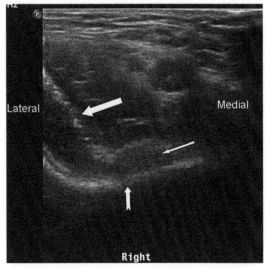

Fig. 21. An 18-year-old female athlete with snapping hip. Transverse sonogram image of the iliopsoas tendon at the level of the acetabular brim during injection of the iliopsoas bursa/tendon sheath show the needle entering from a lateral to medial approach (*large arrow*). The needle tip should be placed adjacent to or just beneath the iliopsoas tendon (*thin arrow*) at the level of the acetabular brim (*notched arrow*) Care should be taken not to inject too caudal, as the hip joint may be inadvertently injected.

sense that inflammation of one will often result in inflammation of the other due to their close proximity.[120]

An accurate diagnosis of the cause of painful snapping hip is essential for deciding on the appropriate treatment. The cause for an individual's hip pain may not be identified until after iliopsoas bursa injection confirms pain relief. Treatment options for the painful snapping iliopsoas tendon include nonoperative management (rest, analgesics, and physical therapy), injection of corticosteroids and anesthetic agents into the iliopsoas bursa (**Fig. 21**), and surgery.[15,121,124–126]

SUMMARY

There are many causes for hip pain in the athlete. Having an understanding of the spectrum of abnormalities around the hip will help with the decision for the appropriate imaging method in the evaluation of these disorders. MR imaging and sonography will aid not only in preoperative planning but in the appropriate selection of patients to undergo hip arthroscopy, which tends to lead to better postoperative results. Although radiographs are the first step in the workup for the painful hip, MR imaging is considered the next imaging test of choice for the evaluation of most common hip abnormalities in athletes, including labral injuries, ligament injuries, osteochondral injuries, fractures, bursitis, and musculotendinous injuries.

REFERENCES

1. Cotten A, Boutry N, Demondion X, et al. Acetabular labrum: MRI in asymptomatic volunteers. J Comput Assist Tomogr 1998;22(1):1–7.
2. Lage LA, Patel JV, Villar RN. The acetabular labral tear: an arthroscopic classification. Arthroscopy 1996;12(3):269–72.
3. Keene GS, Villar RN. Arthroscopic anatomy of the hip: an in vivo study. Arthroscopy 1994;10(4): 392–9.
4. Czerny C, Hofmann S, Urban M, et al. MR arthrography of the adult acetabular capsular-labral complex: correlation with surgery and anatomy. AJR Am J Roentgenol 1999;173:345–9.
5. Lecouvet FE, Vande Berg BC, Malghem J, et al. MR imaging of the acetabular labrum: variations in 200 asymptomatic hips. AJR Am J Roentgenol 1996;167:1025–8.
6. Petersilge CA, Haque MA, Petersilge WJ, et al. Acetabular labral tears: evaluation with MR arthrography. Radiology 1996;200(1):231–5.
7. Hodler J, Yu JS, Goodwin D, et al. MR arthrography of the hip: improved imaging of the acetabular labrum with histologic correlation in cadavers. AJR Am J Roentgenol 1995;165:887–91.
8. Dinauer PA, Murphy KP, Carroll JF. Sublabral sulcus at the posteroinferior acetabulum: a potential pitfall in MR arthrography diagnosis of acetabular labral tears. AJR Am J Roentgenol 2004;183: 1745–53.
9. Kim YT, Azuma H. The nerve endings of the acetabular labrum. Clin Orthop Relat Res 1995; 320:176–81.
10. Mason JB. Acetabular labral tears in the athlete. Clin Sports Med 2001;20(4):779–90.
11. McCarthy J, Noble P, Aluisio FV, et al. Anatomy, pathologic features, and treatment of acetabular labral tears. Clin Orthop Relat Res 2003;406: 38–47.
12. Petersilge CA. MR arthrography for evaluation of the acetabular labrum. Skeletal Radiol 2001;30: 423–30.
13. Van Dyke JA, Holley HC, Anderson SD. Review of iliopsoas anatomy and pathology. Radiographics 1987;7(1):53–84.
14. Jacobson T, Allen WC. Surgical correction of the snapping iliopsoas tendon. Am J Sports Med 1990;18(5):470–4.
15. Lyons JC, Peterson LF. The snapping iliopsoas tendon. Mayo Clin Proc 1984;59(5):327–9.
16. Chandler SB. The iliopsoas bursa in man. Anat Rec 1934;58:235–40.
17. Schaberg JE, Harper MC, Allen WC. The snapping hip syndrome. Am J Sports Med 1984;12(5):361–5.
18. Pfirrmann CW, Chung CB, Theumann NH, et al. Greater trochanter of the hip: attachment of the abductor mechanism and a complex of three bursae-MR imaging and MR bursogrpahy in cadavers and MR imaging in asymptomatic volunteers. Radiology 2001;221(2):469–77.
19. Fernbach SK, Wilkinson RH. Avulsion injuries of the pelvis and proximal femur. AJR Am J Roentgenol 1981;137:581–4.
20. Nishii T, Tanaka H, Sugano N, et al. Evaluation of cartilage matrix disorders by T2 relaxation time in patients with hip dysplasia. Osteoarthritis Cartilage 2008;16(2):227–33.
21. Plotz GM, Brossman J, von Knoch M, et al. Magnetic resonance arthography of the acetabular labrum: value of radial reconstructions. Arch Orthop Trauma Surg 2001;121:450–7.
22. Byrd JW. Labral lesions: an elusive source of hip pain case reports and literature review. Arthroscopy 1996;12(5):603–12.
23. Czerny C, Hofmann S, Neuhold A, et al. Lesions of the acetabular labrum: accuracy of MR imaging and MR arthrography in detection and staging. Radiology 1996;200(1):225–30.
24. Mintz DN, Hooper T, Connell D, et al. Magnetic resonance imaging of the hip: detection of labral and chrondral abnormalities using noncontrast imaging. Arthroscopy 2005;21(4):385–93.
25. Schmidt MR, Notzli HP, Zanetti M, et al. Cartilage lesions in the hip: diagnostic effectiveness of MR arthrography. Radiology 2003;226(2):382–6.
26. Chu CR, Izzo NJ, Papas NE, et al. In vitro exposure to 0.5% bupivacaine is cytotoxic to bovine articular chondrocytes. Arthroscopy 2006;22(7):693–9.
27. Chu CR, Izzo NJ, Coyle CH, et al. The in vitro effects of bupivacaine on articular chondrocytes. J Bone Joint Surg Br 2008;90(6):814–20.
28. Daum WJ. Anesthesia update #21. Use of local anesthetic with the hip arthrogram as a diagnostic aid. Orthop Rev 1988;17(1):123–5.
29. Byrd JW, Jones KS. Diagnostic accuracy of clinical assessment, magnetic resonance imaging, magnetic resonance arthrography, and intra-articular injection in hip arthroscopy patients. Am J Sports Med 2004;32(7):1668–74.
30. Fitzgerald RH. Acetabular labrum tears. Clin Orthop Relat Res 1995;311:60–8.
31. Yoon LS, Palmer WE, Kassarjian A. Evaluation of radial-sequence imaging in detecting acetabular labral tears at hip MR arthrography. Skeletal Radiol 2007;36:1029–33.
32. Ziegert AJ, Blankenbaker DG, De Smet AA, et al. Comparison of standard hip MR arthrographic

imaging planes and sequences for detection of arthroscopically proven labral tears. AJR Am J
Roentgenol 2009;192:1397–400.

33. Llopis E, Cerezal L, Kassarjian A, et al. Direct MR
arthrography of the hip with leg traction: feasibility
for assessing articular cartilage. AJR Am J Roentgenol 2008;190:1124–8.

34. Masi JN, Newitt D, Sell CA, et al. Optimization of
gadodiamide concentration for MR arthrography
at 3T. AJR Am J Roentgenol 2005;184:1754–61.

35. Robben SG, Lequin MH, Diepstraten AF, et al.
Anterior joint capsule of the normal hip and in children with transient synovitis: US study with
anatomic and histologic correlation. Radiology
1999;210(2):499–507.

36. Sofka CM. Ultrasound in sports medicine. Semin
Muscoloskelet Radiol 2004;8(1):17–27.

37. Bencardino JT, Palmer WE. Imaging of hip disorders in athletes. Radiol Clin North Am 2002;40:
267–87.

38. Bergman AG, Fredericson M. MR imaging of stress
reactions, muscle injuries, and other overuse
injuries in runners. Magn Reson Imaging Clin N
Am 1999;7(1):151–74.

39. Boutin RD, Newman JS. MR imaging of sports-
related hip disorders. Magn Reson Imaging Clin
N Am 2003;11(2):255–81.

40. Daffner RH, Pavlov H. Stress fractures: current
concepts. AJR Am J Roentgenol 1992;159:
245–52.

41. Anderson MW, Greenspan A. Stress fractures.
Radiology 1996;199(1):1–12.

42. Lee J, Yao L. Stress fractures: MR imaging. Radiology 1988;169(1):217–20.

43. Deutsch AL, Mink JH, Waxman AD. Occult fractures of the proximal femur: MR imaging. Radiology
1989;170(1):113–6.

44. Shindle MK, Ranawat AS, Kelly BT. Diagnosis and
management of traumatic and atraumatic hip instability in the athletic patient. Clin Sports Med 2006;
25:309–26.

45. Philippon MJ, Kuppersmith DA, Wolff AB, et al.
Arthroscopic findings following traumatic hip dislocation in 14 professional athletes. Arthroscopy
2009;25(2):169–74.

46. Blankenbaker DG, Ullrick SR, Davis KW, et al.
Correlation of MRI findings with clinical findings of
trochanteric pain syndrome. Skeletal Radiol 2008;
37:903–9.

47. Sundar M, Carty H. Avulsion fractures of the pelvis
in children: a report of 32 fractures and their
outcome. Skeletal Radiol 1994;23:85–90.

48. Stevens MA, El-Khoury GY, Kathol MH, et al.
Imaging features of avulsion fractures. Radiographics 1999;19(3):655–72.

49. Pisacano RM, Miller TT. Comparing sonography
with MR imaging of apophyseal injuries of the

pelvis in four boys. AJR Am J Roentgenol 2003;
181:223–30.

50. Abe I, Harada Y, Oinuma K, et al. Acetabular labrum:
abnormal findings at MR imaging in asymptomatic
hips. Radiology 2000;216(2):576–81.

51. Hase T, Ueo T. Acetabular labral tear: arthroscopic
diagnosis and treatment. Arthroscopy 1999;15(2):
138–41.

52. Kelly BT, Williams RJ, Philippon MJ. Hip arthroscopy: current indications, treatment options, and
management issues. Am J Sports Med 2003;31(6):
1020–37.

53. Altenberg AR. Acetabular labrum tears: a cause of
hip pain and degenerative arthritis. South Med J
1977;70(2):174–5.

54. McCarthy J, Busconi B. The role of hip arthroscopy
in the diagnosis and treatment of hip disease.
Orthopedics 1995;18(8):753–6.

55. Schnarkowski P, Steinbach L, Tirman PF, et al.
Magnetic resonance imaging of labral cysts of
the hip. Skeletal Radiol 1996;25(8):733–7.

56. Philippon MJ, Arnoczky SP, Torrie A. Arthroscopic
repair of the acetabular labrum: a histologic
assessment of healing in an ovine model. Arthroscopy 2007;23(4):376–80.

57. Boyd KT, Peirce NS, Batt ME. Common hip injuries
in sport. Sports Med 1997;24(4):273–88.

58. Dorrell JH, Catterall A. The torn acetabular labrum.
J Bone Joint Surg Br 1986;68B(3):400–3.

59. Ikeda T, Awaya G, Suzuki S, et al. Torn acetabular
labrum in young patients. J Bone Joint Surg Br
1988;70(1):13–6.

60. Klaue K, Durnin CW, Ganz R. The acetabular rim
syndrome. J Bone Joint Surg Br 1991;73(3):423–9.

61. Yamamoto Y, Tonotsuka H, Ueda T, et al. Useful-
ness of radial contrast-enhanced computed
tomography for the diagnosis of acetabular labrum
injury. Arthroscopy 2007;23(12):1290–4.

62. Blankenbaker DG, De Smet AA, Keene JS. Classification and localization of acetabular labral tears.
Skeletal Radiol 2007;36:391–7.

63. Leunig M, Werlen S, Ungersbock A, et al. Evaluation of the acetabular labrum by MR arthrography.
J Bone Joint Surg Br 1997;79:230–4.

64. Petersilge CA. Chronic adult hip pain: MR arthrography of the hip. Radiographics 2000;20(S):
S43–52.

65. Magee T, Hinson G. Association of paralabral cysts
with acetabular disorders. AJR Am J Roentgenol
2000;174(5):1381–4.

66. Steiner E, Steinbach LS, Schnarkowski P, et al.
Ganglia and cysts around joints. Radiol Clin North
Am 1996;34(2):395–425.

67. Haller J, Resnick D, Greenway G, et al. Juxtaace-
tabular ganglionic (or synovial) cysts: CT and MR
features. J Comput Assist Tomogr 1989;13(6):
976–83.

68. Kassarjian A, Llopis E, Schwartz RB, et al. Obturator externus bursa: prevalence of communication with the hip joint and associated intra-articular findings in 200 consecutive hip MR arthrograms. Eur Radiol 2009;19(11):2779–82.

69. Saddik D, Troupis J, Tirman PF, et al. Prevalence and location of acetabular sublabral sulci at hip arthroscopy with retrospective MRI review. AJR Am J Roentgenol 2006;187:W507–11.

70. McCarthy J, Noble P, Schuck M, et al. The role of labral lesions to development of early degenerative hip disease. Clin Orthop Relat Res 2001;393: 25–37.

71. Studler U, Kalberer F, Leunig M, et al. MR arthrography of the hip: differentiation between an anterior sublabral recess as a normal variant and a labral tear. Radiology 2008;249(3):947–54.

72. Blankenbaker DG, De Smet AA, Keene JS. Sonography of the iliopsoas tendon and injection of the iliopsoas bursa for diagnosis and management of the painful snapping hip. Skeletal Radiol 2006;35: 565–71.

73. Blankenbaker DG, Tuite MJ. The painful hip: new concepts. Skeletal Radiol 2006;35:352–70.

74. Steinbach L, Palmer WE, Schweitzer ME. Special focus session. MR arthrography. Radiographics 2002;22(5):1223–46.

75. Kelly BT, Weiland DE, Schenker ML, et al. Arthroscopic labral repair in the hip: surgical technique and review of the literature. Arthroscopy 2005;21(12): 1496–504.

76. Farjo LA, Glick JM, Sampson TG. Hip arthroscopy for acetabular labral tears. Arthroscopy 1999;15(2): 132–7.

77. Philippon MJ, Schenker ML. A new method for acetabular rim trimming and labral repair. Clin Sports Med 2006;25:293–7.

78. Sierra RJ, Trousdale RT. Labral reconstruction using the ligamentum teres capitis. Report of a new technique. Clin Orthop Relat Res 2008; 467:753–9.

79. Byrd JW, Jones KS. Traumatic rupture of the ligamentum teres as a source of hip pain. Arthroscopy 2004;20(4):385–91.

80. Delcamp DD, Klaaren HE, Pompe van Meerdervoort HF. Traumatic avulsion of the ligamentum teres without dislocation of the hip. Two case reports. J Bone Joint Surg Am 1988;70(6): 933–5.

81. Fuss FK, Bacher A. New aspects of the morphology and function of the human hip joint ligaments. Am J Anat 1991;192(1):1–13.

82. Gray AJ, Villar RN. The ligamentum teres of the hip: an arthroscopic classification of its pathology. Arthroscopy 1997;13(5):575–8.

83. Byrd JW. The role of hip arthroscopy in the athletic hip. Clin Sports Med 2006;25:255–78.

84. Laorr A, Greenspan A, Anderson MW, et al. Traumatic hip dislocation: early MRI findings. Skeletal Radiol 1995;24(4):239–45.

85. Bencardino JT, Kassarjian A, Palmer WE. Magnetic resonance imaging of the hip: sports-related injuries. Top Magn Reson Imaging 2003;14(2):145–60.

86. Tehranzadeh J, Vanarthos W, Pais MJ. Osteochondral impaction of the femoral head associated with hip dislocation: CT study in 35 patients. AJR Am J Roentgenol 1990;155:1049–52.

87. Newman JS, Newberg AH. MRI of the painful hip in athletes. Clin Sports Med 2006;25:613–33.

88. Newberg AH, Newman JS. Imaging the painful hip. Clin Orthop Relat Res 2003;406:19–28.

89. Palmer WE. MR arthrography of the hip. Semin Muscoloskelet Radiol 1998;2(4):349–62.

90. Weaver CJ, Major NM, Garrett WE, et al. Femoral head osteochondral lesions in painful hips of athletes: MR imaging findings. AJR Am J Roentgenol 2002;178:973–7.

91. King D, Richards V. Osteochondritis dissecans of the hip. J Bone Joint Surg Am 1940;22:327–48.

92. Moorman CT, Warren RF, Hershman EB, et al. Traumatic posterior hip subluxation in American football. J Bone Joint Surg Am 2003;85:1190–6.

93. Bittersohl B, Hosalkar HS, Haamberg T, et al. Reproducibility of dGEMRIC in assessment of hip joint cartilage: a prospective study. J Magn Reson Imaging 2009;30:224–8.

94. Tiderius CJ, Jessel R, Kim YJ, et al. Hip dGEMRIC in asymptomatic volunteers and patients with early osteoarthritis: the influence of timing after contrast injection. Magn Reson Med 2007;57:803–5.

95. Knuesel PR, Pfirrmann CW, Noetzli HP, et al. MR arthrography of the hip: diagnostic performance of a dedicated water-excitation 3D double-echo steady-state sequence to detect cartilage lesions. AJR Am J Roentgenol 2004;183:1729–35.

96. Siepmann DB, McGovern J, Brittain JH, et al. High-resolution 3D cartilage imaging with IDEAL-SPGR at 3T. AJR Am J Roentgenol 2007;189:1510–5.

97. Hardaker WT, Whipple TL, Bassett FH. Diagnosis and treatment of the plica syndrome of the knee. J Bone Joint Surg Am 1980;62(2):221–5.

98. Jee WH, Choe BY, Kim JM, et al. The plica syndrome: diagnostic value of MRI with arthroscopic correlation. J Comput Assist Tomogr 1998; 22(5):814–8.

99. Fu Z, Peng M, Peng Q. Anatomical study of the synovial plicae of the hip joint. Clin Anat 1997;10(4): 235–8.

100. Atlihan D, Jones DC, Guanche CA. Arthroscopic treatment of a symptomatic hip plica. Clin Orthop Relat Res 2003;411:174–7.

101. Blankenbaker DG, Davis KW, De Smet AA, et al. MRI appearance of the pectinofoveal fold. AJR Am J Roentgenol 2009;192:93–5.

102. Ito K, Minka MA, Leunig M, et al. Femoroacetabular impingement and the cam-effect. J Bone Joint Surg Br 2001;83(2):171–6.

103. Notzli HP, Wyss TF, Stoecklin CH, et al. The contour of the femoral head-neck junction as a predictor for the risk of anterior impingement. J Bone Joint Surg Br 2002;84:556–60.

104. Siebenrock KA, Leunig M, Ganz R. Periacetabular osteotomy: the Bernese experience. Instr Course Lect 2001;50:239–45.

105. Ganz R, Parvizi J, Beck M, et al. Femoroacetabular impingement. Clin Orthop Relat Res 2003;417: 112–20.

106. Kassarjian A, Yoon LS, Belzile E, et al. Triad of MR arthrographic findings in patients with cam-type femoroacetabular impingement. Radiology 2005; 236(2):588–92.

107. Stulberg SD, Cordell LD, Harris WH, et al. Unrecognized childhood hip disease: a major cause of idiopathic osteoarthritis of the hip. The Hip Society: The Hip. St. Louis (MO): C.V. Mosby Company; 1975. 212–28.

108. Beall DP, Sweet CF, Martin HD, et al. Imaging findings of femoroacetabular impingement syndrome. Skeletal Radiol 2005;34:691–701.

109. Eijer H, Leunig M, Mahomed MN, et al. Cross-table lateral radiographs for screening of anterior femoral head-neck offset in patients with femoro-acetabular impingement. Hip Int 2001; 11:37–41.

110. Leunig M, Beck M, Kalhor M, et al. Fibrocystic changes at anterosuperior femoral neck: prevalence in hips with femoroacetabular impingement. Radiology 2005;236:237–46.

111. Siebenrock KA, Kalbermatten DF, Ganz R. Effect of pelvic tilt on acetabular retroversion: a study of pelves from cadavers. Clin Orthop Relat Res 2003;407:241–8.

112. Reynolds D, Lucas J, Klaue K. Retroversion of the acetabulum. A cause of hip pain. J Bone Joint Surg Br 1999;81(2):281–8.

113. Rakhra KS, Sheikh AM, Allen D, et al. Comparison of MRI alpha angle measurement planes in femoroacetabular impingement. Clin Orthop Relat Res 2009;467(3):660–5.

114. Lohan DG, Seeger LL, Motamedi K, et al. Cam-type femoral-acetabular impingement: is the alpha angle the best MR arthrography has to offer? Skeletal Radiol 2009;38:855–62.

115. Mardones R, Lara J, Donndorff A, et al. Surgical correction of "cam-type" femoroacetabular impingement: a cadaveric comparison of open versus arthroscopic debridement. Arthroscopy 2009;25(2):175–82.

116. Pelsser V, Cardinal E, Hobden R, et al. Extraarticular snapping hip: sonographic findings. AJR Am J Roentgenol 2001;176:67–73.

117. Allen WC, Cope R. Coxa saltans: the snapping hip revisited. J Am Acad Orthop Surg 1995;3(5): 303–8.

118. White RA, Hughes MS, Burd T, et al. A new operative approach in the correction of external coxa saltans. Am J Sports Med 2004;32(6):1504–8.

119. Janzen DL, Partridge E, Logan M, et al. The snapping hip: clinical and imaging findings in transient subluxation of the iliopsoas tendon. Can Assoc Radiol J 1996;47(3):202–8.

120. Johnston CA, Wiley JP, Lindsay DM, et al. Iliopsoas bursitis and tendinitis. A review. Sports Med 1998; 25(4):271–83.

121. Wahl CJ, Warren RF, Adler RS, et al. Internal coxa saltans (snapping hip) as a result of overtraining: a report of 3 cases in professional athletes with a review of causes and the role of ultrasound in early diagnosis and management. Am J Sports Med 2004;32(5):1302–9.

122. Deslandes M, Guillin R, Cardinal E, et al. The snapping iliopsoas tendon: new mechanisms using dynamic sonography. AJR Am J Roentgenol 2008;190:576–81.

123. Cardinal E, Buckwalter KA, Capello WN, et al. US of the snapping iliopsoas tendon. Radiology 1996;198:521–2.

124. Anderson SA, Keene JS. Results of arthroscopic iliopsoas tendon release in competitive and recreational athletes. Am J Sports Med 2008;36(12): 2363–71.

125. Kouvalchouk JF, Guyot J, Boisaubert B, et al. [Anterior snapping of the hip associated with the ilial psoas]. Rev Chir Orthop Reparatrice Appar Mot 1998;84(1):67–74 [in French].

126. Idjadi J, Meislin R. Symptomatic snapping hip: targeted treatment for maximum pain relief. Phys Sportsmed 2004;32(1):25–31.

The Spectrum of MR Imaging in Athletic Pubalgia

Adam C. Zoga, MD[a],*, Frank E. Mullens, MD, MPH[b],
William C. Meyers, MD, MBA[c]

KEYWORDS

• MR imaging • Sports injury • Musculoskeletal

The term athletic pubalgia has many definitions in the published literature. For imagers, athletic pubalgia is best considered as a clinical syndrome in which groin pain that cannot be attributed to an intrinsic hip lesion occurs during or after specific activities or ranges of motion. Athletic pubalgia can occur at any age, but is most prevalent between the second and the fourth decades, and most reviews indicate that it is more frequent in, but not exclusive to, men. As the term suggests, athletes, in particular, are commonly hampered by activity-related groin pain, although the syndrome can afflict both high-level competitors and recreational enthusiasts or those who participate less often. Lesions precipitating this groin pain are often localized to the pubic symphysis region, but can be as distant as the anterior superior iliac spine or the thigh adductor muscle compartment, and can primarily involve soft tissue, osseous structures, or both. Historically, terms including sports hernia and Gilmore groin have been used to describe some of these lesions, but true hernias are rare in this patient population. Clinically, it is often difficult to localize these lesions and to distinguish athletic pubalgia from groin pain related to hip labral tears or cartilage injuries, creating a diagnostic conundrum for orthopedists, sports medicine physicians, general surgeons, physical therapists, and team trainers.[1–3] Injuries causing athletic pubalgia are particularly common with activities that involve twisting at the waist while running, and sudden, acute directional change and sideways movement, such as football, soccer, baseball, ice hockey, and lacrosse, but some lesions are frequent in distance runners and postpartum women. In one series, nearly half of a cohort of Australian Rules football participants (including umpires) had groin pain, and 77% of this group had osseous edema at the pubic symphysis.[4,5] Athletic pubalgia is not a new phenomenon; a series from 1974 reported that 58% of soccer players had suffered a groin injury, but improved conservative and surgical treatment options have led to the need for more accurate imaging delineation of contributing lesions.[6]

In recent years, imaging contributions to the understanding of anatomic, biomechanical, and pathologic considerations about the pubic symphysis have helped reinforce, or even guide, newer surgical and percutaneous treatments. An athletic pubalgia lesion that might have been considered career ending 10 years ago may be treated successfully today with effective imaging and intervention, allowing for a return to athletic activity. However, many athletes struggle with groin pain for years without ever receiving a clear diagnosis or being offered an effective treatment plan. Confusion among treatment providers can also frequently lead to suboptimal surgeries for presumed hernias or nerve entrapment syndromes. Imaging, and in particular magnetic

[a] Thomas Jefferson University, 132 South 10th Street, 1083A, Philadelphia, PA 19107, USA
[b] Department of Radiology, Musculoskeletal Division, Thomas Jefferson University Hospital, 132 South 10th Street, 1083A, Philadelphia, PA 19107, USA
[c] Department of Surgery, Drexel University College of Medicine, 245 North 15th Street, 7150, Philadelphia, PA 19102, USA
* Corresponding author.
E-mail address: adam.zoga@jefferson.edu

Radiol Clin N Am 48 (2010) 1179–1197
doi:10.1016/j.rcl.2010.07.009

resonance (MR) imaging, should play a primary role in the workup, diagnosis, and treatment of athletic pubalgia.[7-10] This review outlines standard of care, cutting-edge MR imaging techniques for athletic pubalgia, and reviews the spectrum of imaging findings that are encountered in this patient group.

NORMAL ANATOMY

The pubic symphysis is a midline amphiarthrodial articulation with contributions from the left and right innominate bones via the superior and inferior pubic rami, and an intervening articular disk. The medial body of the pubic bone forms its articular surface, which is ovoid and covered by a thin layer of hyaline cartilage. There are transversely oriented subchondral ridges and grooves that, along with the fibrocartilaginous interpubic disk, help protect the joint by dissipating shear forces borne by the innominate bones. The superior and inferior pubic rami merge to form the pubic body 3 to 4 cm from the symphysis, and the upper, anterior margin of the pubic body forms a ridge termed the pubic crest. At the most inferolateral aspect of the pubic crest is an osseous excrescence that serves as an attachment site for the inguinal ligament as well as the caudal rectus abdominis, the pubic tubercle.

Four ligaments, the articular disk, and tendinous attachments contribute to supporting the bony symphysis. The superior pubic ligament extends along the pubic crests, ultimately reaching the superior margin of the pubic tubercles. The arcuate ligament is larger and more caudal, spanning the inferior margin of the symphysis and reaching the inferior borders of the pubic tubercles while blending with the articular disc, the aponeuroses of the gracilis and adductor longus tendon origins, and the caudal attachment of the rectus abdominis muscles. Although difficult to isolate on MR images, the arcuate ligament is almost certainly injured in athletic pubalgia lesions involving the rectus abdominis/adductor aponeurosis. The anterior pubic ligament has a narrow breadth but consists of 2 bundles, the deep one blending with the disk, and the posterior pubic ligament is a gracile structure at the posterior symphyseal margin.[11,12]

Numerous muscle and tendon attachments, both origins and insertions, in the vicinity of the pubic symphysis provide additional dynamic stabilization. The caudal rectus abdominis and the proximal adductor longus blend to form an elongated osseous attachment spanning the region of the pubic tubercle and the anteroinferior pubic body. At cadaveric dissection, a thick and rigid aponeurosis is present in this region, combining elements of the rectus abdominis, adductor longus, pectineus, arcuate ligament, and pubic periosteum. The lateral edge of this aponeurosis is just deep to the posteromedial wall of the superficial inguinal ring, perhaps adding to its integrity. Medially, there is anatomic variability. In some cases, there are distinct left and right rectus abdominis/adductor aponeuroses with a midline soft tissue cleft or raphe, whereas, in others, the left and right aponeuroses merge at midline, forming a thick, platelike structure superficial to the pubic symphysis.

The rectus abdominis inserts caudally at the anterior and anteroinferior regions of the pubic symphysis. The lateral rectus abdominis attachment is in close proximity to the external inguinal ring, which may explain the association with inguinal hernia symptoms. The midline capsule of the pubic symphysis is intimately related to the caudal rectus abdominis attachment as well as the arcuate ligament, a relationship that may explain the association between osteitis pubis and rectus abdominis insertional pathology. Laterally, the origin of the pectineus, and adductor longus and brevis are arrayed anterior to posterior on the undersurface of the lateral pubis and are indistinguishable from the caudal rectus abdominis attachment. This combination of rectus abdominis and adductor fibers, along with the pubic symphysis capsule, arcuate ligament, and anterior pubic periosteum, form a large midline aponeurotic plate. More posteriorly, the gracilis tendons originate lateral to the joint, whereas more cephalad, the external oblique muscles attach lateral to the joint (**Fig. 1**).[13-15]

BIOMECHANICS

The interconnected tendinous and ligamentous attachments around the pubic symphysis play a vital role in pelvic stability. With rotation and extension, the rectus abdominis and adductor longus are relative antagonists; the rectus abdominis muscles elevate the pubic region, whereas the adductor longus myotendinous units exert an anterior inferior force vector. Injury to one muscle or tendon results in a tendency toward injury of the opposing tendon by disrupting normal biomechanics and the anatomic continuity of the tenoperiosteal origins.[8] Subsequently, the pubic symphysis becomes unstable. The investigators believe that it is this instability at the pubic symphysis that most often leads to osteitis pubis and, subsequently, chronic groin pain in many athletes. Once the pubic symphysis region is destabilized, athletes tend to continue activity with abnormal biomechanics. This abnormality can

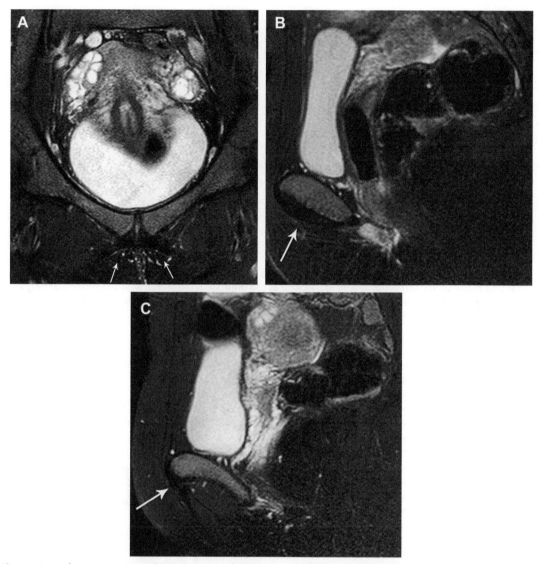

Fig. 1. Normal anatomy. Normal MR imaging of the rectus abdominis/adductor aponeurotic plate and aponeurosis. (*A*) Axial oblique T2 at midline: normal pubic symphysis, aponeurotic plate and bilateral proximal adductor tendons (*arrows*). (*B*) Sagittal T2 at midline: normal rectus abdominis/adductor aponeurotic plate (*arrow*). (*C*) Sagittal T2 several slices lateral to midline: normal rectus abdominis/adductor aponeurosis (*arrow*) with proximal adductor tendon origin inferiorly.

lead to several musculoskeletal injuries around the pelvis, ranging from myotendinous strains to osseous stress fractures and even internal derangements of the hips. When imaging patients with athletic pubalgia, or any activity-related musculoskeletal pelvis injury, it is important to acknowledge these unique biomechanics (**Fig. 2**).[7,16–18]

IMAGING TECHNIQUE

MR imaging is the current standard for evaluation of musculoskeletal pelvic pain. A dedicated

athletic pubalgia protocol is recommended for this specific subset of injury. The patient is generally imaged supine (rarely, prone positioning is needed to minimize respiratory artifact), with an empty bladder. Initially, 3 large field of view sequences are taken using the built-in body coil. A coronal short tau inversion recovery (STIR) sequence is carried out to maximize detection of fluid while maintaining homogeneous fat suppression; this sequence, with its lower resolution, does not detect smaller lesions, but ensures detection of fractures or destructive lesions. A coronal non–fat-suppressed T1-weighted spin echo is

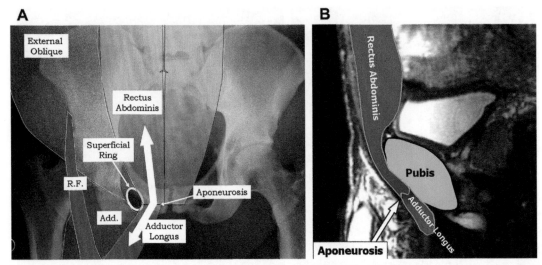

Fig. 2. Biomechanics. (*A*) The points of attachment of the rectus abdominis and adductor muscles and their counterbalancing major vector forces (*large arrows*), as well as the intimate relationship with the superficial ring and the approximate site of the rectus abdominis/adductor aponeurosis. (*B*) Accessory muscles include the rectus femoris (RF) and the secondary adductors and hip rotators (Add.).

performed to evaluate for infiltrative bone marrow process such as metastases, myeloma, or infection. Axial T2-weighted fast spin echo (FSE) fat-suppressed image is performed to assess symmetry of muscles, tendons, bursae, and osseous structures. Following these sequences, a surface receiver coil placed at midline, superficial to the pubic symphysis, is activated, allowing focused imaging of this region with a field of view of 20 to 24 cm. Use of the surface coil and the smaller field of view centered on the rectus abdominis/adductor aponeurosis region markedly increases signal-to-noise ratio.[10] Axial oblique images are then prescribed off a sagittal localizer paralleling the arcuate line of the pelvis, and this sequence is acquired over an 8-cm span centered at midline (**Fig. 3**). These images highlight the caudal rectus abdominis attachments and open the adductor tendon origins.[9] A T2-weighted fat-suppressed FSE true sagittal image is obtained, centered at the pubic symphysis. This sequence evaluates the rectus abdominis/adductor aponeurosis with its periosteal attachments on the anterior and anteroinferior pubic ramus. An athletic pubalgia MR imaging protocol is outlined in **Table 1**.[19–21]

The advantage of the outlined protocol is that it provides specific evaluation for common musculoskeletal causes of groin pain. Furthermore, it allows evaluation for inguinal hernias and nonmusculoskeletal groin pain, and, if not conclusive, can guide further evaluation of these conditions. However, using such an athletic pubalgia protocol

in an inappropriate clinical setting can lead to misdiagnosis of common sources of pelvic pain such as endometriosis, and subtle acetabular labrum tears. Alternative MR protocols may be useful with specific clinical concerns. Intravenous

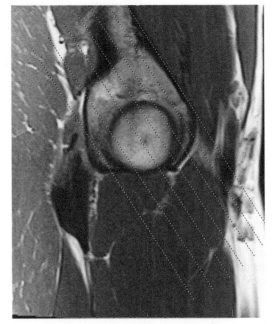

Fig. 3. Coronal oblique plane. Intermediate-weighted sagittal images at the acetabulum shows plane selection for coronal oblique imaging that parallels the arcuate line.

Table 1
Athletic pubalgia MR imaging protocol

Sequence/ Plane	FOV (cm²)	Matrix	Section (cm) Thickness/Gap	TR (ms)	TE (ms)	TI (ms)	BW (kHz)	ETL
Coronal STIR	28 (cover B hips)	256 × 192 2–3	4/1	>2000	20–40	150	8	16
Coronal T1 SE	28 (cover B hips)	256 × 256 1–2	4/1	400–800	Min			16
Axial T2 FSE Fat saturated	28 (cover B hips)	256 × 256 2–3	4/1	>2000	50–60		8	16
Axial oblique PD FSE	20	384 × 384 1–2	3/0.5	3000 (max)	25–30		4	16
Sagittal T2 FSE Fat saturated	20–24	256 × 256 2–3	3/0.5	>2000	50–60		8	16
Axial oblique T2 FSE Fat saturated	20	256 × 192 2–3	3/1	>2000	50–60		8	16

Abbreviations: BW, bandwidth; ETL, echo train length; FOV, field of view; PD, proton density; SE, spin echo; TE, echo time; TI, inversion time; TR, repetition time.

contrast is recommended with any concern for a soft tissue tumor or infection. If the primary consideration is a sliding or intermittent hernia, a rapid, spoiled gradient echo sequence can be acquired during active Valsalva, mimicking the dynamic capabilities of ultrasound. With this technique, positioning the patient prone on the coil can help decrease motion artifact.[22,23]

PATHOLOGY BY MR IMAGING

Using a systematic approach for image review and an athletic pubalgia protocol, MR is a sensitive and specific modality for injuries manifesting as athletic pubalgia. Although concomitant and bilateral lesions are frequently encountered, several dominant and reproducible patterns of imaging findings have been reported. On the high-resolution sequences, osseous and osteochondral structures at the pubic symphysis should be assessed as a joint, and then the imager should use any secondary signs or indicators to identify any possible breach in the tendinous attachments around the symphysis in the region of the pubic tubercles. Inguinal canal structures should be interrogated for hernia, varicocele, and symmetry. The larger field of view sequences should be reviewed for more-remote myotendinous hip flexor

or adductor compartment injuries, apophysites, soft tissue masses, sacroiliac pathology, and any suggestion of internal derangements of the hips.[8,10,19]

The Secondary Cleft

There are 2 clefts that have been described at or near the pubic symphysis. The primary cleft is developmental and is present in 10% of adults in the posterosuperior central portion of the pubic symphyseal disc. At MR imaging, T2 hyperintense signal with a vertical configuration can be present in normal patients at the pubic symphysis in the region of the intra-articular disc representing this primary cleft. A secondary cleft was initially described at fluoroscopy-guided pubic symphysis arthrography, when contrast injected into the region of the primary cleft extended unilaterally inferolateral to the pubic symphysis with a curvilinear configuration. This configuration was adapted to MR imaging, where T2 hyperintense signal extending inferolateral from the symphysis with a similar morphology was termed the MR secondary cleft. In patients with athletic pubalgia, an arthrographic secondary cleft or an MR secondary cleft correlates strongly with the situs and site of pain. Sometimes the secondary cleft extends between the rectus abdominis or adductor tendon attachments and bone, and sometimes it has a subchondral or subapophyseal element, so it is not diagnostic of any single injury, but it is an important observation to make as an indicator of regional injury. A unilateral secondary cleft often reflects an ipsilateral rectus abdominis/adductor detachment, whereas a bilateral MR imaging secondary cleft can indicate a midline rectus abdominis/adductor aponeurotic plate disruption (**Fig. 4**).[24,25]

Osteitis Pubis

As with other fibrous joints, the pubic symphysis is subject to a range of conditions leading to painful inflammatory osteochondral changes and microinstability. The central disc can degenerate, similarly to the knee meniscus or the glenoid labrum, and, with persistent activity, articular surfaces are subject to trauma. Once there is osseous injury, altered biomechanics related to instability of the joint or gait aberrancies can destabilize the anterior pelvis, leading to many of the lesions observed in athletic pubalgia. In this regard, at imaging, the pubic symphysis can serve as a window to athletic pubalgia. In other instances, an initial tear at one of the tendinous attachments can lead to abnormal biomechanics that subsequently damage the symphysis itself, initiating a cycle of musculoskeletal injury.[26]

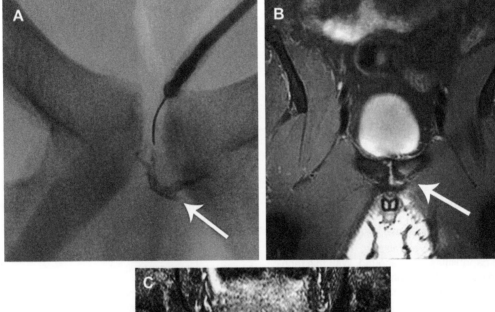

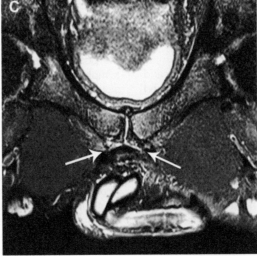

Fig. 4. The secondary cleft. MR imaging of ipsilateral right caudal rectus abdominis/adductor aponeurosis injury. (*A*) Fluoroscopy spot image of a left-sided secondary cleft during a symphyseal injection (*arrow*). (*B*) Coronal oblique T2 fast spin echo fat suppressed image shows an MR secondary cleft to the left in a (*arrow*). (*C*) Coronal oblique T2 FS image shows bilateral secondary clefts at MR imaging (*arrows*).

Osteitis pubis indicates bony injury at the symphysis, and subchondral bone marrow edema in a pattern reminiscent of osteoarthritis is the hallmark MR imaging findings. Marrow edema should be bilateral, but is often asymmetric to the side of pain, and should span the subchondral region of the symphysis from anterior to posterior. This is a distinct pattern from the isolated periosteal or subcortical bony edema anteriorly at the pubic tubercles related to tendinous avulsive stress. Chronic osteitis pubis can manifest with productive changes of osteoarthritis including hyperintense subchondral cysts, hypointense sclerosis, and even subchondral bony resorption. Acute osteitis pubis presents with subchondral bone marrow edema but normal osseous morphology. Often, osteitis pubis at MR imaging is observed in conjunction with perisymphyseal soft tissue lesions including injury at the rectus abdominis/ adductor aponeuroses. In these instances, it can be difficult to establish whether the osteitis pubis was the precipitating lesion, or whether it was a secondary osteoarthritis occurring after the initial soft tissue injury (**Fig. 5**).[8,19,27,28]

Osteitis pubis can occur without rectus abdominis or adductor tendon injury. The pubic symphysis ligaments are often damaged in pregnancy and during childbirth, and postpartum osteitis pubis can result, especially in the setting of postpartum athletic activity. These primary stabilizers can also be injured with pelvic fractures or shear-force traumas across the symphysis, leading to destabilization and, ultimately, osteitis pubis. In the skeletally immature patient, unfused apophyses at the pubic symphysis can be injured, leading to a developmental osteitis pubis (see **Fig. 5**).

Rectus Abdominis/Adductor Aponeurosis Injury

An injury simultaneously involving the caudal rectus abdominis, the adductor longus origin, and the pubic tubercle periosteum or the pubic symphysis capsule is the most frequently encountered lesion on MR imaging in the setting of athletic pubalgia. Most commonly, there is confluent interstitial tearing or detachment of 1 or both rectus abdominis muscles at the level of the symphysis and the adductor longus tendons, often a chronic source of debilitating groin pain.[10,19] However, in the setting of an acute and often extreme trauma, a frank breech can occur between these 2 structures with detachment and subsequent retraction of 1 or both. This spectrum of injury centered at the level of the pubic tubercle has been termed rectus abdominis/adductor aponeurosis lesion.[29] These lesions are frequently unilateral, involving the lateral edge of the caudal rectus abdominis and often leaving a defect in close proximity to the posteromedial wall of a now-patulous superficial inguinal ring. This ipsilateral rectus abdominis/adductor lesion presents with focal tenderness in the region of the superficial ring and the pubic tubercle, and is most likely to reflect the injury sometimes termed sports hernia or sportsman's hernia.[8,17,29–31] MR indicators of this lesion include subenthesial or periosteal bone marrow edema at the site of the rectus abdominis attachment on the pubic tubercle and enlargement or interstitial tearing of the adductor longus origin. There is often a unilateral secondary cleft, and this off-midline injury can be unilateral or bilateral, with or without osteitis pubis. Athletes with this injury are more likely to be treated

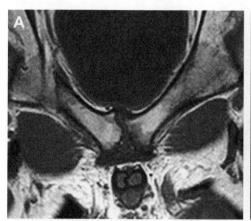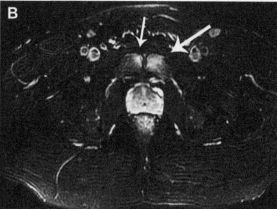

Fig. 5. Osteitis pubis. MR imaging of osteitis pubis. (*A*) Intermediate-weighted axial oblique image of a 20-year-old soccer player shows advanced chronic osteitis pubis with widening of the pubic symphysis, articular surface irregularity, and productive change. (*B*) Axial T2 fat-suppressed turbo spin echo image shows acute, asymmetric osteitis pubis with left (*large arrow*) greater than right (*small arrow*) subchondral bone marrow edema.

surgically than those with isolated rectus abdominis or adductor tendon injuries (**Fig. 6**).[19]

In other cases, rectus abdominis/adductor aponeurosis injuries appear on MR to be centered at the pubic symphysis, extending into the medial edge of both aponeuroses. These midline lesions rarely manifest as distraction between the rectus abdominis and the adductor tendons, but generally exhibit signal suggesting a lifting or delamination of the entire apparatus from the pubic symphysis region, and can be termed rectus abdominis/adductor aponeurotic plate disruption. Both caudal rectus abdominis muscles are involved, spanning midline in a transverse plane and generating confluent, bilateral secondary clefts.[17,29] Osteitis pubis is common with these lesions, and adductor tendinopathy is often asymmetric by MR imaging. Rectus abdominis injury can be symmetric or asymmetric, and may or may not extend to the lateral edges of the aponeuroses, but the consistent finding is a detachment spanning the midline pubic symphysis. Athletes with this lesion rarely return to their preinjury level without surgical repair. Earlier series have reported up to a 4% incidence of contralateral rectus abdominis injury after a unilateral pelvic floor repair, and the investigators believe that this high number may, in part, reflect an initial bilateral lesion (**Fig. 7**).[16]

Rectus Abdominis Strain

The rectus abdominis can be strained anywhere along its course, similar to other abdominal muscles. In the mid- to lower abdomen, the rectus abdominis is often injured in conjunction with the internal or external oblique muscles. This so-called abdominal strain manifests on MR as feathery T2 hyperintensity, with the direction of the hyperintense signal along the muscle bellies reflecting specific muscle involvement. In the lower abdomen and pelvis, rectus abdominis strain is more likely to reflect a rectus abdominis/adductor aponeurosis injury, but can still occur in isolation. The contralateral rectus abdominis serves as an internal and readily available control. Focused attention to the tenoperiosteal caudal rectus abdominis attachment is important in this region because an isolated muscle injury should heal completely with conservative therapy, but an aponeurosis injury can lead to chronic pain and pelvic instability.

Atrophy of the rectus abdominis is frequently encountered with athletic pubalgia, and may represent chronic tendinous lesion, previous rectus abdominis strain, or denervation injury. Two series have documented the situs of rectus muscle atrophy correlated with the side of groin pain, and 1 reported a high incidence of muscle atrophy on the side of previous herniorrhaphy (**Fig. 8**).[8,19,32]

Adductor Syndromes

Several syndromes isolated to the thigh adductor compartment have been described in the sports medicine literature, and adductor origin lesions have been described as a common source of debilitating groin pain in many types of athletes worldwide.[10,18] Injuries can be acute or chronic, and range from acute avulsions at tendon origins to degenerative distal myotendinous junction strains.

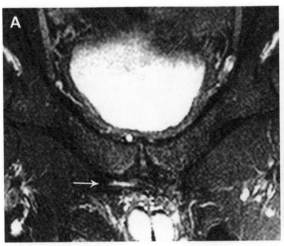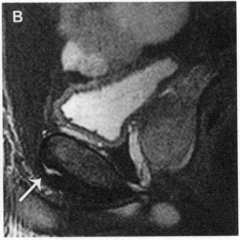

Fig. 6. Ipsilateral aponeurosis lesion. MR imaging of ipsilateral right caudal rectus abdominis/adductor aponeurosis injury. (*A*) Axial oblique T2 FS image shows right-sided abdominis/adductor detachment (*arrow*). (*B*) Sagittal T2 FS image to the right of midline shows right abdominis/adductor detachment (*arrow*).

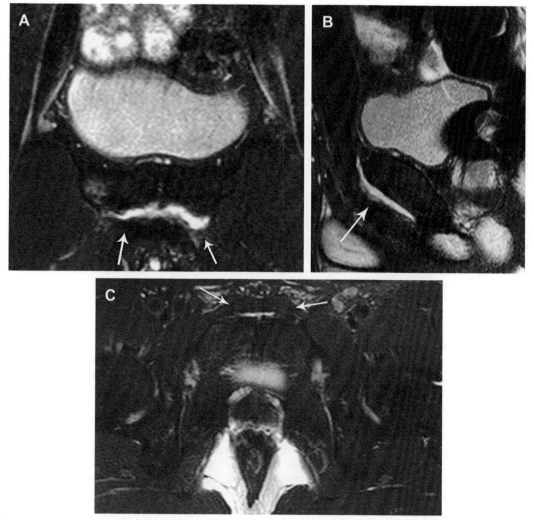

Fig. 7. Midline aponeurotic plate disruption. MR imaging of rectus abdominis/adductor aponeurotic plate disruption. (*A*) Axial oblique T2 FS image shows bilateral secondary cleft (*arrows*) with fluid signal undermining the midline aponeurotic plate consistent with detachment. (*B*) Midline sagittal T2 FS image in a different patient shows midline aponeurotic plate detachment (*arrow*). (*C*) Axial T2 FS (same patient as **Fig. 8**B) image shows bilateral secondary cleft (*arrows*).

Chronic tendinopathies at the proximal adductor are similar to those found elsewhere in the body, with enlargement and hypointensity indicating hypoxic degeneration and even sometimes hydroxyapatite deposition (calcific tendinosis). More acute injuries include osseous or periosteal avulsions and myotendinous or muscle belly strains. MR imaging is useful in characterizing the numerous adductor compartment variants. The adductor longus is often primarily involved with secondary, less severe injury at the adjacent pectineus or adductor brevis. Individual muscles and tendons involved should be delineated in an MR imaging report, along with location along the myotendinous axis and some attempt at grading the

most severe injury. Complete avulsion of the adductor longus with retraction should alert the imager to a likely ipsilateral rectus abdominis injury. An osseous avulsion of the adductor longus can occur in isolation, but almost always leads to a large adductor compartment hematoma.[10,16,19,33]

Discriminating between an isolated adductor avulsive injury and a rectus abdominis/adductor aponeurosis injury can be difficult, and is somewhat subjective. Without question, operative reports from different surgeons have labeled the same lesion as adductor avulsion, rectus abdominis tear with adductor strain, and aponeurosis injury. Therefore, it is important for imagers to acknowledge the intricate anatomy of this region

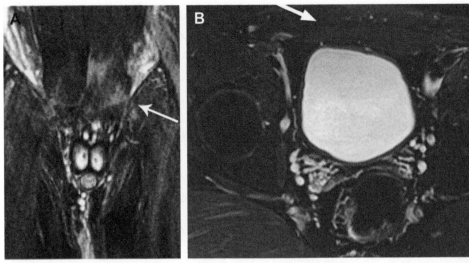

Fig. 8. Rectus abdominis strain. MR imaging of acute and chronic injury to the caudal rectus abdominis muscle. (*A*) Coronal STIR image shows hyperintensity of the distal left rectus abdominis muscle (*arrow*) consistent with grade I strain. (*B*) Axial T2 FS image shows right caudal rectus abdominis muscle atrophy (*arrow*) consistent with chronic injury.

and fully describe the location of the lesion with regard to the pubic symphysis, the pubic tubercle, and the inguinal canal and superficial ring.

A particularly troublesome adductor compartment lesion occurs when an injury at the distal myotendinous junction of an adductor tendon causes rupture of the muscle sheath and herniation of muscle fibers through the subsequent defect, leading to a muscle strain refractory to conventional conservative therapies. This lesion has been termed baseball pitcher/hockey goalie syndrome, although it is not isolated to these athletes or activities. This chronic strain can manifest on MR as focal T2 hyperintense signal at a myotendinous junction with thickening, hypointensity, and nodularity of the sheath adjacent to the myotendinous unit. Distal myotendinous injuries within the adductor compartment are frequently encountered with recurrent groin pain after a pelvic floor repair or adductor tendon release, and surgical debridement may be necessary to facilitate healing (**Fig. 9**).[7,34]

Inguinal Hernias

True hernias are rare in the setting of athletic pubalgia, both on MR imaging and at surgery. The inguinal canals are optimally evaluated on coronal oblique images where they are elongated to show all internal contents. Any persistent herniation should be directly visible on athletic pubalgia MR imaging. The inguinal canals should be symmetric and contain a small amount of fat without enteric visceral structure, fluid, fibrosis, or mass effect.

More frequently encountered are findings suggesting prior herniorrhaphy, ranging from hernia plugs to susceptibility artifact indicating the presence of mesh. Occasionally, refractory groin pain is related to scarring in the inguinal region after multiple previous hernia surgeries. In a more common scenario, there are MR findings indicating previous herniorrhaphy, but there is an ipsilateral rectus abdominis/adductor aponeurosis lesion caudal to the surgical site. This observation reinforces the idea that the term sports hernia may sometimes lead to misdirected surgical procedures. Reinforcing the inguinal wall with mesh may provide transient symptom relief with an aponeurosis injury, but symptoms almost inevitably return as athletic activity is resumed. Nonetheless, a small percentage of patients with athletic pubalgia will have a true inguinal or femoral hernia, so the canals should be examined with each MR imaging review (**Fig. 10**).[8,35,36]

Athletic Pubalgia in Women

MR imaging referrals for athletic pubalgia generally reflect the reported demographic incidence of sports hernia lesions with a young age range and a strong male predominance. Nonetheless, women can sustain any of the injuries described earlier. In our experience, there are a few additional nuances to consider when imaging the female athletic pubalgia patient.

Although women can sustain an ipsilateral rectus abdominis/adductor aponeurosis injury, in the experience of the authors, a midline rectus

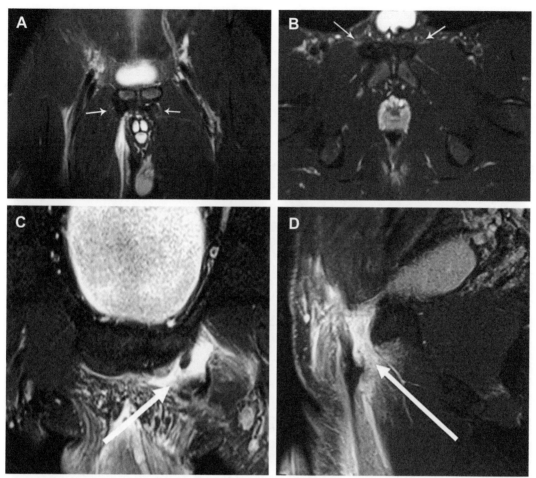

Fig. 9. Adductor syndromes. MR imaging of adductor tendinosis and avulsion. (*A*) Coronal STIR image shows thickening and increased signal within the adductor tendons, left greater than right (*arrows*), consistent with tendinosis. (*B*) Axial T2 FS image shows thickening and increased signal within the adductor tendons, left greater than right (*arrows*), consistent with tendinosis. (*C*) Axial oblique T2 FS image shows complete tear of the proximal left common adductor origin with interposed fluid signal and tendon retraction (*arrow*) in a professional football player. (*D*) Axial T2 FS image shows complete tear of the proximal left common adductor origin with interposed fluid signal and tendon retraction (*arrow*) in a professional football player.

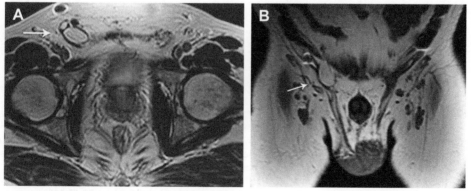

Fig. 10. Inguinal hernia. MR imaging of an inguinal hernia. (*A*) Axial T2 image shows right inguinal hernia (*arrow*). (*B*) Coronal T1 image shows right inguinal hernia (*arrow*).

abdominis/adductor aponeurotic plate disruption is more frequently encountered in the female athlete. This tendency may, in part, reflect anatomic differences between men and women anterior and inferior to the pubic symphysis, where men have more passages through the pelvic floor to allow for passage of genitourinary structures. Pregnancy causes changes in biomechanical forces and vectors throughout the pelvis that can stress the pubic symphysis, its stabilizing attachments, and the sacroiliac joints, leading to osteitis pubis and sacroiliitis. Postpartum osteitis pubis may reflect these forces along with any ligamentous injuries sustained during delivery. Some confounders, including endometriosis, adnexal cysts, and uterine fibroids, are exclusive to

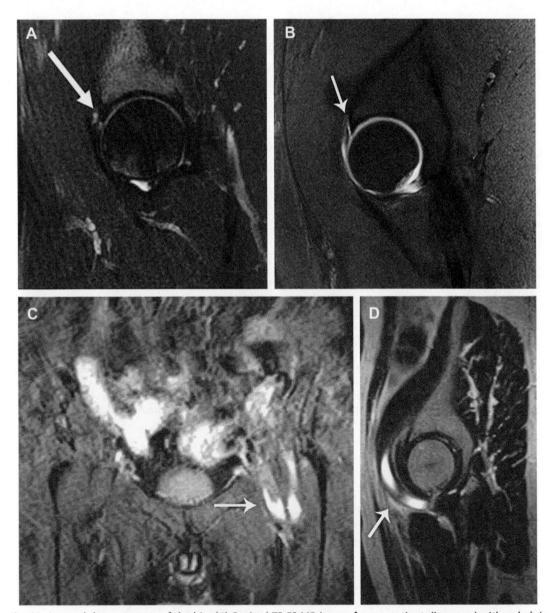

Fig. 11. Internal derangements of the hip. (*A*) Sagittal T2 FS MR image from a patient diagnosed with pubalgia shows an anterosuperior labral tear with associated paralabral cyst (*arrow*) in a runner on noncontrast athletic pubalgia evaluation. (*B*) Sagittal T1 FS direct arthrogram MR image shows anterior labral tear with detachment presenting as groin pain (*arrow*). (*C*) Coronal T2 FS MR image shows fluid surrounding the left iliopsoas tendon consistent with a distal iliopsoas strain and subsequent bursitis (*arrow*). (*D*) Sagittal T2 FS MR image showing a fluid filled, distended iliopsoas bursa (*arrow*).

women. Femoral hernias are more common in women. The spectrum of peripartum-, post-partum-, and pregnancy-related causes of groin pain is not fully described yet, but an imaging approach to women with athletic pubalgia must acknowledge these conditions and the musculoskeletal dangers they pose. Thus, the imager may need a lower threshold for deviating from the standard athletic pubalgia protocol toward contrast examinations or computed tomography and ultrasound studies when histories and initial findings are atypical.[16,29]

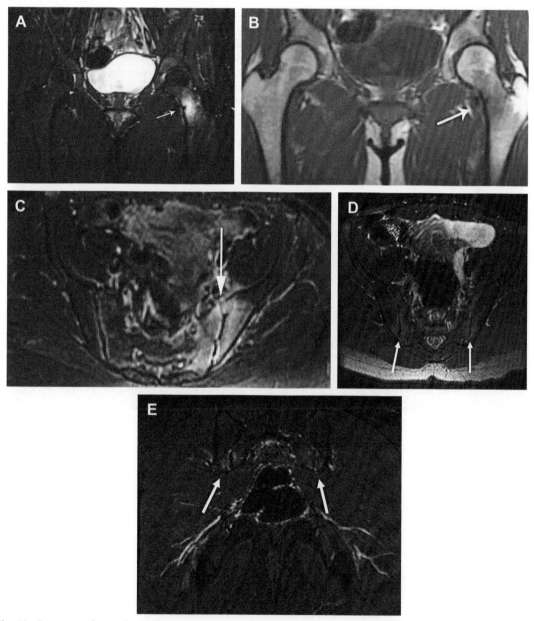

Fig. 12. Osseous and articular pathology. (*A*) Coronal STIR MR image of a typical femoral neck stress fracture presenting as unilateral groin pain in a runner (*arrow*). (*B*) Coronal T1 image shows a compressive aspect to a subacute femoral neck stress fracture (*arrow*). (*C*) Axial T2 FS MR image shows unilateral left sacroiliitis with intense bone marrow edema spanning the left sacroiliac joint in an adolescent athlete following steroid injection for groin pain (*arrow*). (*D*) Axial T2 FS image in a 12-year-old pentathlete shows symmetric bilateral sacroiliac marrow edema (*arrows*). (*E*) Coronal STIR image from the same patient shows findings typical of an early, bilateral sacroiliitis; the patient was ultimately diagnosed with ankylosing spondylitis (*arrows*).

Confounding Pathologies

Given the numerous muscle and tendon attachments about the pelvis, it is not surprising that a myriad of lesions remote from the pubic symphysis can cause pain referred to the groin and thus mimic athletic pubalgia, reinforcing the need for the larger field of view survey sequences in all MR imaging pelvis (and hip) protocols. These sequences are not meant to replace other dedicated pelvis MR imaging protocols, such as dynamic contrast enhanced imaging of the female pelvis or direct MR arthrography of the hip, but they should alert the imager to potential confounding lesions as a cause for groin pain.

Internal derangements of the hip, including synovitis, femoral acetabular impingement, and acetabular labral tears, are a common source of groin pain in the athlete. Although noncontrast MR protocols are insensitive for labral tear, any subchondral marrow edema at the acetabulum, hip effusion, synovial herniation pit, paralabral cyst, or cam-type morphology should be observed on an athletic pubalgia protocol. If there are no lesions in the region of the symphysis on MR, then consideration should be given to a more definitive direct MR arthrographic study of the hip. The iliopsoas tendons and bursae should be assessed for symmetry and abnormal fluid signal, particularly at the level of the iliopectineal eminence, where an externally snapping hip can occur (**Fig. 11**).[37]

Osseous stress injuries frequently present with groin pain. The femoral neck and pubic rami are common locations for such injuries, and stress fracture here can be misdiagnosed as an athletic

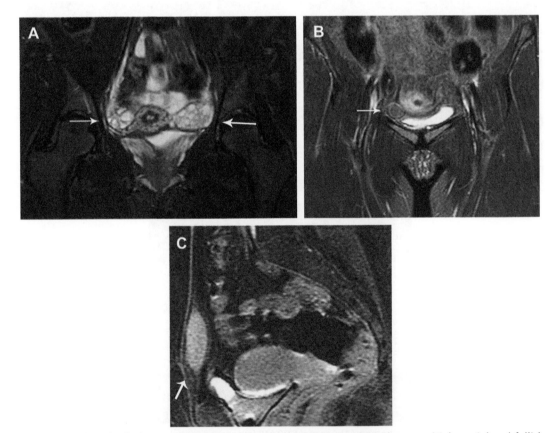

Fig. 13. Visceral and soft tissue pathology. (*A*) Coronal oblique T2 FS image shows multiple peripheral follicles within the ovaries in a 15-year-old female soccer player with groin pain and otherwise normal MR imaging, characteristic of polycystic ovarian disease (*arrows*). (*B*) Coronal oblique T2 FS MR images show an exophytic fibroid to the right (*arrow*), presenting as pain at the rectus abdominis/adductor aponeurosis. (*C*) Sagittal T1 FS image from a pubalgia protocol converted to a pre- and postcontrast mass protocol shows an enhancing, fusiform mass within the lower rectus abdominis muscle that was signed out as a synovial sarcoma within a cesarean section scar after resection (*arrow*).

pubalgia lesion. In the skeletally immature, the triradiate cartilage is a common location for stress injury leading to groin pain exacerbated by activity. At MR, osseous and growth plate stress injuries present as focal T2 hyperintensity on fluid-sensitive, fat-suppressed sequences, often with adjacent soft tissue edema. A superimposed hypointense line confirms a stress fracture. Other osseous lesions that can cause groin pain in the young athlete include osteoid osteoma, Langerhans cell histiocytosis, and the rare aggressive bone tumor (**Fig. 12**).[19,38]

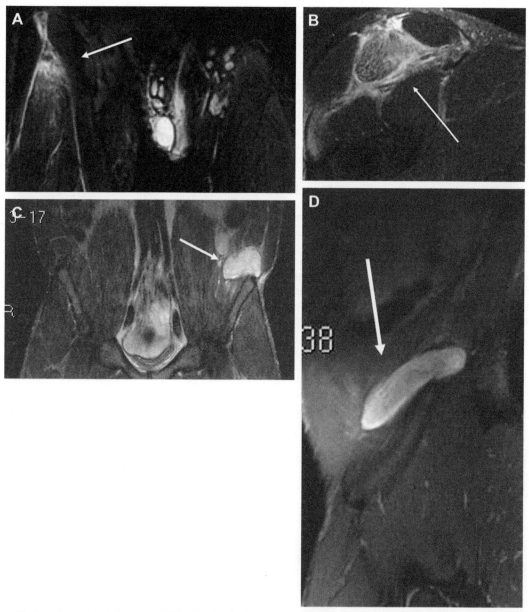

Fig. 14. Muscle strains. (*A*) Coronal STIR shows a high-grade partial tear of the right rectus femoris (*arrow*) that presented as right groin pain in a professional basketball player. (*B*) Axial T2 FS from the same examination confirms a high-grade (grade 2) partial tear of the rectus femoris in cross section (*arrow*). (*C*) Coronal STIR in a collegiate quarterback shows avulsion of the distal left external oblique muscle with an associated large hematoma (*arrow*). (*D*) Sagittal T2 FS from the same patient 5 days after the initial injury shows a hematoma evolving along the plane of the lower external oblique (*arrow*).

Visceral pathology is a particular confounder for athletic pubalgia in young female patients. Ovarian cysts or follicles, endometriosis, adenomyosis, and uterine fibroids can all present with groin pain. Chronic groin pain in a young nonathlete is particularly worrisome, because the musculoskeletal athletic pubalgia lesions discussed earlier are less likely. In this scenario, nerve entrapment syndromes and soft tissue tumors are concerns, and consideration should be given to replacing the athletic pubalgia protocol with a pre- and post-contrast MR pelvis protocol. The lower lumbar spine and sacroiliac joints occasionally serve as a source for referred groin pain, especially in the nonathlete (**Fig. 13**).[16,19]

Muscle strains some distance from the pubic symphysis are common sources of groin pain and should be easily identified on the coronal STIR and axial T2 FSE fat-suppressed sequences of the pelvis. A concomitant pubic symphysis lesion can also be present, so the imager must still review the higher resolution sequences at the symphysis (**Fig. 14**). In the skeletally immature, apophysitis can occur at the anterior inferior iliac spine, the anterior superior iliac spine, or the ischial tuberosities, manifesting as osseous, chondral, and tendinous hyperintensities on fluid-sensitive sequences and apophyseal fragmentation on T1-weighted images. Anterior inferior iliac spine (AIIS) apophysitis at the rectus femoris origin is a common cause of groin pain in the dominant extremity of a young kicking athlete (**Fig. 15**).[32,38]

Postoperative MR Imaging

There are numerous operative therapies aimed at alleviating the symptoms of rectus abdominis/adductor aponeurosis lesions. Persistent or recurrent groin pain after any of these may result from reinjury at a site of repair, but more likely reflects either failure of the procedure or a new injury remote from the repair. The authors have noted that, even after a clinically successful pelvic floor repair, a secondary cleft persists at the site of initial injury. Comparison with preoperative imaging is essential in assessing response to therapy. At the pubic symphysis, after repair of an aponeurosis lesion, imagers should note any improvement or evolution of osteitis pubis, any increase in T2 signal at the secondary cleft, and any new or contralateral lesion. Imaging postoperative patients at 3 tesla may help the imager distinguish between intermediate signal reflecting granulation tissue and fluid signal reflecting recurrent injury in the region of the secondary cleft on T2-weighted sequences, although this theoretic advantage is unproved.

In a small postoperative series, the most common MR finding in athletes with recurrent groin pain was strain pattern at the proximal or distal myotendinous junction of the ipsilateral adductor longus. This injury correlated well with physical examination findings, but its cause remains unclear. In most cases, bone marrow edema at the pubic symphysis had improved, a secondary cleft persisted, and new rectus abdominis/adductor aponeurosis tears in the same

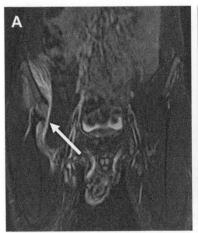
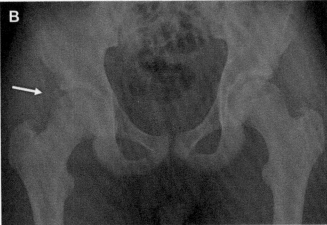

Fig. 15. Apophysitis. (*A*) Coronal STIR image shows apophyseal avulsion at the right AIIS with subenthesial bone marrow edema with associated strain of the proximal rectus femoris and adjacent hematoma (*arrow*). (*B*) Anteroposterior radiograph image from the same patient confirms an osseous avulsion at the skeletally immature right AIIS with caudal retraction of the fragment (*arrow*).

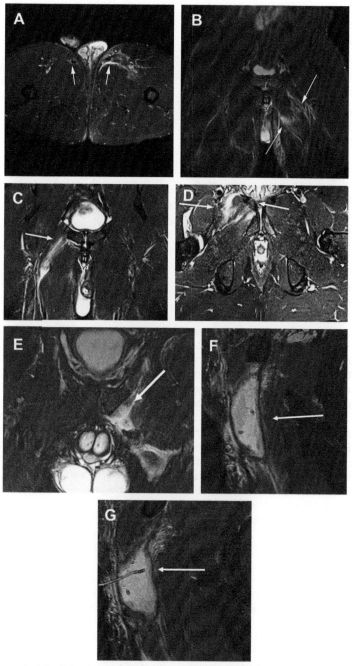

Fig. 16. Postoperative pubalgia. (*A*) Axial T2 fast spin echo fat suppressed shows interstitial edema in the bilateral adductor compartments, left greater than right, centered at the proximal myotendinous junction (*arrows*). (*B*) Coronal STIR delineating myotendinous strains in status after bilateral pelvic floor repair, a condition termed baseball pitcher hockey goalie syndrome (*arrows*). (*C*) Coronal STIR MR image shows a right secondary cleft with detachment of the left rectus abdominis/adductor aponeurosis (*arrow*) and associated right adductor compartment muscle strain in a professional football player status after left-sided pelvic floor repair. (*D*) Axial T2 fast spin echo fat suppressed confirms a new right-sided injury in this athlete with a history of left-sided rectus abdominis/adductor aponeurosis injury and subsequent repair (*arrows*). Contralateral aponeurosis injuries occur in approximately 4% of athletes after unilateral pelvic floor repair. (*E*) Axial oblique T2 FS MR image shows complete avulsion of the left abdominis/adductor aponeurosis with significant retraction of the proximal left adductor tendon (*arrow*). (*F, G*) Follow-up postsurgical T2 FS sagittal images show a complex fluid collection consistent with abscess with drain noted in the collection in (*arrow*). Postsurgical complications increase with the severity of the initial injury.

location were rare. In the setting of a mesh repair, susceptibility artifact generated by the edge of the mesh can occasionally confirm a malpositioned repair (Fig. 16).

SUMMARY

MR imaging has been proved as an essential diagnostic tool in the workup and treatment planning of patients with activity-related groin pain, or athletic pubalgia. Several reproducible injury patterns have been described, and can be consistently demonstrated on MR imaging using a dedicated, noncontrast athletic pubalgia protocol. Osteitis pubis should be recognized on MR and interrogated as a process reflecting joint instability, precipitating an algorithmic assessment of the ligamentous and tendinous attachments about the pubic symphysis. Rectus abdominis/adductor aponeurosis injuries should be identified and characterized as either ipsilateral or midline plate lesions, and frank tears or gaps should be reported. When no lesion is found in the pubic symphysis region, attention should be turned to the regional muscles, tendons, bursae, the visceral pelvis, and, ultimately, the hips. True hernias are rare in the setting of athletic pubalgia, but inguinal canal asymmetries are common and should be noted.

All imaging centers that routinely perform musculoskeletal MR should have a canned athletic pubalgia protocol. Groin pain can occur with a myriad of lesions that would be treated most appropriately by different subspecialtists, and MR imaging can serve as a triage and referral aid in these generally young, athletic patients.[16,34,39,40]

REFERENCES

1. Taylor DC, Meyers WC, Moylan JA, et al. Abdominal musculature abnormalities as a cause of groin pain in athletes. Inguinal hernias and pubalgia. Am J Sports Med 1991;19(3):239–42.
2. Lynch SA, Renstrom PA. Groin injuries in sport: treatment strategies. Sports Med 1999;28:137–44.
3. Brittenden J, Robinson P. Imaging of pelvic injuries in athletes. Br J Radiol 2005;78:457–68.
4. Morelli V, Weaver V. Groin injuries and groin pain in athletes: part 1. Prim Care 2005;32:163–83.
5. Verrall GM, Slavotinek JP, Fon GT. Incidence of pubic bone marrow oedema in Australian rules football players: relation to groin pain. Br J Sports Med 2001;35(1):28–33.
6. Harris NH, Murray RO. Lesions of the symphysis in athletes. Br Med J 1974;4(5938):211–4.
7. Meyers WC, Foley DP, Garrett WE, et al. Management of severe lower abdominal or inguinal pain in high-performance athletes. PAIN (Performing Athletes with Abdominal or Inguinal Neuromuscular Pain Study Group). Am J Sports Med 2000;28: 2–8.
8. Zoga AC, Kavanaugh EC, Omar IM, et al. Athletic pubalgia and the "sports hernia": MR imaging findings. Radiology 2008;247(3):797–807.
9. Albers SL, Spritzer CE, Garrett WE Jr, et al. MR findings in athletes with pubalgia. Skeletal Radiol 2001; 30:270–7.
10. Robinson P, Barron DA, Parsons W, et al. Adductor-related groin pain in athletes: correlation of MR imaging with clinical findings. Skeletal Radiol 2004; 33:451–7.
11. Putschar WG. The structure of the human symphysis pubis with special consideration of parturition and its sequelae. Am J Phys Anthropol 1976;45(3 pt 2): 589–94.
12. Williams A. Thigh. In: Stranding S, editor. Gray's anatomy: the anatomical basis of clinical practice. 39th edition. Edinburgh (Scotland): Elsevier Churchill Livingstone; 2005. p. 1465–7.
13. Gamble JG, Simmons SC, Freedman M. The symphysis pubis: anatomic and pathologic considerations. Clin Orthop Relat Res 1986;203:261–72.
14. Vix VA, Ryu CY. The adult symphysis pubis: normal and abnormal. Am J Roentgenol Radium Ther Nucl Med 1971;112:517–25.
15. Walheim G, Olerud S, Ribbe T. Mobility of the pubic symphysis. Measurements by an electromechanical method. Acta Orthop Scand 1984;55(2):203–8.
16. Meyers WC, McKechnie A, Philippon MJ, et al. Experience with "sports hernia" spanning two decades. Ann Surg 2008;248(4):656–65.
17. Shortt CP, Zoga AC, Kavanagh EC, et al. Anatomy, pathology, and MRI findings in the sports hernia. Semin Musculoskelet Radiol 2008;12(1):54–61.
18. Cunningham PM, Brennan D, O'Connell M, et al. Patterns of bone and soft-tissue injury at the symphysis pubis in soccer players: observations at MRI. AJR Am J Roentgenol 2007;188:W291–6.
19. Omar IM, Zoga AC, Kavanagh EC, et al. Athletic pubalgia and "sports hernia": optimal MR imaging technique and findings. Radiographics 2008;28: 1415–38.
20. Zajick DC, Zoga AC, Omar IM, et al. Spectrum of MRI findings in clinical athletic pubalgia. Semin Musculoskelet Radiol 2008;12:3–12.
21. Joesting DR. Diagnosis and treatment of sportsman's hernia. Curr Sports Med Rep 2002;1:121–4.
22. Garvey JF, Read JW, Turner A. Sportsman hernia: what can we do? Hernia 2010;14(1):17–25.
23. Van den Berg JC, de Valois JC, Go PM, et al. Groin hernia: can dynamic magnetic resonance imaging be of help? Eur Radiol 1998;8:270–3.
24. O'Connell MJ, Powell T, McCaffrey NM, et al. Symphyseal cleft injection in the diagnosis and

treatment of osteitis pubis in athletes. AJR Am J Roentgenol 2002;179:955–9.

25. Brennan D, O'Connell MJ, Ryan M, et al. Secondary cleft sign as a marker of injury in athletes with groin pain. MR image appearance and interpretation. Radiology 2005;235:162–7.

26. Gibbon WW, Hession PR. Diseases of pubis and pubic symphysis. MR imaging appearance. Am J Roentgenol 1997;169:849–53.

27. Kunduracioglu B, Yilmaz C, Yorubulut M, et al. Magnetic resonance findings of osteitis pubis. J Magn Reson Imaging 2007;25(3):535–9.

28. Rodriguez C, Miguel A, Lima H, et al. Osteitis pubis syndrome in the professional soccer athlete. a case report. J Athl Train 2001;36:437–40.

29. Kavanagh EC, Zoga AC, Omar I, et al. MR Imaging of the rectus abdominis/adductor aponeurosis: findings in the 'sports hernia'. proceedings of the American Roentgen Ray Society. AJR Am J Roentgenol 2007;188:A13–6.

30. Caudill P, Nyland J, Smith C, et al. Sports hernias: a systematic literature review. BR J Sports Med 2008;42(12):954–64.

31. LeBlanc KE, LeBlanc KA. Groin pain in athletes. Hernia 2003;7:68–71.

32. Overdeck KH, Palmer WE. Imaging of hip and groin injuries in athletes. Semin Musculoskelet Radiol 2004;8:41–55.

33. Nicholas SJ, Tyler TF. Adductor muscle strains in sports. Sports Med 2002;32:339–44.

34. Zoga AC, Morrison WB, Roth CG, et al. MR findings in athletic pubalgia: normal postoperative appearance and reinjury patterns after pelvic repairs and releases for 'Sports Hernia'. Proceedings of the Radiologic Society of North America. Chicago, 2009.

35. Van den Berg JC, de Valois JC, Go PM, et al. Detection of groin hernia with physical examination, ultrasound, and MRI compared with laparoscopic findings. Invest Radiol 1999;34:739–43.

36. Gullmo A. Herniography: the diagnosis of hernia in the groin and incompetence of the pouch of Douglas and pelvic floor. Acta Radiol Suppl 1980;361: 1–76.

37. Blankenbaker DG, Tuite MJ. The painful hip: new concepts. Skeletal Radiol 2006;35(6):353–70.

38. Kavanagh EC, Koulouris G, Ford S, et al. MR imaging of groin pain in the athlete. Semin Musculoskelet Radiol 2006;10:197–207.

39. Ziprin P, Prabhudesai SG, Abrahams S, et al. Transabdominal preperitoneal laparoscopic approach for the treatment of sportsman's hernia. J Laparaoendosc Adv Surg Tech A 2008;18(5): 669–72.

40. Malycha P, Lovell G. Inguinal surgery in athletes with chronic groin pain: the sportsman's hernia. Aust N Z J Surg 1992;62:123–5.

Imaging Pediatric Sports Injuries: Upper Extremity

Kirkland W. Davis, MD*

KEYWORDS

- Pediatric • Sports medicine • MR imaging • Shoulder
- Elbow • Wrist

The pediatric musculoskeletal system has noteworthy differences from that of the adult. Because of the anatomic and physiologic differences and the differences in training methods and sports participation between children and adults, the pediatric athlete often incurs unique injuries. With more than 30 million children and adolescents engaging in organized sports in the United States each year, athletic activities have become the most common cause of injuries and emergency department visits for adolescents[1] and the fourth most common overall reason for primary care clinic visits for pediatric patients, after well-child visits, otitis media, and upper respiratory tract infections.[2] A compilation of epidemiologic studies on pediatric sports injuries by Caine and colleagues[3] concluded that the highest rates of injury per hour of participation for boys occur in ice hockey, rugby, and soccer, whereas for girls the highest rates are in soccer, basketball, and gymnastics. As children age, the rates of injury become even higher in football, rugby, and soccer because adolescents become heavier, faster, and stronger and in gymnastics, presumably because of the longer training hours leading to more overuse injuries and more difficult routines placing additional stress on the body.[3] Whereas lower extremity injuries are more common in pediatric athletes overall, children engaged in baseball, judo, gymnastics, and snowboarding are more likely to sustain upper extremity injuries.[3]

Sprains, strains, and contusions are reported to be the most common pediatric sports injuries, followed by lacerations, fractures, and inflammatory phenomena.[3] Adolescents are especially vulnerable to injury for several reasons: (1) adolescents typically have an imbalance between strength and flexibility as they grow, (2) pediatric bones become more porous and susceptible to fracture as they lengthen, and (3) it is often during the adolescent period that training schedules increase dramatically and competitions become much more frequent.[4,5]

This article explores the injuries to the upper extremity that are commonly sustained by children and adolescents engaging in athletic activities, focusing not only on the injuries that are unique to the developing musculoskeletal system but also on some "adult" injuries that are commonly seen in the pediatric athlete. This discussion excludes most injuries that are classified as acute trauma, with a few exceptions; specifically, acute Salter-Harris fractures involving the growth plates, long bone fractures, elbow dislocations, and catastrophic injuries are excluded. This article focuses on injuries that commonly undergo imaging workup; they are discussed by the joint/body region, with an initial discussion of overuse injuries. The pediatric gymnast warrants a separate discussion because of the peculiar nature of the stresses that this sport engenders and the pattern of associated injuries. For the purposes of this article, the terms sports and athletics include not only team sports but also athletic training and dance. Although injury patterns often vary depending on whether a patient's physes are open or fused, injuries of the immature and mature skeleton are included in this article

Department of Radiology, University of Wisconsin Hospital and Clinics, University of Wisconsin School of Medicine and Public Health, Madison, WI, USA
* Corresponding author. E3/311 CSC, 600 Highland Avenue, Madison, WI 53792-3252.
E-mail address: kdavis@uwhealth.org

Radiol Clin N Am 48 (2010) 1199–1211
doi:10.1016/j.rcl.2010.07.020

because both are presented to the typical pediatric sports medicine clinic.

OVERUSE INJURIES

Nearly half of all pediatric athletic injuries are overuse injuries.[3] In general, overuse occurs when training demands exceed the body's physiologic ability to compensate.[6] This situation exists amongst novices and elite athletes alike. Overuse injuries are the result of activities that lead to chronic submaximal loading of a tissue.[7] This chronic loading causes microscopic damage to tissues. Normal repair processes are overwhelmed in the face of ongoing stresses. Without adequate time to recover, injuries manifest in many ways.[7,8] Examples of injuries include fatigue stress fractures, apophysitis, fatigue injuries to growth plates, and some muscle and tendon injuries. Specific examples of injuries in the upper extremity include (1) tendinitis of the rotator cuff, proximal biceps tendon, forearm flexor and extensor tendon origins, triceps insertion, and wrist extensor tendons; (2) chronic injuries to the physes of the proximal humerus, distal radius, medial humeral epicondyle, and olecranon process; (3) stress fractures of the olecranon process; and (4) articular cartilage injuries of the lateral elbow.[5,9] Elbow overuse injuries are typical in throwing athletes, whereas wrist overuse syndromes occur with training errors including extended training regimens, repetition of impact, and poor techniques.[9]

Children and adolescents are often at risk for overuse injuries for several reasons, including improper techniques (especially rapid increase in training activities), lack of preseason training, poorly fitting footwear and protective equipment, certain playing surfaces, training errors, the susceptibility of unfused physes, and growth-related muscle weakness and imbalance.[1,7,8,10] The adolescent growth spurt is a particular risk factor for several stress injuries because during the growth spurt (1) bone mineralization lags linear growth, weakening the bone; (2) physeal cartilage is relatively weaker and more susceptible to damage; (3) muscle-tendon tightness results when muscle growth cannot match bone lengthening; and (4) lack of coordination becomes more common with rapid growth spurts.[10–12] Growing cartilage is known to be less resistant to repetitive microtraumas, rendering the cartilage at joint surfaces more prone to shear injuries such as osteochondritis dissecans (OCD), rendering the apophyses more vulnerable to traction apophysitis, and sometimes leading to chronic stress injuries of the epiphyseal physes, namely at the proximal humerus (Little League shoulder) and distal radius (gymnast wrist).[10,13] In addition, many adolescents and even children are training harder than ever and participating in just one sport but year-round. Although this is not a new phenomenon, with reports emphasizing the increase in pediatric overuse sports injuries almost 3 decades ago,[10,14] overuse injuries continue to proliferate.[6]

Another cause for the proliferation of overuse injuries is the continuing shift of childhood athletic activities from free play to organized sports. Overuse injuries are almost exclusive to the organized setting, whereas acute traumatic injuries predominate in free play.[10] With the shift toward organized athletics and the trend toward year-round single-sport involvement, overuse injuries proliferate; time off from all sports and cross-training in different seasons allows the body to recover in ways that it cannot in a sustained single sport. With the focus on a single sport, overuse injuries are intimately related to the specific demands of the individual sport,[14] as described in this article and the accompanying discussion on lower extremity athletic injuries elsewhere in this issue.

GYMNASTICS INJURIES

A gymnast is the prototypical example of the pediatric athlete susceptible to overuse injuries. Gymnastics not only has seen a remarkable increase in popularity starting in the 1970s but also has undergone a change in typical patterns of activity. Gymnasts start intense training at earlier ages (6 years for eventual elite girl gymnasts and 9 years for boys) and train for longer hours at all ages and levels of expertise.[15] Many of the individual disciplines of gymnastics require repeated and sustained weight bearing on the upper extremities in ways that almost no other sport does. Because of this requirement, gymnasts experience a high number of overuse injuries of the upper extremity and most gymnasts suffer at least one significant injury during their career,[15] with 29% of gymnasts having to modify their training regimen each season due to injury.[16] Some gymnastic disciplines also place repeated extreme forces on the low back[15]; overuse injuries of the pediatric spine are discussed elsewhere in this issue. Ankle injuries are also common in gymnastics but are usually acute injuries such as sprains.[15] Male gymnasts suffer more upper extremity injuries than lower extremity injuries, with shoulder injuries exceeding those of the wrist. In the female gymnast, upper extremity injuries are most common in the wrist, followed by the elbow.[15] In fact, in one study, 70% of the female gymnasts complained of wrist pain.[16]

The most common shoulder complaint in male gymnasts is multidirectional instability, whereas female gymnasts rarely suffer shoulder injuries.[16] The elbow of the pediatric gymnast is especially susceptible to OCD of the capitulum and, to a lesser degree, the radial head, with posterior stresses leading to triceps tendon strains and olecranon apophysitis.[16,17] The forearm of pediatric gymnasts is susceptible to acute and stress fractures. Pediatric gymnasts place incredible repeated stresses across the wrist. These forces can lead to chronic stress injuries of the distal physis of the radius, tears of the triangular fibrocartilage and dorsal wrist ganglia, and stress fractures of the scaphoid.[16] Most of these injuries are discussed within the following sections on each joint.

SHOULDER INJURIES

Acute fractures of the shoulder are uncommon in children and adolescents, with the exception of midshaft clavicle fractures, which are among the most common of all childhood fractures.[18–20] One peculiar fracture in the shoulder of adolescent athletes is a fracture at the base of the coracoid process. The coracoid process is a secondary ossification center and has a physis at its base. Before this physis fuses, it is vulnerable to avulsion (Fig. 1). These fractures are seen in athletes who encounter violent collisions of the upper extremity; for instance, football accounts for more than half of these fractures in the United States.[21]

Because stress fractures are rare in the upper extremity, they are covered more extensively in the article on lower extremity elsewhere in this issue. Stress fractures occasionally occur in the proximal humerus as overuse injuries in throwing athletes, including baseball pitchers and javelin throwers, and those involved in rugby, swimming, and racquetball.[22] These injuries can be imaged with MR imaging, bone scan, or computed tomography) and usually heal with conservative treatment.[22] Similarly, stress osteolysis of the distal clavicle is rare in adolescents but can occur in adolescent weight lifters. When present, this entity decreases mineralization of the distal clavicle and causes resorption of its distal tip.[19]

Acute injuries to the muscle-tendon unit (MTU), including muscle or tendon strain, partial and complete tears of the muscle or tendon, and muscle contusions, are less common in the upper extremity than in the lower, but these injuries do occur (Fig. 2). Undoubtedly, there is some pathologic overlap between these acute injuries and more chronic tendinitis, an overuse injury. The clinical literature is replete with discussions of tendinitis in pediatric athletes,[9,19] but these patients rarely require imaging to establish the diagnosis. Imaging is typically reserved for those cases in which more substantial damage to the tendon, such as a partial or complete tear, is suspected. In the shoulder, rotator cuff tendinitis is especially prevalent in overhead athletes, such as swimmers, throwers, and tennis players, often in the setting of posterior impingement (see later discussion) or with multidirectional instability and joint laxity.[7,9,20,23,24] Rotator cuff tendinitis, also reported in racquetball players, causes dull aching in the shoulder, especially with the arm raised overhead.[19]

Regarding the rotator cuff, discrete tears have been thought to be limited to adults, with less than 1% of these injuries occurring in pediatric

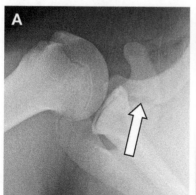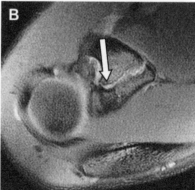

Fig. 1. Coracoid process fracture. (A) Axillary radiograph of the shoulder in a 15-year-old male wrestler demonstrates distraction across the physis at the base of the coracoid process (arrow). (B) Axial fat-suppressed proton density MR image shows high signal intensity across the Salter-Harris I fracture (arrow). There is mild edema in the surrounding soft tissues.

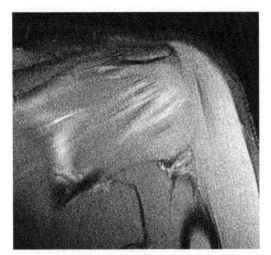

Fig. 2. Muscle strain. Coronal fat-suppressed T2 MR image of the shoulder in a 14-year-old girl who recently had a skiing accident. Feathery high signal intensity interspersed within the infraspinatus muscle fibers indicates muscle belly strain.

patients.[25] Although rotator cuff tears are uncommon in pediatric patients and their true incidence remains unclear, it is now known that they do occur.[20,24] In a review of 103 pediatric shoulder MR images and MR arthrograms at the author's institution, 38 patients underwent arthroscopy, revealing 8 partial thickness and 4 full thickness tears (Davis KW, Kijowski R, Tuite MJ, unpublished data, 2007). In this study, the signs of rotator cuff tear were the same as those in adults; partial thickness tears demonstrated disruptions of a portion of the cuff fibers on either the articular or the bursal surface without a complete gap and full thickness tears demonstrated a communication of the joint space with the subacromial/subdeltoid bursa through the gap (Figs. 3 and 4). Cases of confirmed rotator cuff tears were too few to allow reliable accuracy statistics to be determined for MR imaging/MR arthrography.

One cause of partial thickness rotator cuff tears is thought to be internal impingement, or glenohumeral internal rotational deficit (GIRD). This malady is relatively common in young adult athletes but is being recognized in adolescents also. GIRD occurs in pitchers, quarterbacks, swimmers, and volleyball players related to their long-term overhead athletic activity. Although the theory is evolving, GIRD is thought to be caused by tightness and scarring of the posterior capsule of the glenohumeral joint, which are related to overuse. This tightness leads to abnormal rotation of the humeral head relative to the glenoid when throwing, reducing the internal rotation and forcing the humeral head posteriorly and superiorly. The classic injuries incurred are

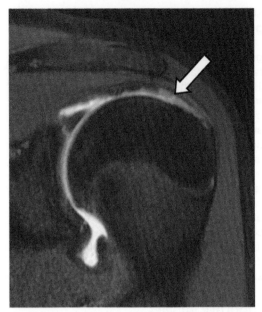

Fig. 3. Partial thickness rotator cuff tear. Coronal fat-suppressed T1 MR arthrogram of a 16-year-old boy who fell snowboarding demonstrates extensive irregularity and defects along the articular surface of the supraspinatus tendon (arrow).

partial thickness articular surface tears of the anterior infraspinatus or posterior supraspinatus, tears of the posterosuperior glenoid labrum, and bare area humeral head cysts.[26]

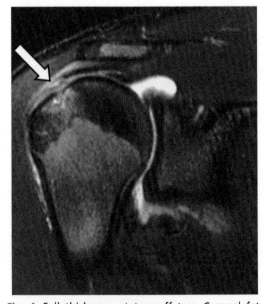

Fig. 4. Full thickness rotator cuff tear. Coronal fat-suppressed T2 MR image in a 16-year-old male hockey player demonstrates fluid signal traversing the thickness of the supraspinatus tendon (arrow), with retraction of a portion of the tendon more medially.

Instability of the glenohumeral joint may take one of the following several forms. Traumatic instability results from anterior shoulder dislocations. Shoulder dislocations are relatively common in adolescents, with 40% of all cases occurring in those younger than 22 years, but the condition is rare in young children, with less than 2% of cases occurring in children younger than 10 years.[25] It is estimated that 65% to 90% of teenagers who experience a shoulder dislocation will have repeat dislocations[27,28] and may present for imaging before surgical correction. MR arthrography is the preferred imaging modality and often demonstrates Bankart tears of the anteroinferior glenoid labrum and Hill-Sachs impaction fractures of the posterosuperior humeral head (**Fig. 5**).[20,25]

Atraumatic instability of the glenohumeral joint, or multidirectional instability (MDI), is explained as a congenital or developmental phenomenon caused by laxity of the glenohumeral capsular ligaments and the capsule in general. MDI becomes symptomatic when sports-related stresses on the joint lead to sensations of instability and/or pain, especially in swimmers and gymnasts.[19,20,28] Findings of MR arthrography are typically limited to a capacious joint capsule (**Fig. 6**). This finding is helpful to arthroscopists, but imaging is often performed to exclude labral tear as the source of pain because labral tears are increasingly common in teenaged athletes.[23,26]

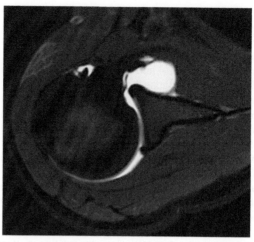

Fig. 6. Multidirectional instability. Axial fat-suppressed proton density MR arthrogram in a 12-year-old female tennis player with clinical shoulder instability demonstrates a patulous capacious capsule.

One chronic shoulder injury to recall is chronic deltoid tendon avulsion that can be related to sports. Donnelly and colleagues[29] reported that in 3 boys with chronic deltoid avulsions, MR imaging demonstrated cortical thickening, irregularity of the deltoid tubercle, and adjacent high T2 signal intensity indicating edema. On MR imaging, the findings may be initially mistaken for a malignant neoplasm but should not demonstrate a true soft tissue mass or cortical destruction. This injury is rare but should be recalled so as to not mistake it for malignancy.

In 1966, Adams[30] reported 5 cases of Little League shoulder, all in adolescent male baseball pitchers. Adams referred to this malady as osteochondrosis, but it is now thought of as a stress injury to the proximal humeral physis. This overuse injury is probably best considered a chronic stress form of a nondisplaced Salter-Harris I fracture and occurs in throwers aged 11 to 16 years, especially baseball pitchers.[7,19] This fracture is thought to result from rotational forces placed on the proximal humeral physis by repetitive pitching (specifically too many pitches per week over many weeks), especially curveballs, and other high-volume throwing activities. Patients describe pain particularly in the follow-through stage of the pitching motion.[4] Recent weight gain and out-of-season throwing also place the pitcher at risk.[7,8,25] This fracture is a classic example of how cross-training (switching sports in different seasons) is advantageous to the pediatric athlete, because switching to a sport that does not stress the arm would allow the physis to recover and probably not sustain this chronic injury.

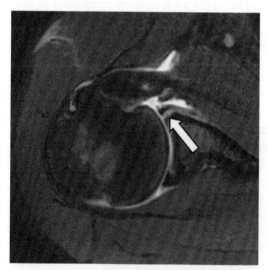

Fig. 5. Labral tear. Axial fat-suppressed proton density MR arthrogram of the shoulder in a 15-year-old boy who had multiple dislocations depicts contrast (*arrow*) extending into a tear of the anteroinferior labrum. This tear is a Bankart labral tear, which is common after shoulder dislocations. The distal subscapularis tendon is quite thickened, presumably from the scars of the multiple dislocations.

Radiographs of patients with Little League shoulder may be normal. When positive for the injury, radiographs demonstrate the physis to be widened, with demineralization, fragmentation, cystic change, and sometimes sclerosis (Fig. 7).[7,25,30] Because the changes may be subtle, the radiographs should be compared with those of the patient's asymptomatic nonthrowing shoulder.[8] MR imaging is not typically performed for this injury, but when performed, it shows widening of the physis, in addition to the increased T2 signal intensity within the physis and occasionally edema in the subchondral bone adjacent to the physis. If the patient is treated appropriately with rest to the throwing arm, Little League shoulder is self-limited and resolves rapidly[30]; appropriate treatment is important, because the proximal humeral physis is responsible for much of the length of the growing humerus.[19]

ELBOW INJURIES

The discussion of elbow injuries in pediatric athletes, especially those who are skeletally immature, centers on a set of maladies grouped under the rubric Little League elbow. About 20% of pitchers aged 10 to 14 years have experienced elbow pain.[31] Little League elbow is an overuse phenomenon resulting from chronic repetitive valgus stresses placed on the elbow by the throwing motion, typically seen in pitchers and quarterbacks who throw more than 200 times per week.[32] This valgus stress occurs during the cocking and acceleration phase of the throwing motion and places tension on the medial side of the elbow and compression on its lateral side.[19,20] These forces, when repeated often

enough, may result in several specific pathologic entities, including traction apophysitis of the medial epicondyle, OCD of the capitulum, loose intra-articular fragments, traction apophysitis of the olecranon, premature closure of the radial physis, and/or overgrowth of the radial head.[7,10] The last 2 injuries have presented rarely in the author's practice and are not described further.

Traction apophysitis describes a condition of irritation and breakdown of the apophyseal physis.[4] As opposed to epiphyses, which occur at the end of the tubular bones and contribute to overall bone length, apophyses do not contribute to overall length and primarily serve as the attachment sites of some tendons to bones. Apophyseal physes represent a weak link in the growing athlete because they are weaker than the bone and the MTU. Certainly, apophyses that are subjected to abrupt extreme forces may displace from the underlying bone, termed an avulsion fracture; however, if the tendon repeatedly subjects the apophysis to chronic submaximal forces, the physis may develop chronic traction apophysitis. Apophyses are especially prone to this condition during periods of rapid growth.[4] Traction apophysitis is thought to result from a series of microavulsions at the bone-cartilage interface[4] and is probably best thought of as a chronic stress reaction or stress fracture of the growth plate, similar to Little League shoulder.

Traction apophysitis of the medial epicondyle is said to be the most frequent component of Little League elbow,[4] although it is encountered less commonly than OCD at the author's institution. The medial epicondyle is the origin of the flexor-pronator tendon group, which places tension on the medial epicondyle when strong valgus forces

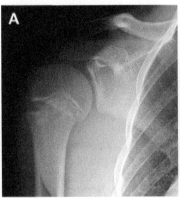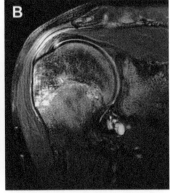

Fig. 7. Little League shoulder. (A) Grashey radiograph of the shoulder in a 13-year-old boy with chronic pain while pitching demonstrates considerable sclerosis, lucency, and irregularity along the proximal humeral physis in this chronic Salter-Harris type I stress injury. (B) Coronal fat-suppressed T2 MR image taken 2 months later demonstrates persistent abnormal high signal intensity along the lateral aspect of the healing physis.

are in effect. This condition afflicts not only pread-olescent and adolescent pitchers who engage in heavy throwing regimens but also tennis players and javelin throwers.[19,33] Radiographs demon-strate variable irregularity of ossification, fragmen-tation, and sclerosis of the apophysis as well as widening and indistinctness of the physis (Fig. 8).[4,18,34] MR imaging demonstrates widening of the physis and increased T2 signal intensity within and possibly adjacent to the physis. The apophysis may be segmented and partially resorbed.[35]

OCD of the capitulum is also a frequent compo-nent of Little League elbow, causing insidious lateral pain and sometimes locking and catching.[36] OCD is a condition in which a layer of subchondral bone and sometimes the overlying articular cartilage become damaged and separate from the underlying bone, whether the fragment displaces or not. Some degree of necrosis of the fragment occurs, but the injury may heal. If the injury worsens, the fragment may eventually break down and displace.[20] OCD of the capitulum is thought to be caused by overuse/repetitive trauma, probably shear and compressive forces that accompany the valgus load. These forces are experienced by overthrowing pitchers and similar athletes, including gymnasts, typically aged 12 to 16 years.[20,31]

Radiography of the elbow is the first step in imaging. Radiography demonstrates a well-

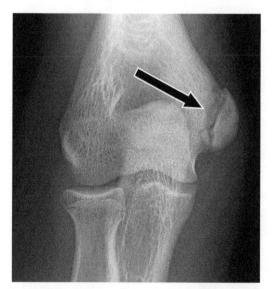

Fig. 8. Little League elbow. Anteroposterior radio-graph of the elbow of a 14-year-old male pitcher with constant medial elbow pain demonstrates widening, lucency, and irregularity along the physis of the medial epicondyle (*arrow*), indicating traction apophysitis.

defined lucent lesion with sclerotic borders,[31] flattening of the articular surface, or fragmenta-tion of the subchondral bone (Fig. 9A); however, some cases may be radiographically occult.[37] Displaced fragments are most commonly located in the olecranon fossa.[37] MR imaging positively identifies these lesions and accurately depicts their size and whether or not there is a displaced fragment.[38] MR imaging demon-strates that the lesion occurs in the anterolateral aspect of the capitulum[25] and is often relied on to help guide surgical intervention. Surgery may be performed in the setting of unstable lesions, which rarely heal, but is largely directed by clin-ical findings of persistent symptoms.[36] On MR imaging, OCD is well demarcated with a linear interface surrounding a crescentic focus of high T2 signal intensity along the articular surface of the subchondral bone anterolaterally. Occasional early cases may show only the focus of the edema and may not have developed the well-defined sclerotic margin yet. MR imaging signs of instability include a rim of high T2 signal intensity surrounding the lesion or cysts under-lying the interface of the lesion with the adjacent normal bone (see Fig. 9B).[25,39] Stable lesions have low T2 signal intensity surrounding the OCD.[39] One must not mistake the pseudodefect of the capitulum, a common normal variant demonstrating a small focus of cartilage absence in the posterolateral capitulum, with OCD, which occurs anteriorly and laterally.[40] OCD of the capitulum more often leads to an inexorable worsening of clinical findings than OCD in the knee, and chronic irregularity of the articular surface and displaced intra-articular fragments are frequent in the elbow.[38] Although surgery often improves the condition, both nonsurgically and surgically treated patients may have chronic pain, premature degenerative arthritis, and loss of terminal extension.[40]

OCD in the elbow may also affect the trochlea. Marshall and colleagues[41] reported a series of os-teochondral lesions of the trochlea, including 3 cases of medial trochlear OCDs, 10 cases of lateral trochlear OCDs, and 5 cases of osteonecro-sis. The lateral trochlear OCD cases occur in a relative vascular watershed, especially in football players, pitchers, and gymnasts. This condition is much less common than OCD of the capitulum and is sparsely reported in the literature. Both cases of lateral trochlear OCD that presented at the author's institution recently occurred in long-time skateboarders (Fig. 10). As with OCD of the capitulum, surgical treatment of trochlear OCD may consist of debridement, microfracture and

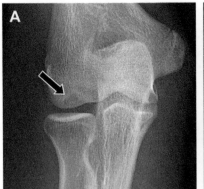
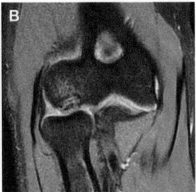

Fig. 9. OCD of the capitulum. (*A*) Anteroposterior radiograph of the elbow in a 16-year-old male pitcher with lateral elbow pain demonstrates a focal lucency in the subchondral bone (*arrow*) surrounded by a rim of sclerosis. (*B*) Coronal fat-suppressed proton density MR image demonstrates a high signal line along the margin of the lesion, indicating instability.

drilling, stabilization with various devices, or even mosaicplasty.[42]

OCD of the capitulum is often confused with Panner disease. Both lesions are best understood as osteochondral lesions of the capitulum. However, Panner disease, classified as an osteochondrosis of the capitulum,[43] usually occurs in children younger than 10 years and involves the entire ossification center,[5,36,38] whereas OCD develops after the age of 10 years and involves only a portion of the capitulum. Panner disease may result in dramatic findings on radiographs, resembling those of Legg-Calvé-Perthes disease of the proximal femoral epiphysis, with fissuring,

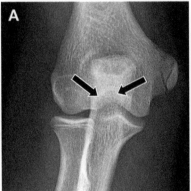
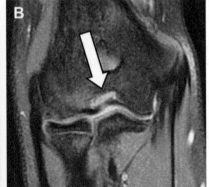
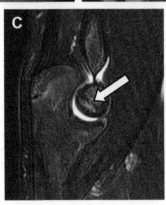

Fig. 10. OCD of the trochlea. (*A*) Anteroposterior view of the elbow in a 16-year-old male skateboarder shows a subtle focal subchondral lucency (*arrows*) along the lateral aspect of the trochlea. (*B*) Coronal fat-suppressed proton density MR image demonstrates high signal intensity in the lesion (*arrow*) surrounded by a thin rim of sclerosis. (*C*) Sagittal T2 MR image also demonstrates the well-defined lesion (*arrow*).

irregularity, fragmentation, and flattening of the epiphysis.[36] However, Panner disease responds well when the affected extremity is rested. Clinical series report good long-term results in the vast majority of patients treated without surgery.[36,38] Some investigators think that Panner disease and OCD exist on a continuum of disordered endochondral ossification, but it remains uncertain if these are distinct entities or not.[36] Nevertheless, their radiographic findings differ, and the prognosis for Panner disease is much better than that for OCD.

Traction apophysitis in the elbow is not limited to the medial epicondyle ossification center. This overuse injury can also affect the olecranon apophysis (Fig. 11). Occasionally mentioned as a component of Little League elbow, traction apophysitis of the olecranon more commonly afflicts high-level gymnasts.[44] Divers, football players, and hockey players have also been diagnosed with olecranon apophysitis.[5,32] Radiographic findings mimic those at the medial epicondyle, with variable degrees of physeal widening and apophyseal indistinctness and fragmentation.[44] Caution must be applied in interpreting the lateral radiograph in children because in young children the normal physis may measure up to 5 mm; by the age of 12 years, though, the physis should be narrow, with serpiginous but congruent apposing borders.[17] Stress fractures are known to occur in the olecranon after physeal closure[44] but may even occur within the olecranon ossification center

before skeletal maturity in baseball pitchers, wrestlers, and gymnasts. When this fracture occurs, radiographs reveal fragmentation and sclerosis of the apophysis and widening of the physis[5,17,31]; undoubtedly, there must be a clinical and radiographic overlap between stress fractures of the apophysis and stress injuries of the physis itself.

The olecranon and medial epicondyle apophyses may suffer avulsions instead of apophysitis. In these instances, the apophysis is displaced, representing an acute Salter-Harris I fracture of the apophyseal physis. These avulsions are acute phenomena, rather than the chronic overuse injuries that traction apophysitis represents, and occur in adolescents as the physis is beginning to fuse. Avulsions more commonly result from violent traumatic events such as a dislocation, whether in the setting of a sports contest or not, rather than as a consequence of normal throwing motion or other normal athletic maneuvers.[25,31,32]

In the older adolescent athlete, the physes are no longer the weak link in the setting of acute trauma or repetitive stresses because they are fused. Fractures may occur, but tendons and ligaments are now the weak link because force is applied to the musculoskeletal system. Tendon ruptures are rare in pediatric patients[45] presumably because they occur in the setting of long-standing chronic tendinopathy,[46] which does not have time to develop before adulthood. However, at least some degree of flexor and extensor tendinopathy, formerly known as medial and lateral epicondylitis respectively, and triceps tendinopathy can develop at the elbow in high-level pediatric

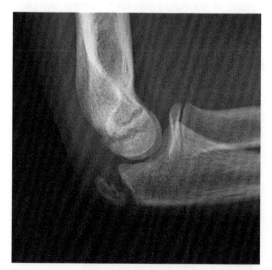

Fig. 11. Repetitive physeal injury of the olecranon. Lateral radiograph in a 13-year-old male pitcher with unremitting elbow pain demonstrates widening of the physis of the olecranon and irregularity and fragmentation of the apophysis. This patient also had traction apophysitis of the medial epicondyle (Little League elbow, not shown).

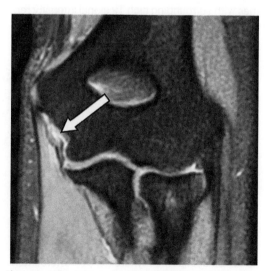

Fig. 12. UCL injury. Coronal fat-suppressed proton density MR image in a 15-year-old girl depicts waviness and partial disruption of the origin of the UCL (*arrow*).

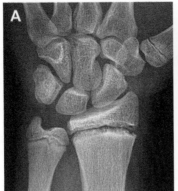
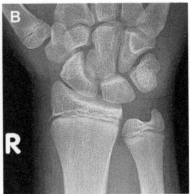

Fig. 13. Gymnast wrist. (*A*) Posteroanterior (PA) radiograph of the left wrist in a 14-year-old male weight lifter with 4 months wrist pain reveals widening, sclerosis, and irregularity of the distal radial physis. (*B*) PA radiograph of the asymptomatic right wrist for comparison.

athletes after physeal fusion.[45] Flexor tendinopathy is more frequent in baseball pitchers and extensor tendinopathy in tennis players, as in adults.[8,18] Tendinopathy about the elbow reflects an incomplete healing response to repetitive trauma/overuse. The underlying pathologic conditions are angiofibroblastic hyperplasia and fibrillary degeneration of collagen, especially involving the flexor carpi radialis and pronator teres medially and the extensor carpi radialis brevis (ECRB) laterally.[8,47] Children may exhibit more microscopic fissuring and tearing than the classic pathologic condition seen in adults, but there are no pathologic studies to support this contention. In any event, radiographic findings are expected to be normal but MR imaging shows thickening and increased signal of the involved tendons, sometimes with surrounding high T2 signal intensity representing peritendinous edema.[47]

Tendon tears about the elbow are rare in the pediatric population, although partial tears of the ECRB have been reported in golfers and tennis players.[45] On the other hand, ligament tears occur more frequently. The anterior band of the ulnar collateral ligament (UCL) is the primary restraint against valgus forces along with the flexor-pronator tendon bundle. With chronic overuse injury in pitchers and similar skeletally mature adolescent athletes, the UCL may undergo stretching, resulting in laxity and pain.[34] Other skeletally mature athletes may have partial or complete tear of the UCL, usually at its origin on the distal surface of the medial epicondyle.[35] MR imaging is especially helpful to define complete UCL ruptures, demonstrating complete disruption of the ligament, fraying and indistinctness of the ligament fibers, and extravasation of the joint fluid.[35] MR imaging of partial thickness UCL tears

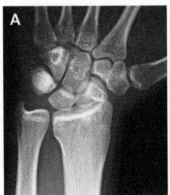
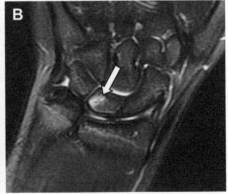

Fig. 14. Ulnar impaction syndrome. (*A*) Posteroanterior radiograph of the wrist in a 13-year-old gymnast with 10 years experience and with wrist pain demonstrates early closure of the distal radial physis and relative shortening of the radius. (*B*) Fat-suppressed coronal MR image shows a normal triangular fibrocartilage but focal edema within the ulnar aspect of the lunate (*arrow*), which is an evidence of early ulnar impaction syndrome related to the patient's positive ulnar variance.

depicts irregularity and poor definition of the ligament fibers at the origin, with intervening high T2 signal intensity (**Fig. 12**), but is less accurate than it is for complete ruptures. MR arthrography is especially helpful in improving the accuracy of detection of partial thickness UCL tears, which typically occur on the internal side (undersurface) of the ligament.[40] Although tears of the elbow lateral collateral ligament (LCL) are relatively common in adults who experience chronic varus stresses, pediatric patients with LCL tears usually have had a dislocation.[40]

WRIST INJURIES

As mentioned earlier, wrist injuries are common in pediatric gymnasts, especially girls. These injuries often have chronic sequelae into adulthood, whether or not the athlete continues the sport in college and beyond. Gymnast wrist generally refers to pain in the wrists of gymnasts, thought to be caused by chronic compressive impact forces, and can reflect several different specific injuries, including overuse injuries of the distal radial physis, tears of the triangular fibrocartilage or rarely the scapholunate or lunatotriquetral ligaments, cartilage damage along the articular surfaces of the distal radius and carpal bones, and dorsal ganglion cysts of the wrist.[48] Most commonly, gymnast wrist refers to injury to the growth plate of the distal physis.[18] This injury is thought to be similar to Little League shoulder and Little League elbow and has a similar radiographic appearance. The physis of the distal radius suffers marked compressive loading during gymnastics routines, especially with the wrist dorsiflexed, applying compression and shearing forces across the physis. As with the injuries of the proximal humeral and medial epicondyle physes, this injury is understood as a chronic stress injury of the physis, basically a nondisplaced Salter-Harris I stress fracture.[49] This injury also occurs in weight lifters and roller skaters.[49] Radiographic changes may include asymmetric widening, haziness, and irregularity of the physis, with variable sclerosis and cystic changes on the metaphyseal side (**Fig. 13**).[49,50] In some patients with the classic clinical findings of gymnast wrist (namely, wrist pain in the setting of gymnastics), radiographs appear normal. In one study, patients with normal radiographic results were able to return to gymnastics and were pain-free after resting for only a few weeks, whereas those with radiographic findings required an average of 3 months of inactivity to heal.[50]

Patients who have substantial injury to the distal radial physis may undergo premature closure of the physis and exhibit a relatively short radius (**Fig. 14**). In essence, these patients have positive ulnar variance and may sustain the various components of ulnar impaction syndrome in their late teenage years and adulthood. This syndrome includes fraying or tearing of the triangular fibrocartilage; damage of the articular cartilage of the lunate, distal radius, and/or triquetrum; and ultimately, tears of the lunatotriquetral ligament and degenerative arthrosis of the involved bones in the end stages.[16] However, full-blown ulnar impaction syndrome with all the components is rare in adolescents. The main component of this syndrome seen in adolescents, other than the positive ulnar variance, is injury to the triangular fibrocartilage,[16] which has also been reported in adolescent basketball players with positive ulnar variance.[51]

Scaphoid fractures are not uncommon in adolescent athletes who fall on an outstretched

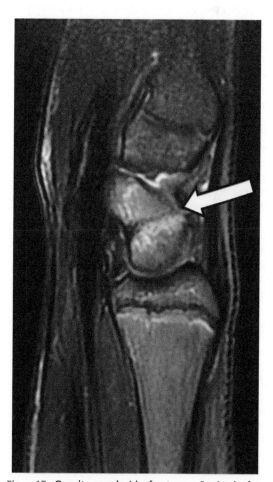

Fig. 15. Occult scaphoid fracture. Sagittal fat-suppressed T2 MR image of the wrist reveals a low signal line across the waist of the scaphoid (*arrow*) surrounded by marrow edema. Radiographs (not shown) were unremarkable.

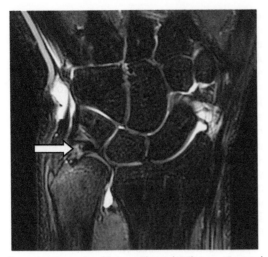

Fig. 16. Triangular fibrocartilage (TFC) tear. Coronal fat-suppressed T2 MR image of the wrist in a 17-year-old male football player who had a hyperextension injury demonstrates irregularity of the peripheral aspect of the TFC. There is fluid signal within the disrupted portions (*arrow*), but the distal ulnar attachment is intact, indicating a partial tear of the TFC.

hand. These fractures are usually nondisplaced and may be occult on radiographs. MR imaging is the best method to detect radiographically occult scaphoid fractures (**Fig. 15**), with a normal MR image having a 100% negative predictive value for scaphoid fracture.[13] MR imaging in this setting also allows examination of the capsular ligaments, which when injured, can masquerade as scaphoid fractures clinically. Bone contusions, in which there is edema in one or more carpal bones and no fracture line on MR imaging, are also common when clinical findings suggest scaphoid fracture.[13] Both MR imaging and ultrasonography are successful in depicting dorsal ganglion cysts of the wrist, which commonly occur in gymnasts and occasionally are symptomatic.

Outside the setting of positive ulnar variance, tears of the scapholunate ligament and triangular fibrocartilage (**Fig. 16**) are rare in pediatric athletes but have been reported.[34] A more common clinical diagnosis is tendinitis of the wrist tendons, especially the extensor tendons, in the setting of overuse.[9] These cases are rarely imaged but would presumably demonstrate the findings of tenosynovitis, including increased T2 signal intensity within the tendon sheath and tendon on MR imaging and increased fluid within the sheath on MR imaging or ultrasonography.[45]

SUMMARY

The continued increase in numbers of children and adolescents participating in organized sports and

the progressive trend toward increased training times and busy competition schedules dictate that more and more overuse injuries of the upper extremity will be encountered. However, acute injuries are not diminishing, and competent radiologists must be familiar with the findings related to both types of injuries. Certain athletic activities result in particular combinations of injuries, such as Little League elbow and gymnast wrist. Familiarity with these injury patterns helps the radiologist to understand the best imaging methods to use and predict the imaging features that these injuries will produce.

REFERENCES

1. Best TM, van Mechelen W, Verhagen E. The pediatric athlete—are we doing the right thing? Clin J Sport Med 2006;16:455–6.
2. Hambidge SJ, Davidson AJ, Gonzales R, et al. Epidemiology of pediatric injury-related primary care office visits in the United States. Pediatrics 2002;109:559–65.
3. Caine D, Caine C, Maffulli N. Incidence and distribution of pediatric sport-related injuries. Clin J Sport Med 2006;16:500–13.
4. Saperstein AL, Nicholas SJ. Pediatric and adolescent sports medicine. Pediatr Clin North Am 1996; 43:1013–33.
5. Maffulli N, Baxter-Jones AD. Common skeletal injuries in young athletes. Sports Med 1995;19: 137–49.
6. Marsh JS, Daigneault JP. The young athlete. Curr Opin Pediatr 1999;11:84–8.
7. Lord J, Winell JJ. Overuse injuries in pediatric athletes. Curr Opin Pediatr 2004;16:47–50.
8. Latz K. Overuse injuries in the pediatric and adolescent athlete. Mo Med 2006;103:81–5.
9. Micheli LJ, Fehlandt AF Jr. Overuse injuries to tendons and apophyses in children and adolescents. Clin Sports Med 1992;11:713–26.
10. Micheli LJ. Overuse injuries in children's sports: the growth factor. Orthop Clin North Am 1983;14: 337–60.
11. Caine D, Maffulli N, Caine C. Epidemiology of injury in child and adolescent sports: injury rates, risk factors, and prevention. Clin Sports Med 2008;27: 19–50, vii.
12. Bright RW, Burstein AH, Elmore SM. Epiphyseal-plate cartilage. A biomechanical and histological analysis of failure modes. J Bone Joint Surg Am 1974;56:688–703.
13. Cook PC, Leit ME. Issues in the pediatric athlete. Orthop Clin North Am 1995;26:453–64.
14. Garrick JG. Sports medicine. Pediatr Clin North Am 1986;33:1541–50.

15. Caine DJ, Nassar L. Gymnastics injuries. Med Sport Sci 2005;48:18–58.

16. Zetaruk MN. The young gymnast. Clin Sports Med 2000;19:757–80.

17. Chan D, Aldridge MJ, Maffulli N, et al. Chronic stress injuries of the elbow in young gymnasts. Br J Radiol 1991;64:1113–8.

18. Auringer ST, Anthony EY. Common pediatric sports injuries. Semin Musculoskelet Radiol 1999;3: 247–56.

19. Gomez JE. Upper extremity injuries in youth sports. Pediatr Clin North Am 2002;49:593–626, vi–vii.

20. Ryu RK, Fan RS. Adolescent and pediatric sports injuries. Pediatr Clin North Am 1998;45:1601–35, x.

21. DiPaola M, Marchetto P. Coracoid process fracture with acromioclavicular joint separation in an American football player: a case report and literature review. Am J Orthop (Belle Mead NJ) 2009;38: 37–9 [discussion: 40].

22. Caviglia H, Garrido CP, Palazzi FF, et al. Pediatric fractures of the humerus. Clin Orthop Relat Res 2005;432:49–56.

23. Kibler WB, Safran M. Tennis injuries. Med Sport Sci 2005;48:120–37.

24. Ireland ML, Andrews JR. Shoulder and elbow injuries in the young athlete. Clin Sports Med 1988; 7:473–94.

25. Emery KH. MR imaging in congenital and acquired disorders of the pediatric upper extremity. Magn Reson Imaging Clin N Am 2009;17:549–70, vii.

26. Sciascia A, Kibler WB. The pediatric overhead athlete: what is the real problem? Clin J Sport Med 2006;16:471–7.

27. Kelly AM, Pappas AM. Shoulder and elbow injuries and painful syndromes. Adolesc Med 1998;9: 569–87, vii.

28. Soprano JV. Musculoskeletal injuries in the pediatric and adolescent athlete. Curr Sports Med Rep 2005; 4:329–34.

29. Donnelly LF, Helms CA, Bisset GS 3rd. Chronic avulsive injury of the deltoid insertion in adolescents: imaging findings in three cases. Radiology 1999;211:233–6.

30. Adams JE. Little league shoulder: osteochondrosis of the proximal humeral epiphysis in boy baseball pitchers. Calif Med 1966;105:22–5.

31. DaSilva MF, Williams JS, Fadale PD, et al. Pediatric throwing injuries about the elbow. Am J Orthop (Belle Mead NJ) 1998;27:90–6.

32. Do T, Herrera-Soto J. Elbow injuries in children. Curr Opin Pediatr 2003;15:68–73.

33. Stanitski CL. Pediatric and adolescent sports injuries. Clin Sports Med 1997;16:613–33.

34. Bernhardt DT, Landry GL. Sports injuries in young athletes. Adv Pediatr 1995;42:465–500.

35. Sugimoto H, Ohsawa T. Ulnar collateral ligament in the growing elbow: MR imaging of normal development and throwing injuries. Radiology 1994;192:417–22.

36. Kobayashi K, Burton KJ, Rodner C, et al. Lateral compression injuries in the pediatric elbow: Panner's disease and osteochondritis dissecans of the capitellum. J Am Acad Orthop Surg 2004;12:246–54.

37. Kijowski R, De Smet AA. Radiography of the elbow for evaluation of patients with osteochondritis dissecans of the capitellum. Skeletal Radiol 2005;34: 266–71.

38. Bowen RE, Otsuka NY, Yoon ST, et al. Osteochondral lesions of the capitellum in pediatric patients: role of magnetic resonance imaging. J Pediatr Orthop 2001;21:298–301.

39. Kijowski R, De Smet AA. MRI findings of osteochondritis dissecans of the capitellum with surgical correlation. AJR Am J Roentgenol 2005;185:1453–9.

40. Tuite MJ, Kijowski R. Sports-related injuries of the elbow: an approach to MRI interpretation. Clin Sports Med 2006;25:387–408, v.

41. Marshall KW, Marshall DL, Busch MT, et al. Osteochondral lesions of the humeral trochlea in the young athlete. Skeletal Radiol 2009;38:479–91.

42. Ansah P, Vogt S, Ueblacker P, et al. Osteochondral transplantation to treat osteochondral lesions in the elbow. J Bone Joint Surg Am 2007;89:2188–94.

43. Ruch DS, Poehling GG. Arthroscopic treatment of Panner's disease. Clin Sports Med 1991;10:629–36.

44. Maffulli N, Chan D, Aldridge MJ. Overuse injuries of the olecranon in young gymnasts. J Bone Joint Surg Br 1992;74:305–8.

45. Azouz EM, Oudjhane K. Disorders of the upper extremity in children. Magn Reson Imaging Clin N Am 1998;6:677–95.

46. Kannus P, Jozsa L. Histopathological changes preceding spontaneous rupture of a tendon. A controlled study of 891 patients. J Bone Joint Surg Am 1991;73:1507–25.

47. Kijowski R, De Smet AA. Magnetic resonance imaging findings in patients with medial epicondylitis. Skeletal Radiol 2005;34:196–202.

48. Mandelbaum BR, Bartolozzi AR, Davis CA, et al. Wrist pain syndrome in the gymnast. Pathogenetic, diagnostic, and therapeutic considerations. Am J Sports Med 1989;17:305–17.

49. Carter SR, Aldridge MJ, Fitzgerald R, et al. Stress changes of the wrist in adolescent gymnasts. Br J Radiol 1988;61:109–12.

50. Roy S, Caine D, Singer KM. Stress changes of the distal radial epiphysis in young gymnasts. A report of twenty-one cases and a review of the literature. Am J Sports Med 1985;13:301–8.

51. Gaca AM. Basketball injuries in children. Pediatr Radiol 2009;39:1275–85.

Imaging Pediatric Sports Injuries: Lower Extremity

Kirkland W. Davis, MD

KEYWORDS

• Pediatric • Sports medicine • Magnetic resonance imaging
• Hip • Knee • Ankle

The number of children and adolescents involved in organized sports and athletic activities continues to increase. There are certainly many positive health and psychological benefits to increasing sports participation in this age group, which should carry on into adulthood as these athletes age. However, one negative factor is the continued increase in the number of athletic injuries suffered by pediatric patients. Of the more than 30 million children and adolescents engaging in organized sports in the United States each year, approximately one-third of school-age children involved in sports sustain an injury requiring medical attention.[1,2] Lower extremity sports injuries, the subject of this article, outnumber upper extremity injuries in pediatric patients.[2] The lower extremity is especially prone to overuse injuries, as opposed to acute traumatic injuries. With the shift of athletic activities and play away from free play and toward organized sports, pediatric overuse injuries have become much more common in the last quarter century.

The developing musculoskeletal system has unique anatomy and physiology. As such, the injuries that skeletally immature patients sustain are often different to those suffered by adult athletes. This article examines the imaging features of injuries sustained by the lower extremities of pediatric athletes. Pediatric sports injuries are most unique in patients with open physes, so this article focuses more on those injuries that are peculiar to the pediatric musculoskeletal system, but includes "adult" injuries where they are relevant to pediatric patients. This article does not address acute traumatic injuries that

are not specific to sports, such as fractures and dislocations, except where particularly relevant. The first major topic is overuse injuries, with general comments and a section on traction apophysitis and stress fractures followed by a discussion of overuse injuries that affect each of the major joints (pelvis/hip, knee, and ankle/foot); the second major topic is acute injuries and other common injuries that do not neatly fit the description of overuse injuries, again addressed by major joints. For the purposes of this discussion, sports and athletics are assumed to include not only standard team and individual organized sports and competitions, but also athletic training and dance.

OVERUSE INJURIES

Nearly half of all pediatric athletic injuries are overuse injuries.[3] Overuse injuries occur when there is repetitive microtrauma to a tissue that outstrips the ability for the body to repair.[2] This process is easy to understand if one considers bones: when activity and stresses on bone are increased, this increases the turnover rate of bone as it adapts to the increased forces. As a normal part of bone physiology, this requires some resorption of bone. If the forces applied are too great, too frequent, and/or too long-standing, assuming they are not great enough to cause a frank fracture, they will result in a stress response or stress fracture in the bone.[4] Other overuse injuries often occur by a similar process of increased activity overwhelming the body's ability to withstand the forces and repair the tissue over the long term.

Department of Radiology, University of Wisconsin Hospital and Clinics, University of Wisconsin School of Medicine and Public Health, 600 Highland Avenue, Madison, WI, 53792-3252, USA
E-mail address: kdavis@uwhealth.org

Radiol Clin N Am 48 (2010) 1213–1235
doi:10.1016/j.rcl.2010.07.004

The pediatric musculoskeletal system is particularly susceptible to overuse injuries for several reasons. Probably most important are that the bones of children and adolescents are relatively weak compared with their young adult counterparts, especially during growth spurts; and there are open growth plates at the end of the long and short tubular bones as well as at apophyses. With the recent trend toward greater youth involvement in organized sports, this susceptibility to overuse has become reality: increasingly demanding training schedules, more active competition schedules, lack of off-season rest time, and limiting young athletes to a single sport year-round without cross training mean that overuse injuries are now common in adolescent and child athletes, when they used to be relatively rare. For instance, a clinical diagnosis of tendinitis used to be considered an affliction of adults. In recent years it has become relatively common for youth athletes to be diagnosed with tendinitis.[2] Tendinitis is a straightforward clinical diagnosis and rarely comes to imaging unless there are atypical features or the patient does not respond to appropriate therapy.

Traction Apophysitis

Although dwarfed by tendinitis (one report of 724 overuse injuries included 585 diagnoses of tendinitis and only 139 of apophysitis),[2] traction apophysitis is relatively common in the setting of overuse. Apophysitis is a diagnosis that is unique to the growing skeleton. Epiphyses occur at the ends of long and short tubular bones and add to the overall length of the bone as their physes continue to produce new bone until skeletal maturity is reached. On the other hand, apophyses are growth centers that serve as attachment sites for some tendons, and are often referred to as secondary growth centers.[5] Apophyses also have physes at their interface with the rest of the bone, and just as the epiphyseal physis can be a weak link in a long bone, often suffering a Salter-Harris fracture, the apophyseal physis is a weak link also. Apophyses may be the subject of a major force and may displace; this is termed an avulsion fracture. However, when the forces placed by a tendon on an apophysis are submaximal but repeated and chronic, an overuse injury known as traction apophysitis may result. This injury is especially common during phases of rapid growth, whereas tendinitis is more likely to result from the same forces in a patient who is in a slow growth stage.[2] Pathologically, traction apophysitis represents an accumulation of microscopic avulsions along the apophyseal physis with secondary inflammatory changes attempting to repair the damage but being overwhelmed by the unremitting chronic stresses.[2,6] Traction apophysitis essentially is a stress fracture of the apophyseal physis, analogous to a nondisplaced Salter-Harris I injury. These injuries cause tenderness and swelling, and result in painful motion/gait.[5] Specific apophyses that commonly undergo traction apophysitis are addressed in the joint-based discussions that follow.

Stress Fractures and Stress Responses

Stress fractures were uncommon in youth athletes before the time when repetitive training for sports became widespread; nowadays they are common.[4,7] The classic description of how a fatigue stress fracture occurs is outlined above. In addition to this concept of increasing forces overwhelming the remodeling process, muscle fatigue in the face of increasing exercise loads may contribute to the formation of stress fractures by altering movement patterns. This process changes the typical distribution of stress and concentrates it at focal sites that are not prepared to withstand the load.[4] As in adults, about half of stress fractures in pediatric patients occur in the tibia, but the fibula (20%) and pars interarticularis of the lumbar spine (15%) comprise the majority of the remaining cases in pediatric athletes, with the femur (3%), metatarsals (2%), and tarsal navicular (2%) accounting for relatively few cases.[4]

Radiographs are the first radiologic study undertaken when stress fracture is suspected. When positive, radiographs demonstrate focal periosteal reaction and occasionally endosteal cortical thickening and/or a lucent fracture line in the cortex. However, only about 10% of radiographs are positive initially, as findings take from 2 to 12 weeks to manifest.[4] Magnetic resonance (MR) imaging has become the imaging method of choice to confirm or exclude stress fractures when radiographs are negative.[8] MR imaging is more precise than bone scintigraphy and allows discrimination of stress fractures from other bone insults, such as osteoid osteoma, osteomyelitis, neoplasm, and ligamentous injury with secondary osseous reaction.[4] Fredericson and colleagues[9] developed an MR imaging grading system for tibial stress fractures that has been clinically validated. Grade 1 injuries exhibit high T2 signal along the periosteum of the tibia, with no signal abnormality present within the bone marrow. Grade 2 injuries add abnormal high T2 marrow signal to the findings, but have no abnormal T1 signal in the marrow. With grade 3 injuries, there is also abnormal low T1 signal within the marrow (**Fig. 1**). Finally, grade 4 injuries

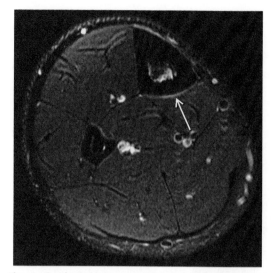

Fig. 1. Grade 3 stress response. Axial fat-suppressed T2 magnetic resonance (MR) image of the leg demonstrates high signal within the marrow and along the periosteum of the tibial shaft (*arrow*). T1 MR image (not shown) demonstrated low signal in a similar pattern in the marrow. Without cortical signal abnormality, this represents a Grade 3 stress response.

include all these findings but add abnormal signal within the cortex, typically a fracture line but sometimes a broader, less linear area of abnormal signal (**Fig. 2**). In common parlance, injuries of grades 1 to 3 are referred to as "stress responses" or "stress reactions" and grade 4 injuries are considered "stress fractures." Increasing grade of stress injury in the tibia reflects increasing severity of injury and often directs the level of restriction of activity recommended to the athlete. Kijowski and colleagues[10] evaluated the radiographs of 86 patients with MR imaging scans demonstrating

tibial stress injuries. The radiographs with periosteal reaction that corresponded to the patient's maximal point of pain correlated with high-grade stress injuries, usually grade 4 (stress fracture). This finding may obviate MR imaging when radiographs of the tibia are positive, as the patient can be treated for stress fracture with confidence as opposed to a low-grade stress response.

Most tibial stress fractures are focal injuries that occur in the proximal third of the bone, typically along the posterior medial side. The injury clinically referred to as "shin splints" is a longer segment injury, purportedly an enthesopathy that encompasses up to half the length of the bone.[11] Shin splints only exhibit periosteal signal abnormality on MR imaging and no abnormal signal within the marrow space.

An important, albeit rare, type of tibial stress fracture occurs in the anterior cortex of the middle third of the bone. This anterior tibial stress fracture occurs in teenagers and young adults involved in sports with frequent leaping, especially basketball.[12,13] On radiographs these injuries are all visible, exhibiting a definite transverse lucent line through the anterior cortex and considerable cortical hypertrophy around the line.[12] The importance of recognizing this type of stress fracture lies in its clinical course. These stress fractures do not heal after a few weeks of simple immobilization; they require longer periods of inactivity and often must undergo surgical excision and bone grafting to heal (**Fig. 3**).[12,14] Before the importance of these injuries was understood, it was common for them to progress to complete fractures on resuming practice following a period of immobilization or rest.[12,14] These stress fractures are considered delayed union stress fractures,[13] and the resistance to healing despite conservative treatment

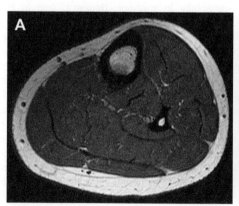
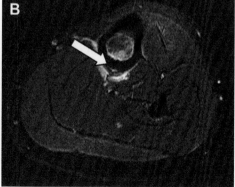

Fig. 2. Stress fracture. T1 (*A*) and fat-suppressed T2 (*B*) axial MR images of the leg demonstrate low T1 and high T2 signal within the marrow of the tibial shaft. There is abnormal signal within the cortex also (*arrow*), indicating this is a grade 4 stress injury, called a "stress fracture."

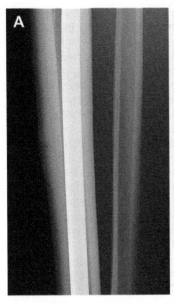
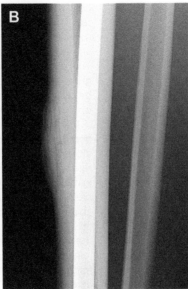

Fig. 3. Stress fracture of the anterior tibial cortex. (*A*) Coned down lateral view of the leg in an 18-year-old football player demonstrates a focal transverse stress fracture line in the anterior cortex with considerable cortical thickening. This lesion still has not healed after intramedullary nailing 6 months ago, and the patient was unable to resume practice. (*B*) Similar coned down lateral radiograph after definitive treatment with excision of the stress fracture bed and bone grafting. The injury healed without incident and the patient returned to practice and competition.

is thought to relate to the fact that the anterior cortex of the tibia is under tension, rather than the posterior proximal or distal cortex, which is where most tibial stress fractures occur and which is under compression.[13,14]

As already mentioned, fibular stress fractures are also relatively common in pediatric athletes. Woods and colleagues[15] studied a series of 20 patients with fibular stress injuries. Fourteen of these occurred in the distal third of the bone, and again all those with corresponding radiographic abnormalities had MR imaging findings that included abnormal signal within the cortex. Cortical signal was linear in only 1 case and globular in 8.[15] Foot and ankle stress fractures usually occur in dancers and distance runners, especially within the metatarsals, and sesamoid stress fractures have been reported in runners, ballet dancers, and soccer and field hockey players.[4] Stress fractures of the tarsal navicular are rare in this age group but are ominous as they are prone to nonunion.[16] Femoral neck stress fractures, relatively common in adults, are rare in most reports on pediatric stress fractures. However, they do occur,[17] and in one report comprised 5 of 53 stress fractures occurring in pediatric athletes.[18] As described earlier, the Fredericson grading system for stress injuries has been clinically validated for the tibia, for which it was developed, but has not been validated for the rest of the skeletal system. One should be judicious in applying this system to other bones: the pathophysiology of other bones is necessarily different because of differences in mechanics and load bearing, and the clinical relevance of specific findings in the tibia may

not directly translate to treatment paradigms for other bones. For this reason, when observing any signs of stress injury to bones other than the tibia, the author calls them "stress fractures" but delineates the specific findings so the sports physician can fashion a treatment regimen to suit the patient. One must be especially cautious about labeling a stress injury of the femoral neck anything but a stress fracture, because a femoral neck stress fracture that is not appropriately treated and progresses on to complete fracture is a catastrophe.

Overuse Injuries of the Hip

One of the chronic hip injuries that lead to pain in pediatric athletes is traction apophysitis, described generally above. Pelvic apophysitis results in dull, activity-related pain near the hip, especially in runners, dancers, and in hockey, lacrosse, and football players.[1] Any of the pelvic apophyses may be involved by traction apophysitis, but it is probably most common at the iliac crest (in runners), anterior superior iliac spine, anterior inferior iliac spine, and ischial tuberosity, at the attachment sites of the abdominal oblique muscles, the sartorius, the rectus femoris, and the hamstring tendons, respectively.[6,19] On radiographs, the physis may have a normal appearance or appear mildly widened, but not displaced.[1] At the ischial tuberosity, the apophysis may not be ossified yet, in which case traction apophysitis will cause the margins of the bone to appear irregular and sclerotic, with lucent defects (**Fig. 4**).[20] MR imaging of traction apophysitis in the pelvis reveals abnormally increased T2 signal in the

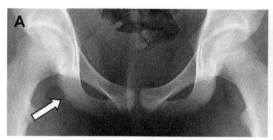
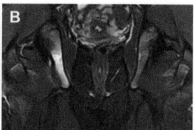

Fig. 4. Ischial apophysitis. (*A*) Coned down anteroposterior (AP) radiograph of the pelvis in a 15-year-old female runner with right hip pain demonstrates cortical irregularity and resorption at the right ischium (*arrow*). (*B*) Coronal short-tau inversion recovery (STIR) MR image depicts extensive high-signal edema in the right ischium, confirming the diagnosis of traction apophysitis.

bone and sometimes the attached tendon. Ultrasound demonstrates soft tissue thickening about the enthesis and thickening and increased echogenicity of the tendon at the attachment site.[11]

Another overuse injury of the pelvis, osteitis pubis, does not occur in children but is seen in late adolescent runners, fencers, and soccer, hockey, and football players.[19,21] The concepts regarding etiology of osteitis pubis and the broader topic of athletic pubalgia continue to evolve, but osteitis pubis is obviously a chronic overuse injury and likely results from stress related to shear forces from unbalanced traction on the pubic symphysis.[21,22] Osteitis pubis results in a gradual onset of pubic pain related to activity. Radiographs reveal sclerosis and rarefaction of the subchondral bone at the pubic symphysis, as well as erosions and cystic changes. However, it can be difficult to discriminate these abnormalities from normal irregularity and fragmentation at the symphysis in the skeletally immature patient.[19,21]

As already mentioned, tendinitis and other overuse injuries of the tendons were once rarely reported in pediatric patients but have become commonplace. Tendinitis is reported about the hip, especially in the iliopsoas and adductor tendons and the iliotibial band.[2] Snapping hip is an overuse phenomenon now seen more commonly in pediatric athletes. The sensation of snapping is divided into 3 types: external snapping hip usually is caused by the iliotibial band rubbing over the greater trochanter with flexion and extension; internal snapping hip results from the iliopsoas tendon snapping over the iliopectineal eminence during internal rotation and extension of the hip; and intra-articular snapping hip, less common in this age group but becoming more frequent, results from intra-articular fragments or tears of the acetabular labrum.[19] Labral tears are being seen more frequently in pediatric patients. Initial fears about hip arthroscopy inducing osteonecrosis of the femoral head in children have not

been borne out, and symptomatic labral tears and loose bodies in pediatric patients are now treated arthroscopically, as they are in adults (see section on acute injuries of the hip).[23]

Overuse Injuries of the Knee

Anterior knee pain is the most common complaint in the adolescent and preadolescent athlete,[5] and many of these complaints stem from the extensor mechanism. Osgood-Schlatter disease (OSD) is one of the common causes of anterior knee pain in this age group. Most common in 12- to 15-year-old boys and 8- to 12-year-old girls, OSD is a traction apophysitis related to strong forces from the quadriceps mechanism. OSD occurs at the insertion of the patellar tendon on the tibial tuberosity.[24] Repeated jumping, squatting, and/or kneeling leads to OSD, which produces local pain, swelling, and tenderness at the tuberosity.[24] Radiographs reveal irregularity of the apophysis, occasional widening of the physis, and separate bone fragments within the distal tendon near its insertion. Thickening of the tendon will also be present (**Fig. 5**).[24,25] Bone fragments within the tendon are present in 50% of cases.[26] At MR imaging, there is abnormal high signal within and surrounding the tendon on T2-weighted images, and deep infrapatellar bursitis is often present.[6,25] On ultrasonography, the tendon will be thickened and heterogeneous, and may exhibit echogenic bone fragments and increased vascularity (**Fig. 6**). This malady is considered self-limited, but even with reduction in athletic activities, symptoms may take months or years to resolve (typically at skeletal maturity), if they ever do.[24,27]

Sinding-Larsen-Johannson disease (SLJ) is a similar traction apophysitis that affects the origin of the patellar tendon at the inferior pole of the patella in a slightly younger age group.[16,28] Technically not an apophysis, the inferior pole of the patella reacts just like the tibial tubercle when

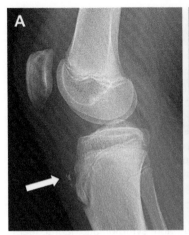
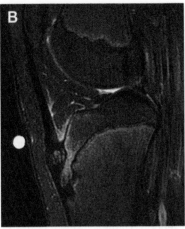

Fig. 5. Osgood-Schlatter disease. (A) Lateral radiograph of the knee in an 11-year-old girl with anterior knee pain and tenderness demonstrates thickening of the distal patellar tendon with an intratendinous bone fragment (*arrow*). (B) Fat-suppressed sagittal T2 MR image confirms edema within the ossicle, tendon, adjacent tibial tubercle, and in the deep infrapatellar recess.

subjected to chronic traction forces by the extensor mechanism, so SLJ is considered a traction apophysitis.[29] The radiographic and MR imaging findings of SLJ are identical to those of OSD, except they occur at the origin of the patellar tendon (**Fig. 7**).[6] For both OSD and SLJ, ossicles within the tendon are not enough to make the diagnosis; there must be soft tissue swelling of the tendon, as bone fragments occasionally may occur at the entheses of the tendon as a normal variant.[30] The situation changes in skeletally mature adolescents, because similar chronic traction phenomena at the inferior pole of the patella result in jumper's knee, which is chronic patellar tendinitis.[16,26] MR imaging findings include thickening and high T2 signal in and around the tendon. Partial tears should be sought, as they may change treatment. On ultrasonography, the normal fibrillar echo pattern of the patellar tendon becomes heterogeneous. The tendon will be swollen and may exhibit partial tears (**Fig. 8**).[31]

A vague group of abnormalities referred to as patellofemoral stress syndrome (PFSS) is the most common cause of chronic anterior knee pain in adolescents.[16,28] This group of maladies was once referred to as chondromalacia patellae; however, because many, if not most, of these patients have no substantial cartilage damage, that term should be reserved for pathologic softening of the patellar articular cartilage.[16,26] PFSS causes dull anterior knee pain and typically has no radiographic findings.[16] PFSS can result from overuse or direct trauma, and often relates to poor patellar tracking and/or malalignment of the lower extremity or extensor mechanism.[1] Pain and apprehension are often present, and abnormal stresses and shear forces from the malalignment may lead to eventual cartilage damage, degenerative arthrosis, and recurrent patellar dislocations.[32] Tight quadriceps muscles, iliotibial band, and hamstrings may result in superior and lateral migration of the patella. When radiographs or MR imaging are positive, findings may include patella alta, lateral tilt of the patella, genu valgum, or trochlear dysplasia.[27,32] The latter abnormality is diagnosed when the trochlea is shallow and the sulcus angle, measured on an axial MR image or an axial view of the knee, is greater than 150°. Caution should be exercised, though, as various measurements in the knee, such as the sulcus

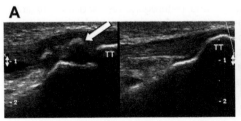
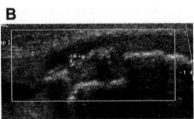

Fig. 6. Osgood-Schlatter disease. (A) Longitudinal side-by-side ultrasonographic images of bilateral knees, with the symptomatic side on the left of the image. The symptomatic side demonstrates the patellar tendon to be thickened and heterogeneous. Densely shadowing bone fragments (*arrow*) are evident. TT, tibial tubercle. (B) Longitudinal Doppler image of the symptomatic knee demonstrates increased vascularity.

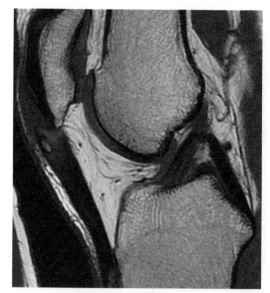

Fig. 7. Sinding-Larsen-Johannson disease. Sagittal proton density MR image of the knee in a 17-year-old male with persistent symptoms despite skeletal maturity. The image demonstrates thickening and increased signal within the proximal patellar tendon just distal to its origin. Intratendinous bone fragment is evident.

angle and patella alta, are often abnormal in asymptomatic knees and normal in patients with PFSS.[32] Excessive lateral pressure syndrome falls under the umbrella of PFSS and demonstrates lateral patellar tilt; with time, cartilage loss results, followed by sclerosis and subchondral cyst formation in the lateral facet of the patella.[32]

Another common overuse condition of the knee is osteochondritis dissecans (OCD). OCD is an

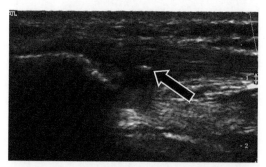

Fig. 8. Patellar tendinopathy. Longitudinal ultrasonographic image of the proximal patellar tendon in a 13-year-old female gymnast with closed physes demonstrates thickening and heterogeneity of the tendon near its origin from the lower pole of the patella. Hyperechoic focus (*arrow*) is thought to be a developing small focus of calcification. Radiographs were not obtained to confirm this finding.

idiopathic acquired pathologic condition that results in delamination and sequestration of a fragment of subchondral bone at the articular surface with its overlying cartilage.[33,34] OCD most commonly affects the knee, dome of the talus, and capitulum at the elbow. OCD of the capitulum is discussed in the accompanying article on pediatric upper extremity sports injuries.

In the knee, OCD affects the posterior lateral (mesial) portion of the medial femoral condyle (MFC) in more than 70% of cases, the central lateral femoral condyle (LFC) in 15% to 20%, and the patella in 5% to 10%.[33] Patellar cases occur almost exclusively in the lower pole, which distinguishes OCD from the upper pole location of dorsal defects of the patella.[35] These lesions present in children, adolescents, and young adults, and are separated into 2 groups: juvenile OCD occurs in patients with completely open physes; adult OCD occurs in patients with closing or closed physes.[36] This distinction is important, as juvenile OCD lesions usually heal without consequence using conservative measures but adult OCD is more likely to become unstable, worsen clinically, require surgical intervention, and lead to premature degenerative arthrosis.[33,37] As with many other overuse injuries, the incidence of OCD of the knee is increasing in pediatric athletes, thought likely to be due to increasing participation in competitive sports.[33] There is not enough evidence to conclusively prove the cause of OCD of the knee, but most investigators believe the root cause is repetitive trauma or shear forces leading to a stress reaction that progresses to a stress fracture in the subchondral bone with components of ischemia. With cessation of impact loading, the lesion may revascularize and heal over time, but continued stresses cause further progression.[33,38,39] End-stage lesions delaminate on a macroscopic level and fragments displace from the bed into the joint.[38] Of the different sites in the knee, OCD occurring in the MFC and trochlea (rare) are most likely to heal.[38] Surgical techniques for OCD include fixation with several devices such as variably threaded screws, K wires, and tacks; picking/microfracture; autologous cartilage implants; and mosaicplasty.[38]

Standard radiographs for investigating the possibility of OCD of the knee include anteroposterior (AP), lateral, and notch views. Lesions in the classic location near the intercondylar notch on the MFC are usually best seen on the notch view.[40] The lesion is an oval or lenticular radiolucency along the articular surface, often filled with a central fragment(s) of bone (**Fig. 9**).[36] One must be careful when evaluating these lesions in the youngest patients, as young children often have

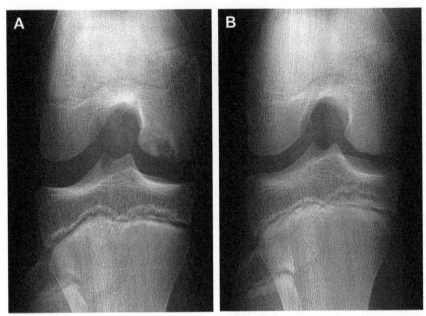

Fig. 9. Osteochondritis dissecans (OCD). (*A*) Notch view of the knee in a 12-year-old girl with chronic knee pain demonstrates the OCD lesion along the mesial aspect of the medial femoral condyle. This consists of an oval lucent zone with an in situ bone fragment. (*B*) Five months later, after conservative therapy, the lesion has completely healed.

a normal variant of ossification of the posterior condyles, with intact overlying cartilage but with irregularity and apparent fragmentation of the articular bone that is not pathologic.[41]

MR imaging is helpful to evaluate the size and location of the fragment and disruption of the overlying articular cartilage, to search for displaced intra-articular fragments, and to evaluate for signs of instability.[42] Determining whether a lesion is unstable is of critical importance[40]: although surgeons will use clinical progression and the skeletal maturity status to guide many decisions to operate, those decisions are influenced if MR imaging demonstrates the lesion to be stable or unstable. In adult OCD, MR imaging signs of instability include a T2 high-signal rim around the lesion, cysts underlying the lesion, multiple breaks in the subchondral bone plate at the margins of the lesion, and a second rim of low T2 signal surrounding the lesion. If there are displaced intra-articular fragments or if the bed of the lesion demonstrates a hole or gap, the lesion obviously is unstable. Presumably because they have greater propensity to heal, juvenile OCDs have a couple of slightly more stringent criteria to suggest instability: the high-signal T2 rim must be as bright as fluid, not just relatively bright as in adult cases; or cysts underlying the lesion must be multiple or greater than 5 mm to indicate instability of juvenile OCD (**Figs. 10** and **11**).[43] Size of lesions also

carries import: smaller lesions are more likely to heal, and in one report on OCD, 10 of 12 lesions larger than 160 mm^2 resulted in a poor outcome.[36]

A final topic to consider in overuse injuries of the knee is bipartite patella. Many patients have

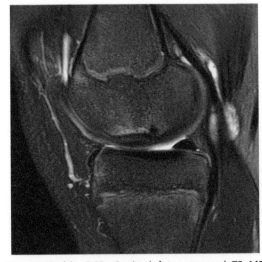

Fig. 10. Stable OCD. Sagittal fat-suppressed T2 MR image in an 11-year-old boy with knee pain demonstrates an OCD lesion on the weight-bearing surface of the MFC. The sclerotic margin is partly undermined by high T2 signal, but it is not as bright as fluid. In this skeletally immature patient, this is likely stable.

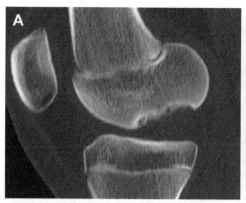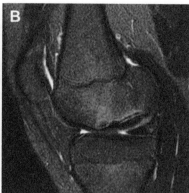

Fig. 11. Unstable OCD. (*A*) Sagittal computed tomography (CT) image demonstrates a large OCD lesion with surrounding sclerosis. The distal femoral physis is nearly completely fused, classifying this lesion as an adult OCD. (*B*) Sagittal fat-suppressed T2 MR image depicts high T2 signal undermining the lesion along its deep surface. Despite the fact that the signal is not as bright as fluid, because this patient is almost skeletally mature this lesion is predicted to be unstable.

normal variants of the patella in which there are 2 (or more) ossification centers that never demonstrate osseous bridging. These bipartite patellae have a fibrocartilaginous synchondrosis along the interface between the pieces. In the normal state, these multipartite patellae are not symptomatic; however, when subject to chronic stresses from the pull of the quadriceps mechanism or if acutely traumatized, they may become chronically painful. These mobile, symptomatic bipartite patellae will eventually demonstrate degenerative changes along the interface, indicating the painful abnormal motion. The smaller secondary ossicle in bipartite patellae is usually in the superior lateral corner (75%), but may occupy the lateral margin (20%) or occasionally the lower pole.[26]

Overuse Injuries of the Ankle and Foot

Although athletic ankle injuries are more commonly acute,[16] overuse injuries do occur at the ankle and foot. One of these lesions is the osteochondral lesion of the talus (OLT). The terminology for these lesions has evolved, formerly including OCD and osteochondral fractures. OLTs are thought of as transchondral fractures resulting from tangential shearing forces[44] or repetitive microtrauma,[45] are common in high-impact and running sports, and are seen in association with ankle sprains.[46] Although OLTs occasionally occur after an acute inversion ankle sprain, more commonly they occur months after the initial injury or after a series of ankle sprains. OLTs are most common in boys in their second decade and occur along either the medial or lateral edge of the talar dome.[47] Radiographic findings may be subtle,

but demonstrate a focal rounded lucent zone underlying the articular surface of the medial or lateral talar dome (**Fig. 12**).[44] At MR imaging, these lesions resemble OCD in the knee or elbow, with a well-defined lesion of subchondral bone that may have high signal in its midst on T2 images. Focal defects of the overlying articular cartilage are frequent on MR imaging but sometimes difficult to see because of the high resolution required to depict well the thin ankle cartilage. MR imaging signs of instability include displaced intra-articular

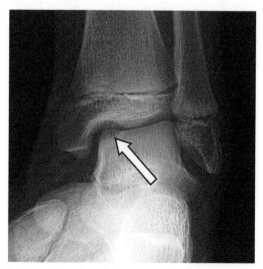

Fig. 12. Osteochondral lesion of the talus (OLT). Mortise radiograph of the ankle in an 11-year-old female dancer demonstrates a focal, lenticular lucency in the medial talar dome (*arrow*).

fragments, cartilage defects more than 5 mm wide, cysts underlying the lesion, and linear high T2 signal undermining more than 5 mm of the OLT (**Fig. 13**).[45]

Although tarsal coalition is not an injury per se and is not induced by athletic activity, it usually becomes symptomatic in adolescents as they increase their sports involvement. Coalition is a failure of segmentation of 2 ossific centers in utero. In the foot, coalition commonly occurs between the anterior process of the calcaneus and the navicular or between the talus and calcaneus, typically at the middle subtalar facet. The abnormal connection may consist of bone, cartilage, or fibrous tissue. Secondary signs on radiographs may include a talar beak, which is an abnormal excrescence of bone just proximal to the articular surface of the talar head; elongation of the anterior process of the calcaneus, referred to as the "anteater sign"; or a poorly defined middle subtalar facet. Computed tomography (CT) is the preferred modality for establishing the diagnosis. As the tarsals become fully ossified and the youth sustains more extensive athletic activity, the coalition becomes symptomatic because of abnormal stresses placed across the abnormal union.[45] These cases may demonstrate surrounding degenerative sclerosis and cysts on CT scans or osseous edema at MR imaging (**Fig. 14**). Tarsal coalition should be suspected in an adolescent athlete suffering recurrent ankle sprains or recurrent distal fibular physeal fractures.[48]

A similar scenario of traumatic irritation and recurrent discomfort may occur in pediatric athletes with accessory navicular syndrome. An accessory navicular is a normal variant ossicle that occurs along the medial pole of the tarsal navicular. Type I accessory naviculars are small ossicles contained within the distal portion of the tibialis posterior tendon; type II are larger ossicles onto which this tendon inserts. Type II accessory naviculars have a synchondrosis with the underlying navicular bone. Pain may be the acute result of trauma to this region, but if the synchondrosis is repeatedly stressed by tension from the posterior tibial tendon it may become chronically irritated and symptomatic; this is analogous to a traction apophysitis. CT and MR imaging scans show changes similar to those of coalition, with sclerosis and subchondral cysts at CT and osseous and soft tissue edema at MR imaging (**Fig. 15**).

There is some overlap of true traction apophysitis entities in the foot and ankle with cases of osteochondrosis, which is a term for disordered endochondral ossification that becomes symptomatic. Sever disease is a common overuse traction apophysitis at the calcaneal tuberosity[49] that causes exquisite tenderness at the attachment of the Achilles to the apophysis.[50] This apophysitis usually occurs in 10- to 13-year-olds with tight Achilles tendons and plantar fasciae who have undergone recent growth spurts and concurrent increases in activity.[34,51] Sever disease may lead to fragmentation and sclerosis of the apophysis and widening of the physis (**Fig. 16**), but these findings are often present to a similar degree in asymptomatic preadolescents.[49] As such, there are no reliable radiographic signs of Sever disease, and this diagnosis is a purely clinical one. Even MR imaging often demonstrates moderate high T2 signal in the calcaneal apophysis in asymptomatic youths, so MR imaging also is not diagnostic.[52] Iselin disease is a similar traction apophysitis that occurs at the attachment of the peroneus brevis tendon onto the fifth metatarsal base apophysis in runners.[51] Radiographs are typically normal,[16] but may demonstrate enlargement or fragmentation of the apophysis and widening of the physis.[53]

The 2 common osteochondroses of the foot are Köhler disease and Freiberg infraction. Köhler disease occurs in the tarsal navicular of active 5- to 9-year-old children.[49] Radiographic findings

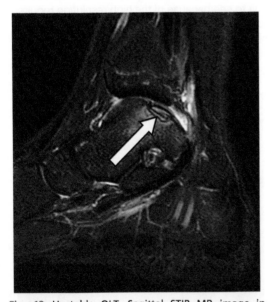

Fig. 13. Unstable OLT. Sagittal STIR MR image in a 13-year-old female gymnast who suffered an ankle sprain 2.5 years ago and has endured chronic pain for the last 2 years. There is a demarcated, well-defined osteochondral fragment in situ along the posterior medial talar dome. (*Arrow*) High signal/fluid between the fragment and the remainder of the talus strongly suggests instability.

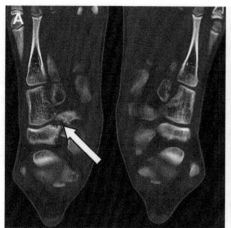
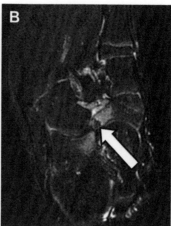

Fig. 14. Nonosseous tarsal coalition. (*A*) CT scan of the feet in a 10-year-old female gymnast with recent onset of foot pain demonstrates juxtaposition of the anterior process of the right calcaneus with the lateral talus (*arrow*), with no true osseous bridge. The irregularity, sclerosis, and cyst formation along the interface indicates degeneration related to abnormal stresses being placed across the coalition. The left side is normal. (*B*) Oblique axial STIR MR image of the right foot demonstrates mostly low-signal material in the osseous gap at the coalition site (*arrow*), indicating that the coalition is largely fibrous. Surrounding soft tissue and osseous edema confirms the abnormal stresses being placed on this symptomatic calcaneonavicular coalition.

include sclerosis, fragmentation, and narrowing of the navicular; however, similar findings are considered a normal variant when asymptomatic, so symptoms must be present to make this diagnosis.[49,54] Köhler disease is usually self-limited, with good results despite minimal intervention. Freiberg infraction typically occurs in the second or third metatarsal head of 12- to 15-year-old athletic girls, and is related to repetitive stress. Freiberg infraction is considered to be either a stress fracture or stress-induced osteonecrosis, and results in flattening and sclerosis of the metatarsal head and occasional fragmentation.[49,54]

As mentioned earlier, tendinitis is uncommon in the pediatric athlete but is being seen with increasing frequency. In the pediatric foot and ankle, Achilles tendinitis is probably the most common tendinitis that comes to medical attention. Whereas traction apophysitis predominates during growth spurts, tendinitis is more prevalent during periods of relatively slow growth. Achilles tendinitis is usually seen in runners who have recently increased their training regimen or who have poorly fitting shoes.[16,29] This is a straightforward clinical diagnosis and rarely requires imaging.

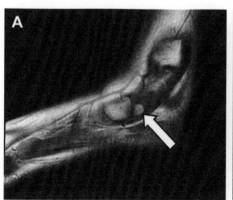
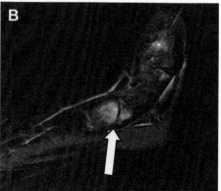

Fig. 15. Accessory navicular syndrome. (*A*) Sagittal T1 MR image of the medial foot in a 13-year-old female soccer player with worsening medial foot pain and tenderness demonstrates a type II accessory navicular (*arrow*). (*B*) Sagittal STIR MR image exhibits high-signal edema within the accessory ossicle and the adjacent navicular, confirming the clinical suspicion of accessory navicular syndrome (*arrow*).

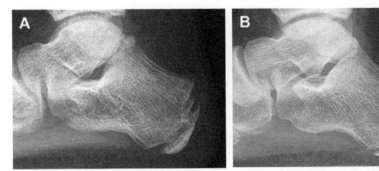

Fig. 16. Sever disease. (*A*) Lateral radiograph of the calcaneus in a 12-year-old boy with heel pain. There is relative osteopenia of the calcaneus, with irregularity and subtle fragmentation along the physis of the calcaneal apophysis, with some sclerosis. This patient had clinical documentation of bilateral Sever disease. (*B*) Lateral view of the same calcaneus 1 year later shows interval growth while the calcaneus has returned to normal.

Additional chronic overuse injuries that may afflict the teenage athlete are the ankle impingement syndromes. Anterior impingement is caused by osseous hypertrophy along the anterior tibia and dorsal talus, usually related to repeated extreme dorsiflexion in dancers and gymnasts. Anterolateral impingement may be present in soccer players and other athletes with recurrent ankle sprains. These athletes may develop the "meniscoid lesion," an irregular thickening of the anterolateral ankle capsule causing pain between the fibula and talus. The most common cause of posterior impingement in this age group is os trigonum syndrome. In this syndrome the os trigonum, a common normal variant ossicle at the posterior aspect of the talus, suffers a chronic impaction/impingement injury in dancers, gymnasts, and divers (**Fig. 17**).[48]

ACUTE INJURIES

This section includes not only truly acute injuries but those that are common but difficult to classify as acute or chronic overuse injuries.

Of course, acute muscle and tendon injuries occur in the pediatric athlete, though not as commonly as in adults. Strains and tears may occur within muscle bellies, and are probably most common in the hamstrings.[34] Muscle strains are diagnosed clinically when there is muscle pain but no loss of strength or motion. When there has been loss of strength or motion, at least partial tearing is implied. At MR imaging, muscle strain demonstrates feathery high T2 signal concentrated along the musculotendinous junction (MTJ) but no disruption (**Fig. 18**). With muscle tears, there is partial or complete discontinuity and hemorrhage in the gap.[55] As in adults, strains

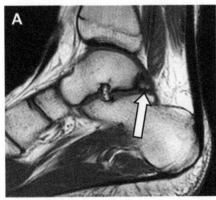
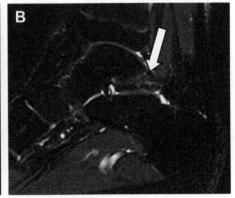

Fig. 17. Posterior impingement. (*A*) Sagittal T1 MR image of the ankle in a 15-year-old boy depicts a small os trigonum (*arrow*). (*B*) Sagittal STIR MR image demonstrates mild edema within the accessory ossicle and the talus, consistent with os trigonum syndrome, the most common cause of posterior impingement in adolescent athletes (*arrow*).

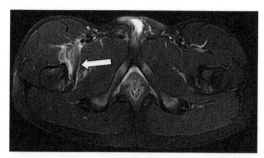

Fig. 18. Musculotendinous injury. Axial fat-suppressed T2 MR image of the hips in a 13-year-old male soccer player with right hip injury. There is feathery interstitial T2 high signal within the distal fibers of the iliopsoas with some disruption of fibers, indicating partial tear of the muscle (*arrow*).

may involve the tendon also, as well as partial and complete tears. Tendon strains demonstrate increased T2 signal within and around the tendon on MR imaging and tears exhibit loss of continuity of tendon fibers. On ultrasonography, tendon injuries cause focal thickening, increased heterogeneity of the expected fibrillar pattern of the tendon, and sometimes increased flow on Doppler imaging. Focal tears interrupt the fibrillar pattern with anechoic or hypoechoic defects.

In sports, the most common location for a muscle contusion is in the quadriceps ("Charley horse").[34] Focal feathery high T2 signal will be present on MR scans but not necessarily concentrated at the MTJ. Sometimes trauma to muscle results in eventual formation of myositis ossificans, which is essentially a focus of hemorrhage and muscle damage that ossifies. Up to one-third of these patients do not recall a history of trauma. Recall of trauma is especially helpful in diagnosis, as these lesions may resemble soft tissue sarcomas on MR scans and at pathology. At MR imaging, the mass acutely contains heterogeneous high T2 signal that will develop a low-signal rim as time passes, eventually forming true bone.[55] When examining muscle masses, one must keep this diagnosis in mind so as to not come to the false diagnosis of sarcoma.

Acute Injuries of the Hip

Most acute injuries around the hip are soft tissue injuries such as muscle contusions.[28] However, osseous avulsions are the most common acute hip injury in the adolescent athlete to present for diagnostic imaging.[6] In this age group, an avulsion is a displaced fracture of an apophysis through its physis. Apophyses are under tension from the tendons attached to them. When there is a sudden passive stretch or more commonly an active

contraction across an apophysis, the apophysis may separate from the underlying bone and retract with the tendon.[19,22] This process occurs because the apophyseal physis is the weakest link in the muscle-tendon-bone complex.[56] There are occasional reports of chronic avulsions in which no inciting event is recalled; presumably these are due to chronic traction from repeated submaximal trauma.[22] As such, undoubtedly there is some overlap between acute avulsions and chronic traction apophysitis. In the pelvis, apophyseal avulsions are most common in teenage sprinters, kickers, hurdlers, and those athletes who perform "splits."[19]

These injuries cause sudden pain and are recognized on radiographs as displacement of an apophysis (**Fig. 19**).[57] Avulsions are usually visible on radiographs because they almost always occur after the cartilaginous apophysis has begun to ossify but before the physis is fused: that is, they occur in adolescents.[22,58] However, the displacement of fragments can be subtle and require attention to detail. Avulsion of the anterior inferior iliac spine may require oblique views such as the frog-leg view to be recognized.[59] The displacement will be visible on MR imaging scans and the gap will be filled with high T2 signal.[56,57] Ultrasonography demonstrates the widened physis also, and can be compared with the asymptomatic side. Hypoechoic or mixed echogenic edema or hemorrhage is evident in the gap, and there usually is hyperemia when Doppler imaging is applied.[56] In a report of 203 avulsions that occurred in patients

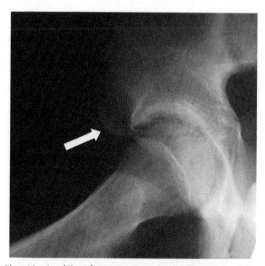

Fig. 19. Avulsion fracture. Frog-leg radiograph of the hip in a 13-year-old boy with recent injury and acute hip pain demonstrates separation of the anterior inferior iliac spine (AIIS) apophysis from the adjacent ilium (*arrow*). Oblique imaging such as this is often necessary to demonstrate AIIS avulsions.

11 to 17 years old, Rossi and Dragoni[58] noted that 109 involved the ischial tuberosity (hamstring origin), 45 occurred at the anterior inferior iliac spine (straight/direct head of the rectus femoris), 39 at the anterior superior iliac spine (sartorius), 7 at the pubic symphysis (hip adductors), and 3 at the iliac crest (abdominal obliques). Soccer (74) and gymnastics (55) were the most frequent sports involved. Involvement of the pubic symphysis does not usually result in a discrete fragment, as with other avulsions, but demonstrates irregularity of the body of the pubic bone on one side.[60] Avulsions of the lesser trochanter (iliopsoas tendon insertion) and greater trochanter (gluteus medius and minimus, external rotators) are rare in this age group.[22]

Another acute osseous injury of the hip is referred to as a "hip pointer." This condition is a contusion of the iliac crest that results in subperiosteal edema but rarely requires imaging.[22] Yet another acute injury in the vicinity of the hip is called "thigh splints." This injury represents a partial adductor tendon avulsion from the posterior medial margin of the proximal half of the femur. The injury starts as an acute event but may persist when it goes unrecognized and untreated.[61] MR imaging demonstrates periosteal reaction at the attachment site of the adductor longus, adductor brevis, or the adductor magnus to the femoral shaft, often with edema in the marrow space but no soft tissue mass or fracture line.[61]

Acute tears of the acetabular labrum and adjacent cartilage defects are thought to be rare in children but occasionally are seen in the teenage athlete. As with adults, labral tears demonstrate contrast filling a crack in the labrum at MR arthrography, typically anteriorly and laterally (Fig. 20). In this age group, degenerated labral tears with grossly morphologically abnormal labral shape would not be expected to occur unless there is significant hip dysplasia.

Acute Injuries of the Knee

Pediatric knee injuries include several conditions that are unique to the immature skeleton, but this article first addresses lesions that are seen in a broad range of ages: ligament injuries and meniscus tears. Although medial and lateral collateral ligament injuries are rare in the pediatric athlete,[11,50] tears of the anterior cruciate ligament (ACL) have become relatively common with the increased extent of athletic activity over the last few decades.[62] Posterior cruciate ligament (PCL) injuries are uncommon in pediatric patients, and are not discussed further here other than to say MR imaging is helpful in diagnosing this injury,

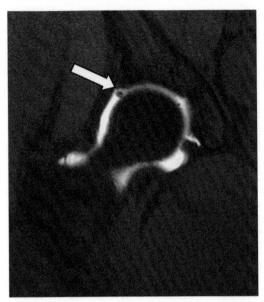

Fig. 20. Acetabular labral tear. Coronal fat-suppressed T1 MR arthrogram image of the hip in a 14-year-old female soccer goalie with ongoing hip pain demonstrates contrast extending between the labrum and the acetabulum (*arrow*).

whether it occurs as an osseous avulsion of the tibial attachment of the PCL or a tear in the PCL substance.[63]

There has long been a dogma that ACL injuries manifest as tibial spine avulsions (Fig. 21) in skeletally immature patients and that "midsubstance" tears, that is, tears of the tendon and not osseous avulsions, occur in teenagers after their physes close.[11,27,64] However, with the continued increase in participation of children and adolescents in organized sports, a marked increase in overall ACL injuries has become evident in this group, including midsubstance tears in the patient with open physes.[65] Complete ACL tears (48%) outnumbered partial tears (26%) and avulsions of the tibial spine (26%) in one study of pediatric ACL injuries[66]; however, all types of injury should be sought, as there is growing evidence that even higher grade partial ACL tears result in significant instability and poor outcome, if left untreated.[67–69] Fortunately, surgical evidence is mounting that ACL reconstructions can be performed in the setting of open physes without affecting growth, allowing aggressive treatment for even children with ACL tears and resulting in improved outcomes.[64,65,69] MR imaging criteria for diagnosing ACL tears should be the same as in adults (Fig. 22A), but at least one study emphasized that discontinuity of fibers was not a very sensitive finding, and that abnormal signal and

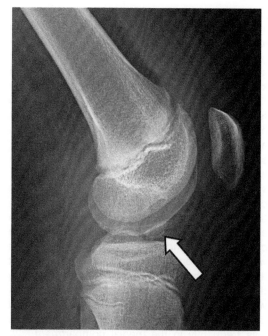

Fig. 21. Tibial eminence avulsion. Lateral radiograph of the knee in an 11-year-old boy who twisted his knee demonstrates a bone fragment anterior to the tibial spine (*arrow*). In younger patients, this avulsion fracture may occur in lieu of an intrasubstance tear of the anterior cruciate ligament (ACL).

reliable in the pediatric population.[66] Classic kissing contusions of the posterior lateral tibial plateau and the midportion of the LFC are pathognomonic for ACL tears in adults,[71] but characteristic lateral compartment contusions in pediatric patients indicate ACL tears only 33% to 72% of the time.[71,72] Regarding the question of whether an absent ACL without edema implies a chronic tear or congenital absence, Manner and colleagues[73] showed that patients with congenitally absent cruciate ligaments demonstrate morphologic abnormalities (hypoplasia) of the intercondylar notch of the distal femur and the tibial eminence. If the bones look normal, ACL absence indicates a chronic tear.

It is well known that, among adolescent athletes with fused physes, ACL tears are much more common in girls than in boys.[74] Definitive conclusions about the cause of this discrepancy are lacking, but evidence points to several factors: anatomic and physiologic features such as differing sizes of the intercondylar notch, relative laxity of ligaments, muscle strength discrepancies, and differences in lower extremity alignment; hormonal factors such as estrogen levels and their variations during the menstrual cycle; environmental factors such as different footwear and playing surfaces; and even physiologic differences such as muscle activation patterns, landing techniques, and foot strike patterns all may play a role.[74–76]

lack of parallelism with Blumensaat's line were more sensitive.[70] Of importance is that secondary signs of ACL tears, especially kissing contusions in the lateral compartment, are helpful but not as

Meniscal tears, once thought to be rare in this population, have now become more common.[77] MR criteria for diagnosing tears in pediatric

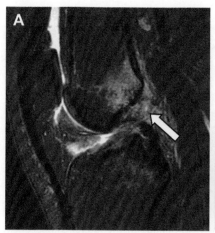
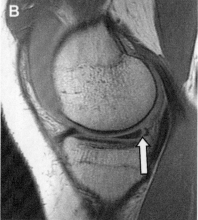

Fig. 22. ACL tear with concomitant meniscal tear. (*A*) Sagittal T2 MR image in a 17-year-old female soccer player with closed physes demonstrates high signal interspersed throughout the expected location of the ACL. The fibers are discontinuous proximally (*arrow*) and they do not parallel Blumensaat's line distally. (*B*) In this proton density MR image in the same patient, there is abnormal vertical linear intermediate signal in the periphery of the posterior horn of the medial meniscus (*arrow*), a classic finding of a traumatic posterior horn meniscal tear.

menisci are the same as in adults: linear increased signal (on proton density sequences) that contacts an articular surface (**Fig. 22**B), abnormal morphology, and displaced fragments indicate meniscal tears.[78] Intrameniscal high signal that does not contact the articular surface of the menisci is frequent in children and is of no consequence. This signal is thought to reflect the increased vascular supply of the pediatric meniscus.[79] Parameniscal and intrameniscal cysts are rare in children and adolescents, but they do occur. As in adults, when present they indicate a high likelihood of meniscal tear.[80]

The accuracy of MR imaging in diagnosing tears of pediatric menisci and ACLs remains a controversial issue. Some investigators continue to discourage knee MR imaging in this population, citing studies that describe poor MR accuracy for diagnosing these injuries and reduced performance of MR imaging compared with clinical examination, compared with arthroscopy as the gold standard.[81–84] However, more recent and better designed studies using improved equipment show that accuracy for pediatric knee MR imaging is approaching that for adults. In a small study, Lee and colleagues[70] reported 95% sensitivity and 88% specificity for ACL tears. Another small study reported 100% sensitivity and 89% specificity for meniscal tears in 26 subjects who underwent arthroscopy.[85] A more recent study that included 156 subjects, 59 of whom went to surgery, reported 92% sensitivity and 87% specificity for the medial meniscus, 93% sensitivity and 95% specificity for the lateral meniscus, and 100% accuracy for the ACL.[86] Given the increasing

propensity for youth to injure their knees, increasing demands of patients and their parents for return to sport, and improving imaging equipment and accuracy, MR imaging has earned a role in the workup of many pediatric sports knee injuries.

In children younger than 10 years, meniscal tears remain rare except in those patients who have discoid menisci.[42] The discoid meniscus is an atavistic variant in which the meniscus is wider and thicker than usual, and extends across the weight-bearing surface of the tibial plateau.[78,87] Variations include the complete (slab) type, which covers the tibial plateau and is attached to the tibia; incomplete (wedge) type, which is also attached to the tibia but does not cover the entire compartment; and Wrisberg ligament type, in which the meniscus covers the plateau but attaches to the ligament of Wrisberg and not the tibia.[87] The incidence of discoid menisci varies with population studied, but occurs in the lateral compartment about 2% of the time and 10 times less frequently in the medial compartment.[88] A discoid meniscus is diagnosed when the transverse width of the meniscal body on a mid-coronal MR image exceeds 14 mm.[89] Because the abnormal meniscus is subject to increased stresses, especially as youth become more involved in athletics, tears and cystic degeneration are common.[88] Both tears and degeneration can be painful. Discoid menisci often contain diffuse intrameniscal signal. Whether linear or globular, when this signal contacts the articular surface of a discoid meniscus, it is usually torn (**Fig. 23**).[90]

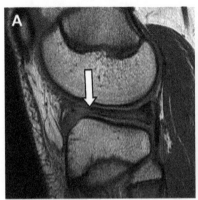
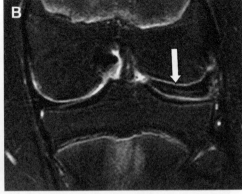

Fig. 23. Torn discoid meniscus. (*A*) Sagittal proton density MR image of the lateral compartment of the knee demonstrates the meniscus to cover almost the entire tibial plateau. Extensive abnormal signal within the meniscus strongly suggests tear, confirmed anteriorly where the signal contacts the articular surface of the meniscus (*arrow*). (*B*) Fat-suppressed coronal MR image shows that the slab type discoid meniscus covers the entire lateral plateau and far exceeds the cutoff of 15 mm for maximum transverse width, indicating discoid meniscus (*arrow*).

Baker cysts, which are extensions of joint fluid between the semimembranosus and medial gastrocnemius tendons posteromedially, are occasional findings at MR imaging of the pediatric knee. In one study, Baker cysts were present in 6.3% of pediatric knee scans. One may wonder if a Baker cyst portends an intra-articular condition, such as meniscal tear, ACL tear, or rheumatoid arthritis, as it often does in adults. In children this is not the case, as most patients with Baker cysts exhibit no other pathology.[91,92] In one study, 25 Baker cysts were associated with no ACL or meniscal tears, and positive findings included only 2 cases of OCD, 1 case of septic arthritis, and 1 case of juvenile chronic arthritis.[91]

Another common acute injury in the adolescent knee is transient dislocation of the patella (TDP), typically occurring between the ages of 14 and 20 years.[93] The mechanism of injury is through twisting the mildly flexed knee medially with the foot planted, causing the quadriceps mechanism to pull the patella laterally.[94] Almost all of these dislocations spontaneously relocate, and the nature of the injury is unsuspected before imaging in approximately half of patients.[32] Radiographs always demonstrate a large effusion, and an axial view of the patella sometimes will demonstrate a medial avulsion of the patella.[5] MR imaging usually is diagnostic because of the classic pattern of injuries related to the lateral dislocation. At some point between dislocation and relocation, the patella and LFC impact each other, and cause contusions in the inferomedial patella and peripheral LFC in 81% of cases (Fig. 24).[95] Injury to the medial soft tissue restraints is just as frequent in TDP,[95] but it is now known that the medial retinaculum is less important than the medial patellofemoral ligament (MPFL), which provides 50% to 80% of the medial restraint to the patella.[93] The MPFL can be difficult to discern. It takes its origin from the medial femur between the adductor tubercle and the medial epicondyle. The MPFL travels anteriorly along the deep surface of the vastus medialis obliquus (VMO) to attach to the upper half of the medial patella.[96] MPFL tears are common after TDP, and usually occur at the femoral attachment. Because the normal MPFL often is difficult to identify, direct identification of torn MPFL fibers is not possible in many tears; instead, one often relies on the secondary signs of substantial edema at the origin, lack of identification of an intact MPFL, and elevation of the VMO by traumatic edema (Fig. 25).[96]

When evaluating MR scans of patients with TDP, one must search for cartilage defects of the medial patellar facet or lateral trochlea, which occur in up to 72% of cases.[93] Impacted fractures of the

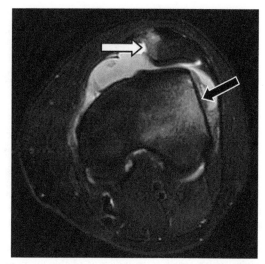

Fig. 24. Transient dislocation of the patella (TDP). Axial fat-suppressed T2 MR image of the knee in a 13-year-old female volleyball player with a history of recurrent patellar dislocations demonstrates the patella to be normally located. However, there are cardinal signs of recent transient dislocation, including a large effusion and high-signal contusions of the medial patella (*white arrow*) and peripheral lateral femoral condyle (*black arrow*). In fact, the inferior medial patella demonstrates an impaction fracture, shown to be specific for TDP in one study. Also note the dystrophic, flattened trochlear groove.

inferior medial border of the patella are specific for TDP.[96] In addition, a shear fracture may affect the LFC, knocking off a long, thin piece of articular cartilage and bone that may lie loose within the joint.[97] Surgeons need to know about these injuries and also should be alerted to possible predisposing factors, such as patella alta and trochlear dysplasia (shallow sulcus).[93]

The acute counterparts to SLJ and OSD affecting the proximal and distal ends of the patellar tendon are patellar sleeve avulsions and tibial tubercle avulsions. Patellar sleeve avulsions occur from an acute jumping injury in patients aged 8 to 12 years.[30] Radiographs reveal anterior soft tissue swelling and a small fragment of bone avulsed from the inferior tip or anterior inferior portion of the patella.[30] It is important to know that these osseous fragments sometimes represent the tip of the iceberg, with a much larger cartilage fragment unseen on the radiographs (Fig. 26). MR imaging is an important tool to identify the size of the cartilage fragment; when large, surgical reduction and fixation is recommended.[98] Tibial tuberosity avulsions occur in adolescent male jumpers who are near skeletal maturity. The typical patient will report an acute event causing the injury. Sharp fragments are visible and elevated on radiographs.[6]

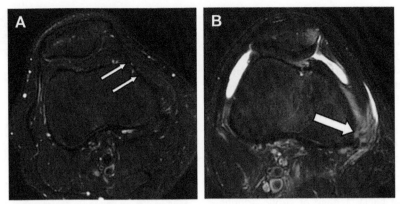

Fig. 25. Medial patellofemoral ligament (MPFL). (*A*) Axial fat-suppressed T2 MR image depicts the normal low-signal MPFL (*arrows*) underlying the vastus medialis obliquus (VMO) muscle. This ligament is often more difficult to identify. (*B*) Axial fat-suppressed T2 MR image in a 13-year-old boy (different patient to the one in *A*) demonstrates disruption of the fibers of the MPFL at its origin (*arrow*). There is considerable high-signal fluid in the vicinity, which serves as an indicator of this injury even when the ligament fibers are indiscernible, and this edema/hemorrhage often elevates the VMO.

Acute Injuries of the Ankle and Foot

Acute athletic injuries to the foot and ankle are very common, and rival those of the knee for most frequent in pediatric athletes. Most of these injuries consist of ankle sprains and sprain equivalents. Although soft tissue and osseous contusions and acute fractures (including juvenile Tillaux and triplane fractures of the distal tibia, as well as a host of fractures of the tarsals, metatarsals, and digits) may occur, they are not considered here. An important comment regarding contusions in the pediatric foot is that one must exercise caution when interpreting

focal high T2 marrow signal of the tarsal bones. Pediatric patients often demonstrate small islands of residual red marrow in the tarsal bones, especially peripherally, mimicking contusions or other pathologic causes of marrow edema.[99]

Ankle sprains and sprain equivalents are quite common in the pediatric athlete. As with other parts of the body, before the distal fibular physis closes it is a weak link compared with ligaments and bones. The pediatric patient with open physes who suffers an ankle inversion injury often exhibits a Salter-Harris I or II fracture of the distal fibular physis. This injury is the most common fracture

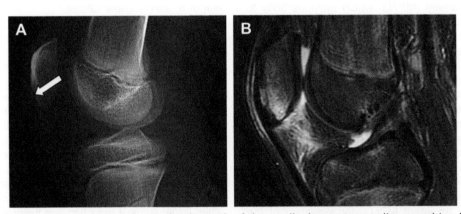

Fig. 26. Patellar sleeve avulsion. (*A*) Lateral radiograph of the patella demonstrates a linear avulsion fragment (*arrow*) along the anterior surface of the inferior pole of the patella with associated overlying soft tissue swelling. These fractures often involve the most distal surface of the inferior pole also. (*B*) Sagittal fat-suppressed T2 MR image reveals high-signal edema within the inferior pole of the patella and the surrounding soft tissues. This patient has ossified nearly all his cartilage; in patients with substantial patellar growth cartilage still unossified, MR imaging is crucial to demonstrate the extent of the injury and guide surgery.

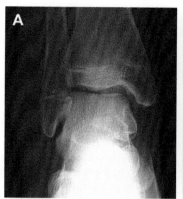
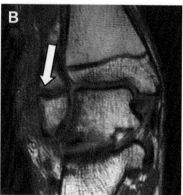

Fig. 27. Distal fibular physeal injury. (A) AP radiograph of the ankle demonstrates considerable lateral soft tissue swelling. The lateral physis appears slightly wide, but this may be a normal appearance. Although radiologists often seek radiographs of the contralateral side for comparison, many primary care and sports medicine physicians assume this is a Salter-Harris I fracture of the physis. In this case, the patient also underwent MR imaging. The coronal T1 image (B) demonstrates widening of the physis (arrow), confirming Salter-Harris I fracture.

in pediatric sports but typically causes only lateral soft tissue swelling on radiographs (Fig. 27).[51,100] When widening of the physis is questioned, the radiologist may request a comparison view of the other ankle, but many clinicians consider this to be a Salter-Harris I injury in the appropriate clinical setting whether or not the radiographs demonstrate any displacement.[51] The important step is to exclude a more serious injury or additional findings such as an OLT. Another type of fibular fracture one may occasionally see is an avulsion of the lateral surface of the distal fibula. This condition occurs when a severe ankle injury causes the superior peroneal retinaculum to avulse from the fibula, and indicates that the peroneal tendons will be free to subluxate.[29]

As the physes close, the adolescent athlete does not seem any less prone to inversion and plantar flexion injuries. The result at this age mirrors that in adults. Ankle sprains cause injury to the anterior talofibular ligament, whether a sprain, partial tear, or complete tear. If the injury is severe, the calcaneofibular ligament also may be injured (Fig. 28).[51] "High ankle sprains," in which the syndesmotic ligaments are injured, are not commonly reported in pediatric athletes.

Tendon injuries are described in the section on general acute injury and are not discussed in depth here. However, it is relevant to note that Achilles tendon tears are rare in the pediatric athlete.[30] With the increasing demands placed on the competitive pediatric athlete, turf toe is becoming seen more often.[51] In this lesion, there is partial or complete rupture of the plantar plate of the first ray, at the plantar surface of the metatarsophalangeal joint.

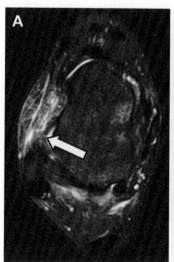
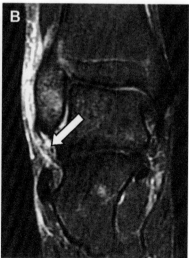

Fig. 28. Lateral ankle ligament injuries. (A) Axial fat-suppressed T2 MR image in a 13-year-old female soccer player with a severe ankle sprain demonstrates thickening and disruption of the anterior talofibular ligament (arrow) with surrounding high-signal edema. (B) Coronal fat-suppressed proton density image depicts similar disruption of the calcaneofibular ligament (arrow).

MR imaging with high-resolution coils can demonstrate this injury, as can ultrasonography.

SUMMARY

The continued increase in numbers of children and adolescents participating in organized sports and the progressive trend toward increased training times and busy competition schedules suggest that radiologists will see more and more overuse injuries of the lower extremity. Acute injuries are not diminishing, though, and competent radiologists must be familiar with the findings related to both types of injuries. Traction apophysitis occurs at all the major joints of the lower extremity, with OSD and SLJ of the extensor mechanism being quite common. The common sites of pelvic avulsions deserve special attention on radiographs, including the ischial apophysis, anterior superior iliac spine, and anterior inferior iliac spine. Acute injuries of the ACL and menisci are being seen more commonly in this age group; with current MR equipment, accuracy for detecting these lesions should approach that in adults. Transient dislocation of the patella is not suspected clinically in about half of the patients: the characteristic patterns of injury at MR imaging make this diagnosis straightforward. In skeletally immature patients, ankle sprains may manifest as Salter-Harris I or II injuries of the distal fibular physis; however, often the only radiographic finding is soft tissue swelling. Familiarity with these injury patterns will help radiologists provide the best service to injured pediatric athletes and to colleagues in the pediatric sports medicine clinic.

REFERENCES

1. Frank JB, Jarit GJ, Bravman JT, et al. Lower extremity injuries in the skeletally immature athlete. J Am Acad Orthop Surg 2007;15:356–66.
2. Micheli LJ, Fehlandt AF Jr. Overuse injuries to tendons and apophyses in children and adolescents. Clin Sports Med 1992;11:713–26.
3. Caine D, Caine C, Maffulli N. Incidence and distribution of pediatric sport-related injuries. Clin J Sport Med 2006;16:500–13.
4. Coady CM, Micheli LJ. Stress fractures in the pediatric athlete. Clin Sports Med 1997;16:225–38.
5. Ryu RK, Fan RS. Adolescent and pediatric sports injuries. Pediatr Clin North Am 1998;45:1601–35, x.
6. Auringer ST, Anthony EY. Common pediatric sports injuries. Semin Musculoskelet Radiol 1999;3:247–56.
7. Ecklund K. Magnetic resonance imaging of pediatric musculoskeletal trauma. Top Magn Reson Imaging 2002;13:203–17.
8. Heyworth BE, Green DW. Lower extremity stress fractures in pediatric and adolescent athletes. Curr Opin Pediatr 2008;20:58–61.
9. Fredericson M, Bergman AG, Hoffman KL, et al. Tibial stress reaction in runners. Correlation of clinical symptoms and scintigraphy with a new magnetic resonance imaging grading system. Am J Sports Med 1995;23:472–81.
10. Kijowski R, Choi J, Mukharjee R, et al. Significance of radiographic abnormalities in patients with tibial stress injuries: correlation with magnetic resonance imaging. Skeletal Radiol 2007;36:633–40.
11. Carty H. Children's sports injuries. Eur J Radiol 1998;26:163–76.
12. Beals RK, Cook RD. Stress fractures of the anterior tibial diaphysis. Orthopedics 1991;14:869–75.
13. Rettig AC, Shelbourne KD, McCarroll JR, et al. The natural history and treatment of delayed union stress fractures of the anterior cortex of the tibia. Am J Sports Med 1988;16:250–5.
14. Green NE, Rogers RA, Lipscomb AB. Nonunions of stress fractures of the tibia. Am J Sports Med 1985;13:171–6.
15. Woods M, Kijowski R, Sanford M, et al. Magnetic resonance imaging findings in patients with fibular stress injuries. Skeletal Radiol 2008;37:835–41.
16. Bernhardt DT, Landry GL. Sports injuries in young athletes. Adv Pediatr 1995;42:465–500.
17. Meaney JE, Carty H. Femoral stress fractures in children. Skeletal Radiol 1992;21:173–6.
18. Micheli LJ. Overuse injuries in children's sports: the growth factor. Orthop Clin North Am 1983;14:337–60.
19. Hotchkiss BL, Engels JA, Forness M. Hip disorders in the adolescent. Adolesc Med State Art Rev 2007;18:165–81, x-xi.
20. Kozlowski K, Campbell JB, Azouz EM. Traumatised ischial apophysis (report of six cases). Australas Radiol 1989;33:140–3.
21. Waite BL, Krabak BJ. Examination and treatment of pediatric injuries of the hip and pelvis. Phys Med Rehabil Clin N Am 2008;19:305–18, ix.
22. Paletta GA Jr, Andrish JT. Injuries about the hip and pelvis in the young athlete. Clin Sports Med 1995;14:591–628.
23. Berend KR, Vail TP. Hip arthroscopy in the adolescent and pediatric athlete. Clin Sports Med 2001;20:763–78.
24. Gholve PA, Scher DM, Khakharia S, et al. Osgood Schlatter syndrome. Curr Opin Pediatr 2007;19:44–50.
25. Rosenberg ZS, Kawelblum M, Cheung YY, et al. Osgood-Schlatter lesion: fracture or tendinitis? Scintigraphic, CT, and MR imaging features. Radiology 1992;185:853–8.
26. Stanitski CL. Knee overuse disorders in the pediatric and adolescent athlete. Instr Course Lect 1993;42:483–95.

27. Davids JR. Pediatric knee. Clinical assessment and common disorders. Pediatr Clin North Am 1996;43: 1067–90.

28. Lyon RM, Street CC. Pediatric sports injuries: when to refer or x-ray. Pediatr Clin North Am 1998;45: 221–44.

29. Wojtys EM. Sports injuries in the immature athlete. Orthop Clin North Am 1987;18:689–708.

30. Gaca AM. Basketball injuries in children. Pediatr Radiol 2009;39:1275–85.

31. Roberts CS, Beck DJ Jr, Heinsen J, et al. Review article: diagnostic ultrasonography: applications in orthopaedic surgery. Clin Orthop Relat Res 2002;401:248–64.

32. Elias DA, White LM. Imaging of patellofemoral disorders. Clin Radiol 2004;59:543–57.

33. Kocher MS, Tucker R, Ganley TJ, et al. Management of osteochondritis dissecans of the knee: current concepts review. Am J Sports Med 2006; 34:1181–91.

34. Saperstein AL, Nicholas SJ. Pediatric and adolescent sports medicine. Pediatr Clin North Am 1996;43:1013–33.

35. Edwards DH, Bentley G. Osteochondritis dissecans patellae. J Bone Joint Surg Br 1977;59: 58–63.

36. De Smet AA, Ilahi OA, Graf BK. Untreated osteochondritis dissecans of the femoral condyles: prediction of patient outcome using radiographic and MR findings. Skeletal Radiol 1997;26:463–7.

37. Sales de Gauzy J, Mansat C, Darodes PH, et al. Natural course of osteochondritis dissecans in children. J Pediatr Orthop B 1999;8:26–8.

38. Micheli L, Curtis C, Shervin N. Articular cartilage repair in the adolescent athlete: is autologous chondrocyte implantation the answer? Clin J Sport Med 2006;16:465–70.

39. Hefti F, Beguiristain J, Krauspe R, et al. Osteochondritis dissecans: a multicenter study of the European Pediatric Orthopedic Society. J Pediatr Orthop B 1999;8:231–45.

40. Wall E, Von Stein D. Juvenile osteochondritis dissecans. Orthop Clin North Am 2003;34:341–53.

41. Gebarski K, Hernandez RJ. Stage-I osteochondritis dissecans versus normal variants of ossification in the knee in children. Pediatr Radiol 2005;35: 880–6.

42. Sanchez R, Strouse PJ. The knee: MR imaging of uniquely pediatric disorders. Magn Reson Imaging Clin N Am 2009;17:521–37, vii.

43. Kijowski R, Blankenbaker DG, Shinki K, et al. Juvenile versus adult osteochondritis dissecans of the knee: appropriate MR imaging criteria for instability. Radiology 2008;248:571–8.

44. Schoenberg NY, Lehman WB. Magnetic resonance imaging of pediatric disorders of the ankle and

45. foot. Magn Reson Imaging Clin N Am 1994;2: 109–22.

45. Patel CV. The foot and ankle: MR imaging of uniquely pediatric disorders. Magn Reson Imaging Clin N Am 2009;17:539–47, vii.

46. Latz K. Overuse injuries in the pediatric and adolescent athlete. Mol Med 2006;103:81–5.

47. Harty MP, Hubbard AM. MR imaging of pediatric abnormalities in the ankle and foot. Magn Reson Imaging Clin N Am 2001;9:579–602, xi.

48. Chambers HG. Ankle and foot disorders in skeletally immature athletes. Orthop Clin North Am 2003;34:445–59.

49. Pommering TL, Kluchurosky L, Hall SL. Ankle and foot injuries in pediatric and adult athletes. Prim Care 2005;32:133–61.

50. Stanitski CL. Pediatric and adolescent sports injuries. Clin Sports Med 1997;16:613–33.

51. Pontell D, Hallivis R, Dollard MD. Sports injuries in the pediatric and adolescent foot and ankle: common overuse and acute presentations. Clin Podiatr Med Surg 2006;23:209–31, x.

52. Vallejo JM, Jaramillo D. Normal MR imaging anatomy of the ankle and foot in the pediatric population. Magn Reson Imaging Clin N Am 2001;9: 435–46, ix.

53. Canale ST, Williams KD. Iselin's disease. J Pediatr Orthop 1992;12:90–3.

54. Vanhoenacker FM, Bernaerts A, Gielen J, et al. Trauma of the pediatric ankle and foot. JBR-BTR 2002;85:212–8.

55. Tuite MJ, DeSmet AA. MRI of selected sports injuries: muscle tears, groin pain, and osteochondritis dissecans. Semin Ultrasound CT MR 1994; 15:318–40.

56. Pisacano RM, Miller TT. Comparing sonography with MR imaging of apophyseal injuries of the pelvis in four boys. AJR Am J Roentgenol 2003; 181:223–30.

57. Dillon JE, Connolly SA, Connolly LP, et al. MR imaging of congenital/developmental and acquired disorders of the pediatric hip and pelvis. Magn Reson Imaging Clin N Am 2005; 13:783–97.

58. Rossi F, Dragoni S. Acute avulsion fractures of the pelvis in adolescent competitive athletes: prevalence, location and sports distribution of 203 cases collected. Skeletal Radiol 2001;30:127–31.

59. Sundar M, Carty H. Avulsion fractures of the pelvis in children: a report of 32 fractures and their outcome. Skeletal Radiol 1994;23:85–90.

60. Schneider R, Kaye J, Ghelman B. Adductor avulsive injuries near the symphisis pubis. Radiology 1976;120:567–9.

61. Anderson SE, Johnston JO, O'Donnell R, et al. MR Imaging of sports-related pseudotumor in children: mid femoral diaphyseal periostitis at insertion site

of adductor musculature. AJR Am J Roentgenol 2001;176:1227–31.

62. Soprano JV. Musculoskeletal injuries in the pediatric and adolescent athlete. Curr Sports Med Rep 2005;4:329–34.

63. Pandya NK, Janik L, Chan G, et al. Case reports: pediatric PCL insufficiency from tibial insertion osteochondral avulsions. Clin Orthop Relat Res 2008;466:2878–83.

64. Mohtadi N, Grant J. Managing anterior cruciate ligament deficiency in the skeletally immature individual: a systematic review of the literature. Clin J Sport Med 2006;16:457–64.

65. Bales CP, Guettler JH, Moorman CT 3rd. Anterior cruciate ligament injuries in children with open physes: evolving strategies of treatment. Am J Sports Med 2004;32:1978–85.

66. Prince JS, Laor T, Bean JA. MRI of anterior cruciate ligament injuries and associated findings in the pediatric knee: changes with skeletal maturation. AJR Am J Roentgenol 2005;185:756–62.

67. Aichroth PM, Patel DV, Zorrilla P. The natural history and treatment of rupture of the anterior cruciate ligament in children and adolescents. A prospective review. J Bone Joint Surg Br 2002;84:38–41.

68. Graf BK, Lange RH, Fujisaki CK, et al. Anterior cruciate ligament tears in skeletally immature patients: meniscal pathology at presentation and after attempted conservative treatment. Arthroscopy 1992;8:229–33.

69. McCarroll JR, Rettig AC, Shelbourne KD. Anterior cruciate ligament injuries in the young athlete with open physes. Am J Sports Med 1988;16:44–7.

70. Lee K, Siegel MJ, Lau DM, et al. Anterior cruciate ligament tears: MR imaging-based diagnosis in a pediatric population. Radiology 1999;213:697–704.

71. Snearly WN, Kaplan PA, Dussault RG. Lateral-compartment bone contusions in adolescents with intact anterior cruciate ligaments. Radiology 1996;198:205–8.

72. Coursey RL Jr, Jones EA, Chaljub G, et al. Prospective analysis of uncomplicated bone bruises in the pediatric knee. Emerg Radiol 2006; 12:266–71.

73. Manner HM, Radler C, Ganger R, et al. Dysplasia of the cruciate ligaments: radiographic assessment and classification. J Bone Joint Surg Am 2006;88: 130–7.

74. Benjamin HJ. The female adolescent athlete: specific concerns. Pediatr Ann 2007;36:719–26.

75. Huston LJ, Greenfield ML, Wojtys EM. Anterior cruciate ligament injuries in the female athlete. Potential risk factors. Clin Orthop Relat Res 2000; 372:50–63.

76. Hewett TE, Myer GD, Ford KR. Anterior cruciate ligament injuries in female athletes: part 1, mechanisms and risk factors. Am J Sports Med 2006;34:299–311.

77. Cook PC, Leit ME. Issues in the pediatric athlete. Orthop Clin North Am 1995;26:453–64.

78. Al-Otaibi L, Siegel MJ. The pediatric knee. Magn Reson Imaging Clin N Am 1998;6:643–60.

79. Takeda Y, Ikata T, Yoshida S, et al. MRI high-signal intensity in the menisci of asymptomatic children. J Bone Joint Surg Br 1998;80:463–7.

80. VanderWilde RS, Peterson HA. Meniscal cyst and magnetic resonance imaging in childhood and adolescence. J Pediatr Orthop 1992;12:761–5.

81. Stanitski CL. Correlation of arthroscopic and clinical examinations with magnetic resonance imaging findings of injured knees in children and adolescents. Am J Sports Med 1998;26:2–6.

82. Kocher MS, DiCanzio J, Zurakowski D, et al. Diagnostic performance of clinical examination and selective magnetic resonance imaging in the evaluation of intraarticular knee disorders in children and adolescents. Am J Sports Med 2001;29:292–6.

83. McDermott MJ, Bathgate B, Gillingham BL, et al. Correlation of MRI and arthroscopic diagnosis of knee pathology in children and adolescents. J Pediatr Orthop 1998;18:675–8.

84. Zobel MS, Borrello JA, Siegel MJ, et al. Pediatric knee MR imaging: pattern of injuries in the immature skeleton. Radiology 1994;190:397–401.

85. King SJ, Carty HM, Brady O. Magnetic resonance imaging of knee injuries in children. Pediatr Radiol 1996;26:287–90.

86. Major NM, Beard LN Jr, Helms CA. Accuracy of MR imaging of the knee in adolescents. AJR Am J Roentgenol 2003;180:17–9.

87. Davidson D, Letts M, Glasgow R. Discoid meniscus in children: treatment and outcome. Can J Surg 2003;46:350–8.

88. Ryu KN, Kim IS, Kim EJ, et al. MR imaging of tears of discoid lateral menisci. AJR Am J Roentgenol 1998;171:963–7.

89. Araki Y, Yamamoto H, Nakamura H, et al. MR diagnosis of discoid lateral menisci of the knee. Eur J Radiol 1994;18:92–5.

90. Stark JE, Siegel MJ, Weinberger E, et al. Discoid menisci in children: MR features. J Comput Assist Tomogr 1995;19:608–11.

91. De Maeseneer M, Debaere C, Desprechins B, et al. Popliteal cysts in children: prevalence, appearance and associated findings at MR imaging. Pediatr Radiol 1999;29:605–9.

92. Lang IM, Hughes DG, Williamson JB, et al. MRI appearance of popliteal cysts in childhood. Pediatr Radiol 1997;27:130–2.

93. Beasley LS, Vidal AF. Traumatic patellar dislocation in children and adolescents: treatment update and literature review. Curr Opin Pediatr 2004;16:29–36.

94. Sanders TG, Morrison WB, Singleton BA, et al. Medial patellofemoral ligament injury following acute transient dislocation of the patella: MR

findings with surgical correlation in 14 patients. J Comput Assist Tomogr 2001;25:957–62.

95. Zaidi A, Babyn P, Astori I, et al. MRI of traumatic patellar dislocation in children. Pediatr Radiol 2006;36:1163–70.

96. Elias DA, White LM, Fithian DC. Acute lateral patellar dislocation at MR imaging: injury patterns of medial patellar soft-tissue restraints and osteochondral injuries of the inferomedial patella. Radiology 2002;225:736–43.

97. Swischuk LE, Hernandez JA, Hendrick EP, et al. Lateral femoral condylar shearing fractures. Emerg Radiol 2003;10:19–22.

98. Bruijn JD, Sanders RJ, Jansen BR. Ossification in the patellar tendon and patella alta following sports injuries in children. Complications of sleeve fractures after conservative treatment. Arch Orthop Trauma Surg 1993;112:157–8.

99. Shabshin N, Schweitzer ME, Morrison WB, et al. High-signal T2 changes of the bone marrow of the foot and ankle in children: red marrow or traumatic changes? Pediatr Radiol 2006;36:670–6.

100. Metzl JD. Sports-specific concerns in the young athlete: soccer. Pediatr Emerg Care 1999;15:130–4.

Sports-Related Injury of the Pediatric Spine

Bradley A. Maxfield, MD

KEYWORDS

• Pediatric • Sports-related injuries • Spine • MR imaging
• Nuclear medicine • Spondylolysis

Acute and chronic injuries to the spine represent a very serious concern for young athletes and their parents, coaches, trainers, and physicians. Acute spinal injuries can be catastrophic, and chronic injuries can sharply limit participation, performance, and enjoyment of youth sports.

The manifestation of both acute and repetitive spinal injury in the pediatric population is distinct from that in adults. Lesions common among child athletes, such as spondylolysis, are seen far less frequently in their adult counterparts. Common adult patterns of injury may be uncommon in children and adolescents. The unique mechanics of the growing spine are responsible for these differences. Like with sports injuries that occur elsewhere in the body, periods of rapid growth are when adolescent athletes are at highest risk for spine injury.[1,2]

Participation in sports increases risk for low back pain in children and adolescents.[2,3] Young athletes have a significantly higher risk of spondylolysis, making the workup of these patients with low back pain unique from their adult counterparts.[4] Acute traumatic injuries to the spine, although rare, are a major cause of death and disability in child athletes. Ligamentous and muscular injuries without fracture occur frequently in pediatric patients, significantly increasing the role of MR imaging.

ACUTE SPINAL INJURIES

Acute spinal injury is fortunately rare in youth sports; however, these injuries can be catastrophic. Cervical cord injury can result in quadriplegia or death. Injury to the thoracic and lumbar spine can result in paraplegia. Morbidity and mortality from spinal injuries are less common than traumatic brain injury in child athletes. Traumatic spinal injuries are estimated to occur in 5 to 15 participants per 100,000.[5] The risk of acute spinal injury is increased in sports that involve athlete-to-athlete contact, sports that mechanically increase athlete velocity, and sports that involve elevation above the playing surface. Sports at higher risk for acute spine injuries include motor sports, cycling, diving, skiing, football, ice hockey, wrestling, and gymnastics.[6–13] The rate of significant spinal injuries in contact sports increases steadily with age and ability level. The increased size and speed of participating athletes dramatically increases the energy of collisions on the playing field.[14] In football, for example, there is almost no incidence of severe spinal injury at the Pop Warner level. Collisions occur, but athlete strength and speed is low. The rate of catastrophic spine injury increases steadily from junior high to high school, through college, and beyond.

CERVICAL SPINE INJURIES

The cervical spine is composed of seven vertebrae separated by cartilage discs and supported by multiple ligaments and surrounding musculature. These structures, aligned in a normal lordotic curve, are capable of dissipating significant energy in flexion, extension, rotation, and axial loading. Normal range of motion of the cervical spine is higher at all levels in younger children compared with adolescents and adults. The point of maximal mobility is located higher in the cervical spine in younger children. In children younger than 8 years, maximal mobility is centered in the upper cervical spine, from the C1 through C3 vertebrae,[15] which

Section of Pediatric Radiology, Department of Radiology, University of Wisconsin School of Medicine and Public Health, Clinical Science Center MC 3552, 600 Highland Avenue, Madison, WI 53792–3252, USA
E-mail address: bmaxfield@uwhealth.org

Radiol Clin N Am 48 (2010) 1237–1248
doi:10.1016/j.rcl.2010.07.006

corresponds to higher risk for upper cervical injuries in this population.[16] The level of maximal mobility steadily descends, reaching the mid cervical spine, during the ages of 8 to 12 years. In adolescence, maximal mobility of the cervical spine descends to the C5 through C6 vertebrae, where it remains into adulthood.

Radiographs are the primary tools for initial evaluation of suspected cervical spinal injury. Anteroposterior, lateral, and odontoid views are indicated for children of ages at which most sports injuries occur. Patients with radiographic abnormalities and those with high-risk mechanism of injury require CT scanning with coronal and sagittal reformatting. CT is superior to radiographs and MR imaging for the detection and delineation of spinal fractures. MR imaging is useful to evaluate suspected muscular and ligamentous injury and injury to the spinal cord.

Flexion injuries of the cervical spine result in stretching of the posterior spinal muscle groups and interspinous ligaments. Muscle tears (**Fig. 1**) and ligamentous tears and sprains (**Fig. 2**) result when the maximal elasticity is exceeded. In flexion, compression of anterior elements occurs, which can result in compression fracture of the vertebral bodies (**Fig. 3**). Cervical flexion results in straightening of the cervical lordosis, which results in a significant decrease in the capacity of the vertebral column and surrounding tissue to dissipate axial energy. Flexion, combined with axial loading, is frequently implicated in severe cervical spine injury in contact sports.[8,17] When maximum energy dissipation is exceeded in this position, the spine will buckle in flexion. This high-energy buckling results in burst fractures of the vertebral bodies, with retropulsion of vertebral body fragments into the spinal canal, or subluxation with the potential for severe cord injury (**Fig. 4**). Combined rotational forces can result in more severe subluxation secondary to increased disruption of supporting tissue.

Flexion fractures occur most commonly at the C5 and C6 vertebral levels in adolescents but may be higher in younger children. Helmet-first football tackles, known as *spearing*, are the most frequent example of this mechanism of injury. Rules banning spearing at the high school and college levels, enacted in the mid-1970s, dramatically reduced the rate of cervical spine injuries. Hockey players checked to the ice and impacting the boards with the top of the helmet is another mechanism of axial loading in flexion that has resulted in severe cord injury and death. Axial loading injuries can also occur in gymnastics, diving, and cheerleading.[13,17,18] Common risk factors in these sports include violent collisions,

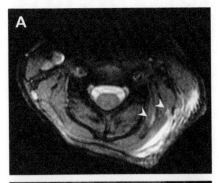

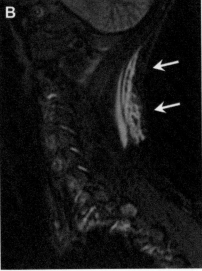

Fig. 1. Ten-year-old male football player injured when his facemask was twisted to the left and his neck was forcibly flexed. Axial T2 star-weighted gradient echo image (*A*) shows tears of the right erector spinae muscles (*arrowheads*). Sagittal fat-saturated T2-weighted image (*B*) shows overlying hematoma (*arrows*).

mechanical increases in acceleration, and elevation of the athlete above the playing surface.

The large range of motion in extension makes the cervical spine vulnerable to hyperextension injury.[5] The range of motion in hyperextension injury is not physically limited until the occiput meets the upper back. In flexion, maximal motion of the spine is physically limited by the chin contacting the upper chest, and the relative strength of the posterior cervical soft tissues provides more resistance. The anterior cervical soft tissues are less robust than the posterior tissues, providing relatively less resistance to forced hyperextension (**Fig. 5**). Cervical hyperextension injuries in pediatric sports result from falls, whiplash injuries, and blows to the anterior head. As in flexion injuries, the addition of rotational forces

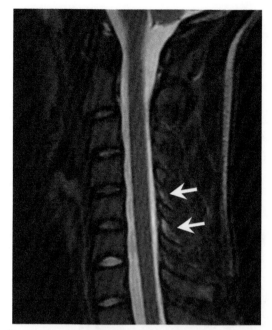

Fig. 2. Thirteen-year-old male football player injured in a helmet-to-helmet collision. He had concussive symptoms and complained of neck pain and paresthesia. Sagittal fat-saturated T2-weighted image shows high signal in the interspinous ligaments at the C4 through C5 and C5 through C6 vertebrae (*arrows*).

to hyperextension results in more instability and increases the risk of neural injury. Just as in flexion injuries in American football, rule changes can also be highly effective in preventing hyperextension

injuries. Significant reductions in cervical spine injuries, many resulting from hyperextension, were seen after restriction of the "high tackle" in South African youth rugby.[19]

THORACOLUMBAR SPINE INJURIES

Acute fractures of the thoracolumbar spine occur less commonly than cervical injuries. They are also less likely to result in catastrophic spinal cord injury. Compression fractures are the most common thoracolumbar fractures seen in young athletes (**Fig. 6**). Mechanisms of injury include axial loading, hyperflexion, and hyperextension. Axial loading is often precipitated by falls landing in a sitting position, often with combined hyperflexion. This mechanism is seen in gymnastics, diving, and jumping sports. Thoracic and lumbar spinal fractures also occur with violent collisions in contact sports such as ice hockey, football, and rugby. Avulsion fractures of the posterior elements can occur in the thoracic and lumbar spine during acute trauma or training. Avulsion of the spinous process of the C7 or T1 vertebrae, known as a *clay-shoveler fracture*, is seen in gymnasts, football linemen, and weightlifters (**Fig. 7**). Avulsion and impingement injury is also seen in the lumbar spinous and transverse processes, commonly in dancers, divers, and gymnasts.

DISK HERNIATION

Acute disk herniation is significantly less common in young athletes than in adults. The clinical presentation can be less clear in children, who often lack sciatica. Unique to the adolescent spine

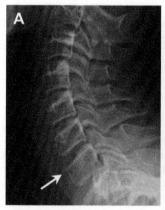
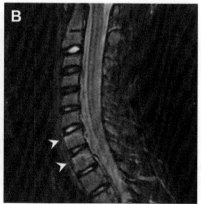

Fig. 3. Fifteen-year-old male hockey player who fell and struck the boards with his helmet. Lateral radiograph of the cervical spine (*A*) shows anterior compression of the C7 vertebral body (*arrow*). Sagittal short tau inversion recovery (STIR) images (*B*) show edema in the C7 and T1 vertebral bodies with mild upper endplate compression (*arrowheads*).

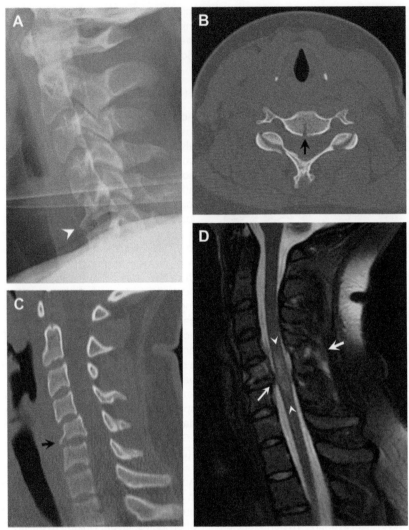

Fig. 4. Fifteen-year-old female swimmer who was practicing dives and struck the bottom of the pool. She initially had complete loss of motion of her extremities with minimal return of function en route to the hospital. Lateral radiograph of the cervical spine (*A*) shows anterior compression of C5 (*white arrowhead*). Axial CT image (*B*) shows a splitting fracture of C5 in the sagittal plane (*black arrow*). Sagittal reconstructed CT image (*C*) shows a flexion teardrop fracture of the anterior inferior edge of C5 (*black arrowhead*) with posterior displacement of the C5 vertebral body. Sagittal fat-saturated T2-weighted MR image (*D*) show spinal cord edema from the C4 through C6 vertebrae (*white arrowheads*). Disruption of the posterior longitudinal ligament and posterior interspinous ligaments is present at the C4 through C5 and C5 through C6 vertebrae (*white arrows*).

is intervertebral disk herniation associated with avulsion fracture of the apophyseal ring (Fig. 8).[20] The apophyseal ring forms at approximately 5 years of age and completely fuses with the vertebral body between 18 to 20 years of age. The attachment of the apophyseal ring to the annulus fibrosis by the Sharpey's fibers is stronger than the fibrocartilage junction with the vertebral body. The apophyseal ring is similarly firmly attached to the posterior longitudinal ligament. When a fracture occurs through the growing cartilage, the ossified fragment remains attached to the annulus and posterior longitudinal ligament. Unlike in the adult population, in whom degenerative changes to the annulus are seen in disk disease, adolescent disk protrusion is more often secondary to destabilization of the annulus from apophyseal injury (Fig. 9).

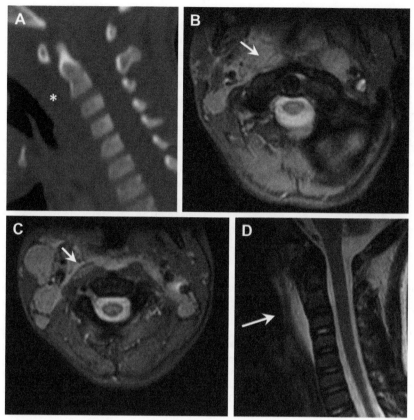

Fig. 5. Six-year-old male soccer player who slipped on a soccer ball while running, falling in a sitting position with hyperextension of his neck. CT shows (A) abnormal thickness of the prevertebral soft tissue (*asterisk*) but no fracture. Axial T2 MEDIC (multiecho data image combination) images (B–C) show signal abnormality in the right longus colli and longus capitus muscles indicating a partial muscle tear (*arrows*). Sagittal fat-saturated T2-weighted images (D) show a related prevertebral hematoma (*arrow*).

SPONDYLOLYSIS

Low back pain is a common complaint among adolescent athletes across various sports. Back pain can impair performance and limit participation. The origin of back pain in young athletes is significantly different from that in adults, requiring a differing radiologic approach to workup. The most striking difference is the high incidence of symptomatic spondylolysis. Spondylolysis is a defect of the pars interarticularis of the vertebral posterior elements. Spondylolysis was classified by Wiltse and colleagues[21] in 1976 (Table 1). These type II (isthmic) lesions are the subtype seen as sports-related injuries in pediatric athletes. Among adolescent athletes with a chief complaint of low back pain, 47% have spondylolysis, compared with an incidence of only 5% in adult controls.[4]

Because of the high incidence of spondylolysis in child athletes with back pain, early imaging of the lumbar spine is very important for diagnosis and treatment. Plain radiographs of the lumbar spine are useful primary tools in the diagnosis of spondylolysis. Four views of the lumbar spine, including anteroposterior, lateral, and bilateral oblique images, are recommended for the evaluation of suspected spondylolysis. Bilateral oblique images offer the best direct visualization of the pars interarticularis. In the oblique projection, the posterior elements of the lumbar vertebrae mimic the profile of a Scottish terrier or "Scottie dog" (Fig. 10). Spondylolysis seen on oblique radiographs is likened to a collar or a break in the dog's neck (Fig. 11). Approximately 20% of pars defects are seen only on oblique radiographs. A spot lateral view centered at the lumbosacral junction can also increase sensitivity (Fig. 12).

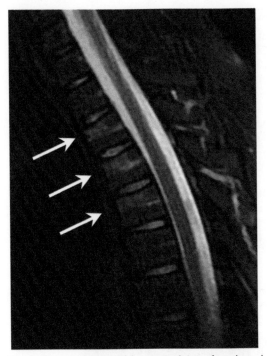

Fig. 6. Fourteen-year-old boy complains of neck and back pain after a fall during a basketball game. Sagittal fat-saturated T2-weighted image shows edema in the upper endplates of the T2 through T4 vertebrae (*arrows*).

Lateral views of the lumbar spine are also useful to detect and grade associated spondylolisthesis. Radiographs are also sensitive to unilateral pars defects. In addition to direct visualization of the lesion, sclerosis of the contralateral pedicle can be seen as a result of stress from a unilateral pars defect. This finding is often seen on the anterior view, where the pedicles can be directly compared for symmetry (**Fig. 13**).

Spondylolysis may occur at any vertebral level, but 85% to 95% of pediatric lesions occur at the L5 vertebra. L4 spondylolysis represents 5% to 15% of pediatric spondylolysis. Pars defects above the L4 vertebra are uncommon. Spondylolysis can be unilateral or bilateral. Patients with unilateral spondylolysis may acquire a defect on the contralateral side from mechanical stress (**Fig. 14**). Spondylolisthesis, forward displacement of the vertebral body on the level below, is more common when pars defects are bilateral (**Fig. 15**).

The Meyerding classification is used to grade spondylolisthesis based on the severity of the translation (**Table 2**).[22] Isthmic spondylolysis is considered to be secondary to mechanical stress on the lumbar posterior elements. In athletes, mechanical stress may occur from repetitive microtrauma, acute shearing forces, acute loading forces, or a combination. Spondylolysis is seen at a increased rate

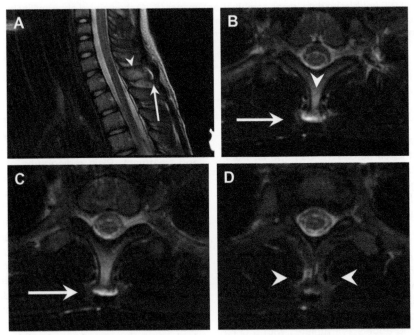

Fig. 7. Fifteen-year-old male swimmer who has had upper back pain since a weight training session. Sagittal T2-weighted fast relaxation fast spin echo (FRFSE) (*A*) and axial T2-weighted FRFSE (*B–D*) show avulsion of the tip of the T1 spinous process (*arrows*). Edema is seen in the proximal aspect of the spinous process and surrounding tissue (*arrowheads*).

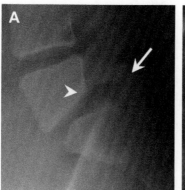
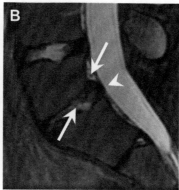

Fig. 8. Fifteen-year-old male football lineman with low back pain. He is also a base drummer in a marching band. Lateral radiographs of the lumbar spine (*A*) show bilateral spondylolysis of the L5 vertebra (*arrow*) with grade 1 spondylolisthesis of L5 on S1. An abnormal contour of the posterior aspect of the inferior endplate of L5 is also seen (*arrowhead*). Sagittal fat-saturated T2-weighted MR image (*B*) shows associated posterior ring apophyseal separation at the lower endplate of the L5 vertebra (*arrow*) with L5-S1 disk herniation (*arrowhead*).

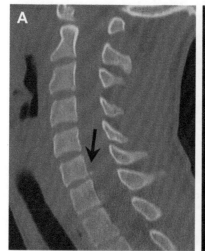
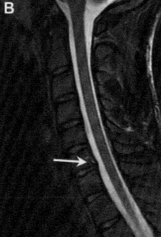

Fig. 9. Apophyseal ring injury. Sagittal CT reconstructed image (*A*) shows a bulging C5-6 disk and posterior displacement of a fragment of the posterior apophyseal ring. Sagittal fat-saturated T2-weighted image (*B*) shows fluid between the vertebral body and the elevated posterior longitudinal ligament (*arrow*).

Table 1
The Wiltse, Newman, and Macnab classification of spondylolysis

Type I	Dysplastic	Congenital deformity of the posterior arch
Type II	Isthmic	Lesions of the pars interarticularis with three subtypes: Type IIA: Lytic fatigue fracture of the pars Type IIB: Elongated but intact pars Type IIC: Acute fracture of the pars
Type III	Degenerative	From longstanding intersegmental instability
Type IV	Traumatic	From fractures in areas of the bony hook other than the pars
Type V	Pathologic	Generalized or local bone disease

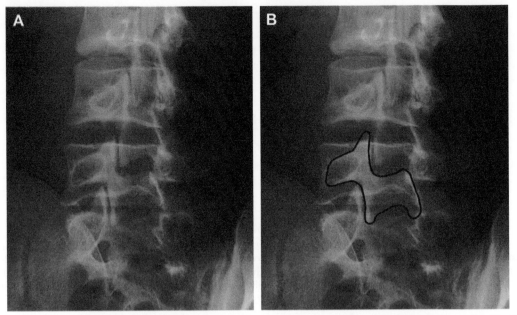

Fig. 10. Oblique radiograph of the lumbar spine (*A*) showing normal posterior elements of L5 and the "Scottie dog" silhouette (*B*).

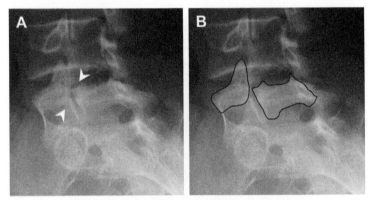

Fig. 11. Spondylolysis. Oblique radiograph of the lumbar spine (*A*) shows spondylolysis in the right pars interarticularis of L5 (*arrowheads*). The broken neck of the "Scottie dog" (*B*).

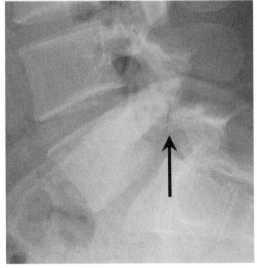

Fig. 12. Spondylolysis. Coned lateral radiograph of the lumbosacral junction shows spondylolysis of the pars interarticularis of L5 (*arrow*).

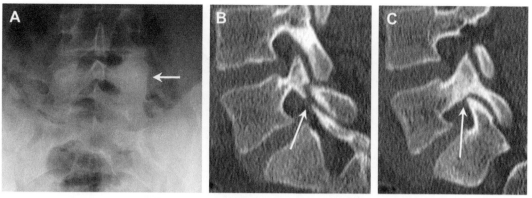

Fig. 13. Fourteen-year-old male football player with low back pain. Anteroposterior radiograph of the lumbar spine (*A*) shows sclerosis of the pedicle of L5 on the left (*arrow*). Sagittal reformatted CT images (*B*) confirm unilateral spondylolysis on the right and (*C*) stress reaction with sclerosis of the pars interarticularis and pedicle on the left (*arrows*).

among athletes participating in many common youth sports, including soccer, football, gymnastics, swimming and diving.[12,13,23,24] Repetitive loading and repeated flexion and extension are implicated in most sports with higher rates of spondylolysis. The powerful kicking motion in soccer rapidly ranges the lumbar spine through extension to hyperflexion while asymmetrically loading and rotating the lumbar vertebrae.[25] Gymnastic training and competition places significant stress on the lower back. Positional stressors in gymnastics include hyperextension, hyperflexion, and

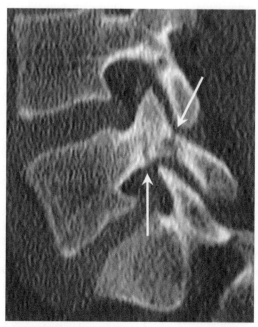

Fig. 14. The patient from Fig. 13 was imaged 6 months later after experiencing continued pain despite bracing and physical therapy. Sagittal reformatted CT images showed new stress fractures of the pars interarticularis and pedicle on the left (*arrows*).

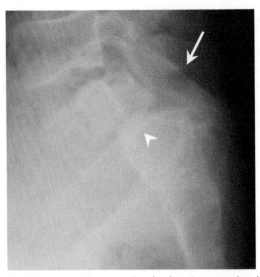

Fig. 15. Fifteen-year-old male high jumper with worsening back pain. Lateral radiographs of the lumbar spine show bilateral spondylolysis of L5 (*arrow*). L5 has slipped anteriorly relative to S1 between 50% and 75% of the vertebral diameter (*arrowhead*); this is classified as Meyerding grade 3 spondylolisthesis.

hyperlordosis. Additionally, frequent axial loading occurs during dismounts. Incidence of spondylolysis in football depends on the position played. The highest rates are seen among linemen, whose powerful blocking results in extension and loading of the lumbar spine on nearly every down.

In pediatric athletes with new symptoms suggesting spondylolysis but normal radiographs, further imaging is indicated. Bone scan with single photon emission CT (SPECT) and CT have historically been the favored secondary imaging modalities. Both CT and bone scan have been shown to be sensitive in the detection of radiographically

occult pars defects. CT shows greater bony detail and alignment but does not provide physiologic information. Increased uptake in the pars, lamina, or pedicle on SPECT bone scan images suggests symptomatic spondylolysis, stress reaction, or stress fracture (**Fig. 16**). SPECT is also used to guide treatment of radiographically diagnosed lesions.[26] Spondylolytic lesions with active uptake on nuclear imaging may better respond to conservative treatment, such as activity restriction or bracing. Radiographic pars defects without uptake on scintigraphy are often asymptomatic. Other origins of the patient's pain should be excluded in these cases (**Fig. 17**). CT and MR imaging are useful to exclude alternate pathology, such as infection or osteoid osteoma.

MR imaging continues to develop as a useful tool in the diagnosis and workup of spondylolysis. MR imaging, although less sensitive in detecting pars lesions, is improving in its ability to detect complete pars defects. It is also useful to detect edema early in the course of stress lesions, in both the pars and the adjacent lamina and pedicles (**Fig. 18**). Although MR signal change is a less direct indication of reparative change than increased uptake on bone scan, MR imaging may be useful in detecting early lesions that better respond to therapy.[27] The lack of ionizing radiation in MR imaging is a distinct advantage over both CT and bone scan.

Table 2 The Meyerding classification of spondylolisthesis	
Grade 1	1%–25% anterior translation
Grade 2	26%–50% anterior translation
Grade 3	51%–75% anterior translation
Grade 4	76%–100% anterior translation
Grade 5[a]	<100% anterior translation

[a] Grade 5 is commonly applied to 100% slip or spondyloptosis, but this was not included in the original description.

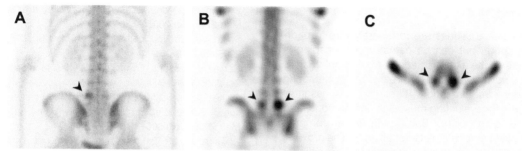

Fig. 16. Sixteen-year-old male football player with low back pain. Tc 99m MDP scintigraphy of the lumbar spine in the posterior projection (*A*) shows abnormal uptake at L5 on the right (*arrowhead*). Coronal (*B*) and axial (*C*) single photon emission CT (SPECT) slices more precisely shows the uptake in the pedicles and pars interarticularis of L5 on the right and less pronounced uptake on the left (*arrowheads*).

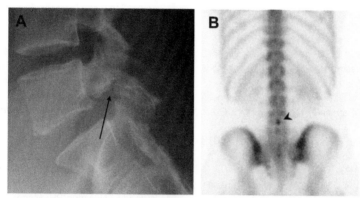

Fig. 17. Sixteen-year-old female diver who had sharp pain posterior low back pain while executing an arching reverse dive. Lateral radiograph of the lumbar spine (*A*) shows spondylolysis at L5 (*arrow*). Tc 99m medronate scintigraphy of the lumbar spine in the posterior projection (*B*) shows no abnormal activity in the region of the pars defects. Abnormal uptake is seen at the tip of the L4 spinous process (*arrowhead*). Clinically the L4 spinous process was very tender to direct palpation. She was diagnosed with "kissing spine" syndrome, or impingement of the spinous processes in positions of hyperflexion.

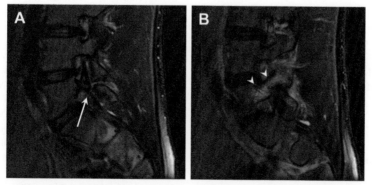

Fig. 18. Fifteen-year-old male football player with back pain during practice. Coronal fat-saturated T2-weighted MR image (*A*) shows spondylolysis on the right (*arrow*). On the left (*B*), abnormal high signal is seen in the pars interarticularis, lamina, and pedicle, consistent with stress reaction (*arrowheads*).

SUMMARY

Acute spinal injuries are fortunately rare in pediatric sports but can be catastrophic. Imaging is integral to the diagnosis and care of spinal trauma. Plain radiographs and CT are critical for detecting vertebral fracture, and MR imaging is an essential adjunct for evaluating muscular, ligamentous, and spinal cord injury. Back pain is a common complaint among athletes of all ages. The growing spine has unique weaknesses that result in a higher rate of detectable radiologic abnormalities. Disk pathology is less common in children, and is often uniquely associated with fracture of the ring apophyses. Spondylolysis is far more prevalent in youth athletes than in their adult counterparts, requiring a different approach to imaging for assessment of adolescent back pain.

REFERENCES

1. Grimmer K, Williams M. Gender-age environmental associates of adolescent low back pain. Appl Ergon 2000;31(4):343–60.
2. Kujala UM, Taimela S, Erkintalo M, et al. Low-back pain in adolescent athletes. Med Sci Sports Exerc 1996;28(2):165–70.
3. Burton AK, Clarke RD, McClune TD, et al. The natural history of low back pain in adolescents. Spine 1996;21(20):2323–8.
4. Micheli LJ, Wood R. Back pain in young athletes. Significant differences from adults in causes and patterns. Arch Pediatr Adolesc Med 1995;149(1):15–8.
5. Proctor MR, Cantu RC. Head and neck injuries in young athletes. Clin Sports Med 2000;19(4):693–715.
6. Mueller F, Cantu RC. NCCSIR eighteenth annual report. National Center for Catastrophic Sport Injury Research: Fall 1982–Spring 2000. Chapel Hill (NC): National Center for Catastrophic Sport Injury Research; 2000.
7. Caine DJ, Maffulli N. Epidemiology of children's individual sports injuries. An important area of medicine and sport science research. Med Sport Sci 2005;48:1–7.
8. Waninger KN. Management of the helmeted athlete with suspected cervical spine injury. Am J Sports Med 2004;32(5):1331–50.
9. Luckstead EF, Patel DR. Catastrophic pediatric sports injuries. Pediatr Clin North Am 2002;49(3):581–91.
10. Maffulli N, Caine D. The epidemiology of children's team sports injuries. Med Sport Sci 2005;49:1–8.
11. Benson BW, Meeuwisse WH. Ice hockey injuries. Med Sport Sci 2005;49:86–119.
12. Stuart MJ. Gridiron football injuries. Med Sport Sci 2005;49:62–85.
13. Caine DJ, Nassar L. Gymnastics injuries. Med Sport Sci 2005;48:18–58.
14. Caine D, Caine C, Maffulli N. Incidence and distribution of pediatric sport-related injuries. Clin J Sport Med 2006;16(6):500–13.
15. Kewalramani LS, Tori JA. Spinal cord trauma in children. Neurologic patterns, radiologic features, and pathomechanics of injury. Spine (Phila Pa 1976) 1980;5(1):11–8.
16. Dietrich AM, Ginn-Pease ME, Bartkowski HM, et al. Pediatric cervical spine fractures: predominantly subtle presentation. J Pediatr Surg 1991;26(8):995–9 [discussion: 999–1000].
17. Torg JS. Epidemiology, pathomechanics, and prevention of football-induced cervical spinal cord trauma. Exerc Sport Sci Rev 1992;20:321–38.
18. Torg JS, Gennarelli TA. Catastrophic Head and Neck Injuries. Adolesc Med 1991;2(1):155–80.
19. Noakes TD, Jakoet I, Baalbergen E. An apparent reduction in the incidence and severity of spinal cord injuries in schoolboy rugby players in the western Cape since 1990. S Afr Med J 1999;89(5):540–5.
20. Peh WC, Griffith JF, Yip DK, et al. Magnetic resonance imaging of lumbar vertebral apophyseal ring fractures. Australas Radiol 1998;42(1):34–7.
21. Wiltse LL, Newman PH, Macnab I. Classification of spondylolisis and spondylolisthesis. Clin Orthop Relat Res 1976;117:23–9.
22. Meyerding H. Spondylolisthesis. J Bone Joint Surg 1931;13:39–48.
23. Giza E, Micheli LJ. Soccer injuries. Med Sport Sci 2005;49:140–69.
24. Nyska M, Constantini N, Cale-Benzoor M, et al. Spondylolysis as a cause of low back pain in swimmers. Int J Sports Med 2000;21(5):375–9.
25. El Rassi G, Takemitsu M, Woratanarat P, et al. Lumbar spondylolysis in pediatric and adolescent soccer players. Am J Sports Med 2005;33(11):1688–93.
26. Bellah RD, Summerville DA, Treves ST, et al. Low-back pain in adolescent athletes: detection of stress injury to the pars interarticularis with SPECT. Radiology 1991;180(2):509–12.
27. Sairyo K, Katoh S, Takata Y, et al. MRI signal changes of the pedicle as an indicator for early diagnosis of spondylolysis in children and adolescents: a clinical and biomechanical study. Spine (Phila Pa 1976) 2006;31(2):206–11.

The Female Athlete

Carol A. Boles, MD[a,*], Cristin Ferguson, MD[b]

KEYWORDS

• Female-specific injury • Anterior cruciate ligament
• Patellofemoral pain syndrome • Female athlete triad

HISTORY

Women have always engaged in some form of athletic activity. Some important milestones give a glimpse of the history of women in athletics. Although the first Olympics were held in 776 BC, women were excluded from those games, both in competition and as spectators. As an alternative, every 4 years women competed in a foot race set up for various age groups.[1] Spartans, being known for their military power, believed that it was important to have strong, healthy, active women so that their sons would be strong soldiers. Girls received an education and participated in sports with the boys.[2] The first female to win an Olympic event was Kyniska, a Spartan princess. She was the owner of the 4-horse chariot team that won the race (the 8-mile tethrippon). The owners, not the charioteers, were considered the winners. As a woman, she was not permitted to accept her prize in person.

In 1567 Mary, Queen of Scots, an avid golfer, was chastised by the church for playing golf a few days following the murder of her second husband.[3] The first professional female athlete was the British boxer, Elizabeth Stokes, who won 3 guineas in 1722.[4] In 1900, 22 women participated in the Olympic Games (the second of the modern Olympics) in Paris, playing tennis, golf, and croquet.[5] The official international Olympic Committee Web site, http://www.olympic.org, lists Margaret Ives Abbott as a gold medal winner for the United States (golf) with Marion Jones a bronze (tennis) and Pauline Whittier a silver (golf). Charlotte Cooper of Great Britain won gold in tennis (singles and mixed doubles).

In the United States, athletic participation by women has increased dramatically over the last several decades. Much of this growth may be attributed to Title IX, which assured funding for women's athletic programs. Since 1972, there has been over a 10-fold increase in sports participation in high school by girls according to data from the National Federation of State High School Associations.

INJURY RISK: MALE VERSUS FEMALE

As sports participation increased, injuries did as well. It became apparent that injury patterns between male and female athletes differed. In general, women are at a greater risk for injuries than men. Of course, when certain injury patterns are isolated, there are some more common in men than women, such as glenohumeral joint instability.[6] There are several reasons for the differences in injury rates. Some are anatomy related, some physiologic. Injuries may be related to sports, either through different mechanics[7] or being related to gender-specific sports. Anterior cruciate ligament (ACL) tears, patellofemoral pain syndrome, chronic ankle sprains, hip pain, stress fractures, back pain, and lateral epicondylitis are more common in the female athlete.[8] However, at least one study has found no difference in injury patterns between men and women competing in comparable sports.[8]

ANATOMIC AND PHYSIOLOGIC DIFFERENCES BETWEEN MAN AND WOMAN

In general, women have shorter and smaller limbs relative to body size; a woman's shorter legs and

[a] Department of Radiology, Wake Forest University Baptist Medical Center, Medical Center Boulevard, Winston-Salem, NC 27157, USA
[b] Department of Orthopedic Surgery, Wake Forest University Baptist Medical Center, Medical Center Boulevard, Winston-Salem, NC 27157, USA
* Corresponding author.
E-mail address: cboles@wfubmc.edu

Radiol Clin N Am 48 (2010) 1249–1266
doi:10.1016/j.rcl.2010.07.015

wider pelvis mean a lower center of gravity. In addition, her wider pelvis may lead to relative varus of hips, increased femoral anteversion, and an increased Q angle, which may predispose to patellofemoral pain syndrome.[9] Females have relatively more laxity of their joints than males, particularly in the knee, ankle, and elbow.[9]

Although females have lesser muscle strength than males, this is due to lower muscle mass while the muscle present functions equally between sexes.[10] Before puberty, boys and girls have similar muscle mass. At puberty, the influence of testosterone in boys leads to greater muscle mass.[11] Weight training does lead to increase in muscle mass for both sexes. The absolute amount is greater in boys, but proportionally the same between sexes.[12] Studies have shown that women have proportionally less muscle mass in the upper extremity than men[11,13] and, similarly, they have a lesser proportional muscle mass in the upper trunk compared with the lower trunk (Fig. 1).[12]

Androgens in men promote greater lean body weight, with the percentage of body fat greater in women (22%–26%) than in men (12%–16%).[14] Given the same body weight, female athletes have a smaller heart, lower diastolic and systolic blood pressure, and smaller lungs, with resultant decreased effectiveness of aerobic activity.[15]

ACL TEARS AND THE FEMALE ATHLETE

Likely the most well-known difference between injury patterns in male and female athletes is the increased incidence of ACL tears, particularly noncontact tears, in female athletes (Fig. 2). This pattern has been studied often and numerous theories for the difference have been proposed, including anatomic and physiologic differences as well as biomechanical and environmental. Most likely the difference is multifactorial; however, no clear unifying concept has been set forth.

This injury is important as it affects not only the athletes' sports participation currently and in the future, but patients who have had an ACL injury have a greater prevalence of osteoarthritis, regardless of treatment and subsequent sports participation.[16] Joint position sense is impaired in the ACL-deficient knee regardless of stability achieved with muscle strengthening.[17] Ten years after injury nearly half of patients have signs of osteoarthritis, and nearly all do after 15 to 20 years.[18]

National Collegiate Athletic Association (NCAA) statistics have repeatedly shown that female athletes are 2 to 8 times more likely to sustain ACL injuries.[19] The tibiofemoral joint is stabilized dynamically by the quadriceps, hamstrings, and triceps surae. The joint is passively stabilized by the joint capsule, medial and lateral menisci, lateral collateral ligament (LCL), iliotibial band, medial collateral ligament (MCL), ACL, and posterior cruciate ligament (PCL). The hamstrings and ACL resist the forward motion of the tibia relative to the femur, but in flexion, the quadriceps also adds to the resisted motion. Likewise, the PCL and quadriceps resist posterior translation of the tibia relative to the femur. The cruciate ligaments also resist hyperextension of the knee joint and internal rotation of the tibia relative to the femur as well as medial and lateral translation.[20]

Anatomy/Physiology

The ACL size is smaller in women than in men even when normalized for body weight.[21] An increased risk of tear relative to ACL size has been demonstrated.[22,23] The ACL consists of 2 somewhat discrete bundles, the anteromedial and the posterolateral. As with the cruciate ligaments, these bundles are named for the tibial attachments.[24–26] The anteromedial bundle is taut in flexion resisting anterior displacement of

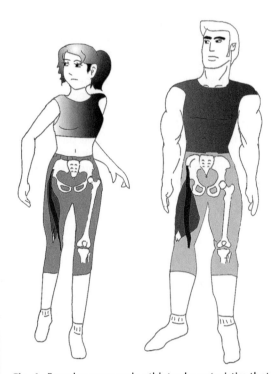

Fig. 1. Female versus male athlete characteristics that may predispose women to some injuries. The female has less upper body strength, and less muscle mass particularly in the vastus medialis obliquus. Also note the wider pelvis, genu valgus, and femoral anteversion and external tibial rotation.

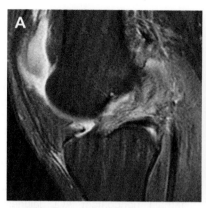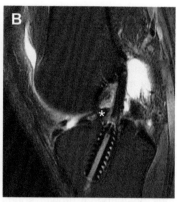

Fig. 2. (*A*) A 17-year-old high school basketball player was going for a loose ball in a game and bent forward, and heard a "pop" in her right knee. Oblique sagittal, fat-suppressed, proton density–weighted MR image (2400/32) reveals the disrupted fibers of the ACL tear. (*B*) Now 19 years old, playing college basketball, she attempted to drive with the ball and felt a "pop" in her right knee. Oblique sagittal, fat-suppressed, proton density–weighted MR (2760/32) demonstrates the intact ACL reconstruction, but a displaced fragment from a medial meniscus bucket-handle tear (*asterisk*).

the tibia between 60° and 90° of flexion.[24] Conversely, the posterolateral bundle is tightened in extension and resists the anterior translation at near full extension.[24] Isolated tears can occur; the anteromedial bundle injured when the knee is in greater flexion and the posterolateral bundle injured in extension.[27,28]

In adolescence, the growing bones about the knee lead to an increase in torque on the knee joint.[29] Boys tend to compensate through increased strength more so than girls.[29,30] As a male grows, femoral condylar width increases as does the femoral condylar notch width. However, females do not have a corresponding increase in condylar notch width.[22] Several studies have reported that those with a narrowed femoral condylar notch have an increased likelihood of and severity of ACL tears.[23,31,32] Others have reported no difference.[33,34]

The Q angle—quadriceps femoris angle—is typically measured on a standing radiograph, as the angle is greatest in full extension.[35] There is variability in the Q angle based on flexion, relaxed or tightened quadriceps muscle, woman or man, supine or standing. The angle is formed by lines connecting the anterior superior iliac spine to the midpoint of the patella and the midpoint patella to the tibial tubercle (**Fig. 3**).[36] The Q angle is greater in women than in men.[37,38] A normal Q angle for women is 17° and for men 14°. A larger Q angle increases lateral pull on the quadriceps muscles, adding medial stress to the knee, which likely increases the risk for ACL tear.[39] Q angles are larger in athletes who sustain an ACL injury than in those who do not.[39] An increased Q angle has been shown to predict future ACL injury risk in some studies,[40] but not in others.[41]

Hormonal factors may play a role. Estrogen receptors are found in human ACL fibroblasts.[42] Furthermore, when estrogen is present, the synthesis of collagen by these fibroblasts is

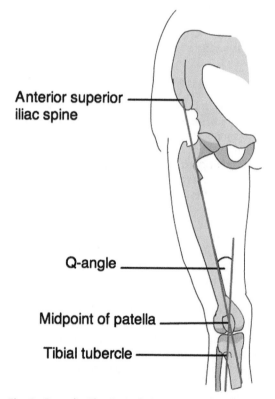

Fig. 3. Q angle. The Q angle is measured by drawing a line between the anterior superior iliac spine and the midpoint of the patella and a second line between the midpoint of the patella and the tibial tubercle. The Q angle is formed between these 2 lines.

reduced, which may decrease strength and thus increase risk of injury.[42,43] High levels of estrogen have also been shown to decrease neuromuscular control of the knee and increase knee laxity.[42,44–46] The greatest injury rate seems to occur during the early and late follicular phases of the menstrual cycle, but the evidence is inconclusive.[47] Other studies have shown no difference during different phases of the menstrual cycle.[48,49] Although the use of oral contraceptives decreases levels of estrogen in females, studies have shown lowered ACL injuries[19,50] or no effect.[51]

Boys have neuromuscular growth spurts proportional to their postpubertal growth spurts whereas girls have a disproportionate increase in height and weight.[29] Females are also more likely to have leg dominance, an imbalance among muscle strength, flexibility, and coordination, which has been associated with increased risk of ACL tear.[52] Coactivation of hamstrings and quadriceps is important to knee dynamic stability.[42] Females have been shown to have quadriceps-dominant contraction during landing and cutting.[52] In addition, women athletes have a low ratio of medial to lateral quadriceps recruitment and increased lateral hamstring firing.[53] These mechanisms compress the lateral joint, open the medial joint, and increase anterior shear force, thus increasing the stress on the ACL.[54]

Biomechanical Factors

Sixty to seventy percent of athletic ACL injuries are noncontact, meaning an indirect force is applied to the ligament.[52,55] The action is frequently during planting, cutting, and landing maneuvers.[56] When force is applied to the knee, the surrounding muscles contract and the knee stiffens, which dissipates the force on the ACL throughout the knee. Muscle stiffness is important in maintaining knee stability and injury prevention.[57] However, flexibility has been shown to increase in women and decrease in men following puberty.[42] Ford and colleagues[58] have shown that hamstring laxity can delay muscle contraction of the hamstrings as well as the cocontraction of the quadriceps during foot strike, increasing the risk of ACL injury. Joint laxity in the knee itself can potentially lead to ACL strain by increasing hyperextension, valgus, and anterior tibial translation.[42] The effect of laxity remains controversial, as studies have reported an association with ACL injuries[23,59] whereas others have not found laxity to be a contributing factor.[60]

Landing from a jump is different between male and female athletes. Females have increased rectus femoris firing and decreased gluteal muscle firing compared with their male counterparts.[61]

Decreased hip/gluteal muscle activation reduces maximal quadriceps and hamstring activation and increases the force placed on the lower extremities.[42,52] Fatigue was also found to affect landing and cutting movements, increasing anterior tibial translation by nearly a third over the nonfatigued athlete.[62] Fatigue contributes to a decrease in knee flexion and an increase in knee varus.[63] No studies have looked at the effect of fatigue on ACL injuries; however, a greater likelihood of injury has been shown during practice as compared with competition.[19]

Hutchinson and Ireland[56] have shown that female noncontact ACL injuries occur during planting and cutting (29%), straight knee landing (28%), or one-step landing with the knee hyperextended (26%). In general, females perform cutting maneuvers in a more erect position than men[64] with decreased flexion at the knee and hip, increased valgus stress at the knee, and greater activation of the quadriceps.[64] The "position of no return," which places the ACL at risk, is an awkward out-of-control landing with the body more upright and the leg in pronation, and the knee in valgus angulation (Fig. 4).[37] Controversy persists as to whether there is a difference in knee flexion during landing between men and women and, if there is a difference, which group has greater flexion or extension.[65–67] However, altering the position during landing or cutting and strengthening programs may actually decrease ACL injuries.[55,64,68]

Anatomic/biometric features of the ankle and hip have also been studied in their relationship to ACL tears. Women have a greater maximum ankle eversion than men, particularly noted during cutting maneuvers, which may increase valgus stress on the knee.[69] Foot pronation, seen with navicular drop, can affect tibial translation and lower extremity alignment, moving the tibia forward and increasing internal tibial rotation.[70,71] Individuals with ACL tears have been shown to have greater navicular drop.[72] Lephart and colleagues[73] has reported that women have greater internal rotation of the hip during landing than male athletes. Gluteus maximus, which controls excessive hip rotation, is less activated in female than in male athletes.[61] Women also tend to land with greater hip adduction and less hip flexion, which may ultimately lead to increased knee valgus, putting strain on the ACL.[42]

Skill Level Differences and Training

The skill level of an athlete has been evaluated with regard to its potential relationship to ACL tears. Using NCAA data and presuming that higher skill

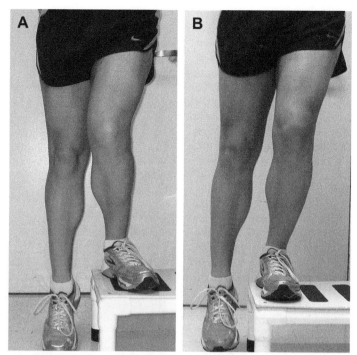

Fig. 4. (A) "Position of no return" that places the ACL at risk during landing or cutting. The left leg has adduction and internal rotation of the hip. The knee is in valgus with external rotation of the tibia, and the foot pronated with weight on the ball of the foot. (B) A safer landing position has flexion at the hip with less or no adduction. The knee is flexed without tibial rotation, and the foot balanced.

levels play at a higher NCAA level, Harmon and Dick[74] reported that there was no difference in ACL injuries based on skill level. However, a study of male soccer players found that injury levels were greater in the more skilled divisions.[75] Although the experience level of female basketball and soccer players has increased over the past several years, ACL injury rates have stayed the same.[76] In addition, despite the awareness and attempts to decrease the rate of ACL tears in men and women, there has been no decrease in the rate of tears.[77]

Environment

Environmental factors may also affect injuries. For example, the altered friction between shoes and surface type may influence movement patterns and either increase or decrease the risk of tear. Drier surfaces increase the friction between the 2 surfaces and have a greater ACL injury rate than a wet surface.[78] Artificial turf and its effect on ACL injury rates remains controversial, with varied studies showing an increase or a decrease injury rate with synthetic turf.[79,80] The shoe, specifically cleat size and pattern, has also been shown to affect rates of ACL injuries.[81] The surface-shoe

combination likely depends on sport, typical planting maneuvers, age of the player, and level of play.[82] Most studies have shown that knee braces are ineffective at preventing ACL injuries[83,84] and that long-term use may actually decrease quadriceps strength.[85,86]

PATELLOFEMORAL PAIN SYNDROME

The patellofemoral joint depends on both static and dynamic stabilization, notably the quadriceps mechanism. Proposed mechanisms for pain include overuse, overload, biomechanical problems, and muscular dysfunction.[87] In addition, inflamed synovium or fat also contribute to anterior knee pain.[88]

Patellofemoral pain syndrome (PFPS) is pain in the retropatellar or peripatellar region of the knee with a stable patella. The diagnosis is made after exclusion of intra-articular pathologies, patellar tendinopathy, peripatellar bursitis, plica syndrome, Sinding-Larsen-Johansson syndrome, and Osgood-Schlatter syndrome.[9,89] PFPS is common in female athletes and there is no one causative etiology. PFPS is part of a spectrum that includes excessive lateral pressure syndrome (ELPS)—exaggerated lateral patellar tilt without subluxation, anterior knee pain, and accelerated lateral patellar cartilage loss; and lateral femoral condyle friction syndrome (LFCFS)—impingement of fat between the patellar tendon and lateral femoral condyle, pain worse with extension, infrapatellar point tenderness, associated with patella alta and lateral patellar tracking. Conservative treatment consists of quadriceps stretches, balanced strengthening, orthotics, proprioceptive training, hip external rotator strengthening, and bracing.[9,87] Most athletes do well when treated conservatively, but some do require surgical intervention. It is this subgroup in which imaging may play a role in determining the exact origin of the pain, and thus the appropriate treatment. The magnetic resonance (MR) findings in LFCFS have been described as localized abnormal fat signal in the inferolateral aspect of the patellofemoral joint, occasionally with some apparent cystic changes (**Fig. 5**).[90]

Epidemiology: Extrinsic Versus Intrinsic

PFPS accounts for approximately 25% of all knee complaints in sports medicine clinics.[91,92] Patellofemoral pain is more common in women than men, accounting for 33% of visits by females versus 18% by males, with an age predilection for the second and third decades of life.[93] The incidence is higher in women than in men, 20% versus 7.4%,[9,93] particularly with regard to running, where it is seen in up to 62% of women and 38% of men.[94] Three major factors contributing to PFPS are: lower extremity and patellofemoral malalignment, quadriceps muscle imbalance and/or weakness, and physical overload of the patellofemoral joint.[9,95]

Biomechanical

Forty years ago, Hughston[96] touted that the primary cause of anterior knee pain was extensor mechanism malalignment. A combination of factors, including a shallow trochlear groove, femoral anteversion, patella alta, increased Q angle, and tibial external rotation contribute to maltracking of the patella. A well-formed trochlear groove allows the patella to maintain its track during motion. The patella is more stable during flexion because of muscular support and less stable during extension and the first 20° of flexion. Patella alta has been associated with recurrent dislocation. Normally the patella engages the trochlea at 20° of flexion, but this occurs later with patella alta and there is overall decreased contact between the patella and trochlea.[35] Because of its unique position in the knee joint, proper tracking requires balanced forces acting

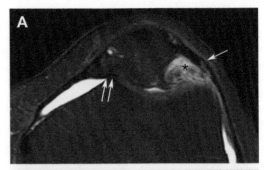

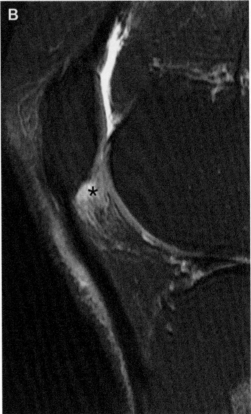

Fig. 5. Lateral femoral condyle pressure syndrome (LFCPS) in a 28-year-old woman. (*A*) Fat-suppressed T2-weighted axial MR image (4600/64) of the knee. The asterisk demonstrates focal signal changes in the fat between the patella and the lateral femoral condyle. She had had a remote lateral retinacular release (*arrow*) and has a medial plica (*double arrow*). (*B*) Sagittal fat-suppressed proton density–weighted MR image (3200/32) of the knee. The abnormal fluid signal is shown in the fat between the patella and lateral femoral condyle (*asterisk*).

on patellar movement, both statically and dynamically. Earl and Vetter[97] graded the etiology into 3 major groups: quadriceps dysfunction, static alignment, and dynamic alignment.

Quadriceps Dysfunction

The primary lateral stabilization of the patella is by the vastus lateralis (VL) via the lateral retinaculum with forces contributed by the biceps femoris, gluteals, and tensor fascia lata transmitted by the iliotibial band. Medial stabilization is from the vastus medialis obliquus (VMO).[98] The medial patellofemoral ligament is the major passive stabilizer, particularly from 0° to 30° of flexion.[35,99] Weakness or delayed firing of the VMO is believed to contribute to lateral tracking.[100,101] However, studies have both supported[102–104] and seemingly disproved[105–107] the relative balance of VMO to VL in PFPS.

Static Malalignment

As already mentioned, the Q angle is the angle formed by the intersection of a line connecting the anterior superior iliac spine and the center of the patella with one from the center of the patella to the tibial tuberosity,[36] and is thought to represent the line force of the quadriceps mechanism so that a larger Q angle reflects greater lateral forces on the patella.[36] However, studies are inconclusive as to the importance of the Q angle in the grand scheme of PFPS.[108]

Static alignment features are femoral neck anteversion, external tibial torsion, and hyperpronation of the foot. Although there is no difference in femoral anteversion between PFPS patients and control subjects,[109,110] femoral anteversion may be a predictor of success of conservative treatment of PFPS.[111] Rather than an independent feature, external tibial torsion may be a compensation for femoral anteversion (feet point laterally with knees forward).[112] Hyperpronation of the foot may be the most important of these features. Hyperpronation causes internal rotation of the tibia during weight placement in gait, preventing the tibia from externally rotating during mid-stance. To compensate, the femur internally rotates to allow the knee to fully lock. This femoral internal rotation during quadriceps firing may increase the lateral forces on the patella as it is compressed against the lateral trochlear groove.[113] There is some support to this theory, as treating PFPS with foot orthotics improves outcomes.[114]

Measurements for patellar maltracking include the tibial tubercle-to-trochlear groove (TT-TG), which is increased from the expected 8 to 15 mm, patellar tilt angle of 20° to 30° (normal <7°), a congruence angle less than 4°, and a decreased sulcus depth from the normal 5 to 7 mm. A trochlear sulcus angle of les than 145° may be considered dysplasia (**Fig. 6**).[35,115] The authors' institution relies mostly on the TT-TG

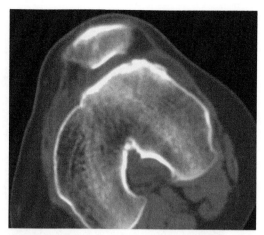

Fig. 6. Dysplasia of the trochlear sulcus. Axial computed tomography (CT) of the knee at the level of the trochlear groove. The sulcus is well over 145°, essentially 180°, in this 28-year-old woman. A subchondral cyst is noted on the lateral femoral condyle with some bony eburnation.

distance. A TT-TG distance of greater than 20 mm is nearly always associated with patellar instability (**Fig. 7**).[116]

Dynamic Malalignment

Clinicians frequently observe a fairly consistent pattern in association with PFPS: excessive contralateral pelvic drop, hip adduction and internal rotation, knee abduction, and tibial external rotation and hyperpronation when patients perform a single-leg squat or step-down (see **Fig. 4**).[117–119] Current thoughts suggest that the lateral tilt of the patella in a non–weight-bearing situation may be physiologic.[120] It is not the patella that is maltracking but rather the femur, which is less well controlled and has greater femoral internal rotation during weight-bearing in PFPS patients compared with controls.[121] Earl and Vetter[97] suggest it is this same motion issue that is also associated with the increased likelihood of ACL tears in the female athlete. Females with PFPS are significantly weakened in isometric hip abduction and external rotation compared with PFPS patients.[122]

ACETABULAR LABRAL TEARS

Although acetabular labral tears were first described in 1957,[123] it has primarily been in the last decade that these injuries have been able to be more clearly evaluated and treated via imaging and hip arthroscopy. The diagnosis often remains difficult because of varied symptoms and changes

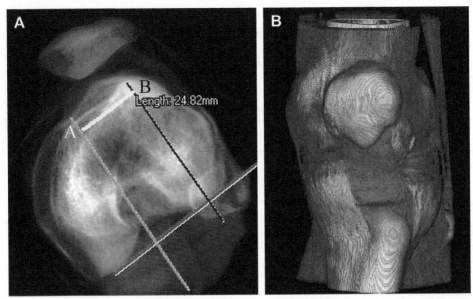

Fig. 7. Tibial tubercle-to-trochlear groove measurement. (*A*) Maximum-intensity projection created from a CT of the knee on a 19-year-old runner. It allows visualization of the tibial tubercle and lowest point of the trochlear groove. Care must be taken to not skew the angle through the knee during reformatting and to identify the correct structures. The trochlear groove low point is A, and the tibial tubercle is B. The distance is measured parallel to a line connecting the posterior aspect of the femoral condyles. In this case, the distance is nearly 25 mm, well above the normal range of 8 to 15 mm. (*B*) Three-dimensional volume reconstruction on the same patient clearly demonstrates the lateral course of the tendon as it courses between the patella and the tibial tubercle.

in nearby structures such as the sacroiliac joints, pelvic floor, and pubis.

The labrum is important to the hip's function. A labrum-free model of the hip demonstrated that contact stress between the femoral head and acetabulum increased up to around 90% compared with a hip with a normal labrum.[124] Athletic activities that require repetitive pivoting motions on a loaded femur have been associated with damage to the acetabular labrum.[123,125] Specific sports, such as soccer, hockey, golf, and ballet, have been linked with labral injury (**Fig. 8**).[126,127] Hip dysplasia, which is more common in women,[128] and femoroacetabular impingement are believed to be initiators of hip disease and osteoarthritis.[129–131] Symptomatic labral tears are more common in women than in men.[126,129,132] Unique to women in the evaluation of groin pain is the possibility of concomitant pelvic floor pain.[133] The obturator externus is thought to be a major cause of pelvic floor pain or deep vaginal pain, and hip abnormalities may lead to abnormal function of this external rotator muscle and possibly pelvic floor pain.[133] With regard to femoroacetabular impingement (FAI), cam-type impingement is more common in young, active male patients with a decreased head-neck

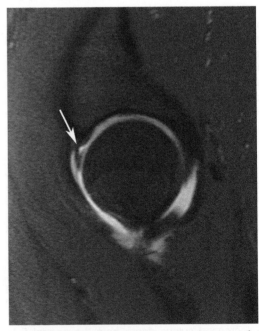

Fig. 8. Labral tear. Sagittal plane, MR arthrogram, fat-suppressed T1-weighted sequence (400/14) in a 15-year-old female karate student demonstrates a tear of the anterior labrum (*arrow*).

offset. Pincer-type impingement is more common in females with excessive femoral head coverage.[134]

Recent reports rate the accuracy of MR arthrography for the diagnosis of labral tears as greater than 95%.[135] Hip injections are successful at localizing pain assumed to have originated from the hip, and are 88% sensitive and 100% specific.[136]

FEMALE ATHLETE TRIAD AND THE MATURING FEMALE ATHLETE

The female athlete triad (FAT) was first described in 1992, and in 1997 a Position Stand by the American College of Sports Medicine characterized the entity as disordered eating, amenorrhea, and osteoporosis.[137] The definition was modified in 2007 to describe the disorder as more of a spectrum than the rigid original definition. Disordered eating is nowadays a spectrum ranging from "optimal energy availability" to "low energy availability +/− eating disorder." Amenorrhea is now a spectrum of "eumenorrhea" to "functional hypothalamic amenorrhea," and osteoporosis is now the spectrum "optimal bone health" to "osteoporosis."[138] Energy availability is the cornerstone of the disorder. More organizations now have Position Stands on FAT, including the American Dietetic Association and the International Olympic Committee.

Although all female athletes are at risk for the triad, sports with an aesthetic component such as ballet, figure skating, and gymnastics, or those sports tied to a weight class, such as tae kwon do, judo, and wrestling, are believed to have a greater risk for athletes to develop FAT. A substantial number of high school athletes (78%) and a surprising number of sedentary students (65%) have one or more components of the triad.[139]

Although athletes with full-blown FAT are fairly uncommon, even one component increases the risk of morbidity in this young female population. A recent study by Torstveit and colleagues[140] found that 46.7% of athletes in sports that stressed leanness had clinical eating disorders compared with 19.8% in non-leanness sports and 21.4% of controls. The 3 disorders in FAT are interrelated through inadequate energy reserves.[137] Those female athletes with disordered eating are more than twice as likely to have menstrual irregularities as those who do not.[139]

Menstrual dysfunction ranges between 6% and 79% in female athletes. This number varies by sport, age, definition and assessment, use of oral contraceptives, training volume, and whether or not subclinical dysfunction is assessed (eg, luteal suppression). This menstrual irregularity is important, as athletes with oligomenorrhea or amenorrhea have significantly lower bone mineral density (BMD) than female athletes who are eumenorrheic.[141,142] However, the return of menstrual function does not equate with return to normal BMD. A study of women taking oral contraceptives had a lower BMD than their noncontraceptive counterparts.[143] Hormonal imbalance also carries a theoretical risk of increased cardiovascular disease.[144]

Osteoporosis is a decreased bone mass and density with an increased incidence or risk of fracture in the postmenopausal woman, as stated by a National Institutes of Health Consensus Group in 2000. BMD is typically assessed by dual-energy X-ray absorptiometry scans and is expressed in standard deviations compared with "normals" based on that of a 20-year-old woman.[145] In the postmenopausal woman, a T score of less than −1.0 is osteopenia and less than −2.5 is osteoporosis. However, these criteria do not apply to the premenopausal female. Assigning normal values for the teenage female is particularly imprecise, as the age of menarche varies greatly. Although cortical bone tends to be preserved, there is a decrease in cancellous bone, increasing the likelihood of some stress fractures, for example, femoral neck, over others such as the tibial shaft.[146,147] Menstrual dysfunction and stress fractures have a positive correlation.[148,149]

The International Society for Clinical Densitometry has proposed using Z scores (comparison to age-matched controls) rather than T scores in premenopausal women.[150] Furthermore, one should not use the term "osteoporosis," but instead should use the phrase "low bone density for chronologic age" in children and "low bone density below expected range for age" if a premenopausal woman. "Osteopenia" should not be used, and "osteoporosis" used only if low BMD with secondary clinical risk factors such as nutritional deficiency, hypoestrogenism, stress fractures, and a low BMD Z score. An example is a case of a 21-year-old female marathon runner. She has a history of multiple stress fractures over the prior 3 years. Bone densitometry is performed. Lumbar spine T score is −2.1 and Z score is −1.7. Left femoral neck T score is −1.5 and Z score is −1.3. Her report should read "low bone density below expected range for age."

In a large study of elite female athletes, 10.2% had a Z score of less than −1.0 and 2% less than −2.0.[151] Other studies of high school athletes reveal Z scores less than −1.0 in 16% to 21% and less than −2.0 in 1% to 4%.[142,152]

Peak bone density is related to that obtained during adolescence. Thus, decreased bone density in the young female is important, as she will likely not be able to regain it and it will be a cause of increased morbidity as she ages.[153] There appears to be a window of time during the development of peak bone mass in which the bone is particularly responsive to weight-bearing physical activity. Impact-loading sports like gymnastics, rugby, and volleyball tend have a more pronounced osteogenic effect than sports without impact loading such as cycling, rowing, and swimming.[154] Because many athletes have higher BMD than their peers, some have suggested further workup to assess for other components of FAT if the Z score is less than −1.0.[155] Others have suggested an increased level of suspicion for FAT in female athletes with stress fractures. Although stress fractures are fairly common in all athletes, the incidence in female Division 1 collegiate athletes is double that of their male counterparts.[156]

As a woman ages, physiologic changes in the bone result in decreased bone mineralization and muscle strength and an increase cardiovascular disease prevalence. Exercise and athletic activity in the aging female population have been shown to be of great benefit, specifically decreasing cardiovascular risk factors.[157] Cardiovascular disease prevalence may decrease by up to 50% in the postmenopausal woman who exercises.[158] Age-related bone resorption becomes more apparent, particularly after the age of 50 years. Progressive resistance training has a more potent effect on bone density than does cardiovascular training.[159] During aging the joint capsules also become stiffer and degenerative changes in cartilage, tendons, ligaments, and vertebral discs develop. In addition, there is a diminished proprioceptive function of these tissues with aging.[160–162]

Muscle may be the most affected by aging, with loss of both muscle mass and functional motor units.[163] Muscle strength is important in bone health. Many studies have documented the positive effect of muscle-strengthening exercises on bone mass in the postmenopausal woman.[164–166] Improved back muscle strength has been shown to decrease the risk of vertebral fractures.[167] The effect of physical activity on bone is site specific. For example, tennis players have up to 33% greater BMD in their dominant humerus, weightlifters greater BMD in the spine and femurs, and swimmers have less BMD in the femoral neck than sedentary people.[168–171] Swimming, despite not being osteogenic, is an excellent athletic activity for an aging woman because improved neuromuscular function decreases fracture risk.[172]

SPORTS-SPECIFIC INJURIES

Many sports have sport-specific injuries more commonly found in the female athlete. For example, cheerleading has a very high female-to-male ratio. Spine injuries, particularly the cervical spine, are a high-morbidity injury and are more often found in cheerleading than other sports. Cheerleading injuries are by far more common in the 12- to 17-year-old age group than those younger. Most injuries are not severe, with sprains and strains being the most common. Serious injuries include fractures and dislocations of the extremities and lumbar and cervical spine (0.04% of all cheerleading injuries), and skull fractures.[173] Half of all catastrophic injuries to female athletes, which include paralysis and death, occur in high school and college cheerleading. The activity is year-round, and most of these injuries occur during maneuvers such as pyramids and partner stunts.[174]

Gymnastics injuries are twice as common during competition than during practice. Half of competition injures and over two-thirds of noncompetition injuries involve the lower extremity. Of note, a gymnast is 6 times more likely to sustain a knee internal derangement during competition than in practice, and almost 3 times as likely to sprain an ankle ligament. Approximately 70% of competition-related injuries are the result of landings in floor exercises or dismounts (Fig. 9).[175] There are more injuries to the back in gymnasts during practice than in competition, however. Intervertebral disc changes in gymnasts are common. MR imaging revealed disc changes in 24% of all gymnasts studied and found the prevalence related to competitive level, with 63% of national or Olympic gymnasts having changes[176]; this is similar to male gymnasts, however.[177] Pars defects, stress fractures of the pars interarticularis, are commonly found in gymnasts as well as in football players and water-skiers.[178]

Ballet dancing is more common among girls and women and the en-pointe foot position is exclusive to the ballerina. This stance may result in posterior impingement (Fig. 10) and fractures of the posterior process of the talus, as well as stress fractures at the base of the second metatarsal.[179] Female runners are more prone to fibular stress fractures. Girls who participate in over 16 hours per week of moderate to vigorous activity are twice as likely to develop stress fractures as those who exercise less than 16 hours per week.[180] Of the high-impact activities, running and gymnastics/cheerleading have been independently associated with an increase in stress fractures.[180]

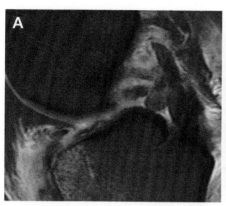
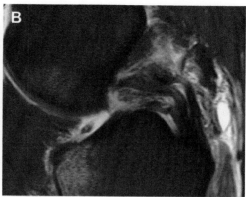

Fig. 9. A 16-year-old gymnast who failed her dismount during her vault in competition, with hyperextension injury. (*A*) Oblique sagittal fat-suppressed T2-weighted MR image of right knee demonstrates a complete disruption of the posterior cruciate ligament (PCL). (*B*) Oblique sagittal fat-suppressed T2-weighted MR image of left knee also demonstrates a complete disruption of the PCL. (*Case Courtesy of* Matt Bowen, MD.)

Female athletes sustain a higher percentage of concussions during games than male athletes regarding comparable sports in the NCAA athletic programs. Women's soccer and men's lacrosse have the highest injury rate of concussions.[181] Base sliding accounts for the vast majority of softball injuries, mainly from rapid deceleration against a stationary base.[182] It has been found that windmill softball pitching also has excessive distraction stresses placed on the throwing shoulder similar to those of the male baseball pitcher (**Fig. 11**). Women softball pitchers are not limited to number of innings pitched nor are pitch counts monitored.

Overuse injuries of the shoulder and elbow in softball pitchers are not infrequent.[183]

Volleyball has one of the fewest injury rates; however, note should be made of "volleyball shoulder." Volleyball shoulder is the second most common overuse injury in the volleyball player and consists of rotator cuff inflammation, impingement, and instability. Thirty-two percent of elite volleyball players develop suprascapular nerve impingement at the region of the spinoglenoid notch, perhaps related in part to the floater serve, which imparts as little spin as possible. To accomplish this, the player stops the overhand

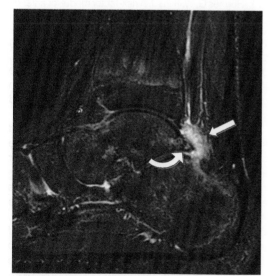

Fig. 10. A 13-year-old ballet student with posterior ankle pain. Sagittal fat-suppressed T2-weighted MR image shows an incomplete os trigonum (*curved arrow*) with adjacent soft tissue edema (*arrow*).

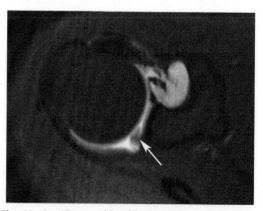

Fig. 11. An 18-year-old softball pitcher with shoulder pain. Fat-suppressed T1-weighted (450/17) postarthrogram MR image of the right shoulder demonstrates abnormal signal in the posterior-superior labrum (*arrow*) with some undercutting of contrast. There is a patulous capsule posteriorly. At arthroscopy, a redundant inflamed labrum was found and debrided, with subsequent marked improvement in her symptoms.

follow-through immediately after striking the ball. This abrupt stop affects the infraspinatus and is associated with hypermobility of the shoulder.[184,185]

SUMMARY

The female athlete is different from the male athlete in several ways. Different sporting activities lead to different injury patterns. However, even with the same athletic activities, anatomic and physiologic differences between the sexes lead to different injuries. In addition, societal norms of aesthetic beauty contribute to the emphasis on appearance of the female athlete. The FAT has the potential to affect the young athlete's health for many years to come. The clinician and the radiologist need to be aware of the varied injury patterns and risks of the female athlete.

ACKNOWLEDGMENTS

Special thanks to Angela Rovnyak for her assistance with the illustrations.

REFERENCES

1. Warren PN. History: a female athletic champion in ancient Olympics. Available at: http://wwwoutsportscom; 2009. Accessed March 30, 2010.
2. Pomeroy SB. Spartan women. New York (NY): Oxford University Press; 2002. Accessed March 30, 2010.
3. Jooste P. The world of Mary, Queen of Scots. Available at: http://www.marie-stuart.co.uk/index.htm; 2007. Accessed March 30, 2010.
4. Available at: http://www.georgianlondon.com/elizabeth-stokes-lady-bare-knuckles; 2009. Accessed March 30, 2010.
5. Available at: http://www.olympic.org. Accessed March 30, 2010.
6. Owens BD, Agel J, Mountcastle SB, et al. Incidence of glenohumeral instability in collegiate athletics. Am J Sports Med 2009;37(9):1750–4.
7. Walsh MS, Bohm H, Butterfield MM, et al. Gender bias in the effects of arms and countermovement on jumping performance. J Strength Cond Res 2007;21(2):362–6.
8. Sallis RE, Jones K, Sunshine S, et al. Comparing sports injuries in men and women. Int J Sports Med 2001;22(6):420–3.
9. Ivkovic A, Franic M, Bojanic I, et al. Overuse injuries in female athletes. Croat Med J 2007;48 (6):767–78.
10. Neptune RR, McGowan CP, Fiandt JM. The influence of muscle physiology and advanced technology on sports performance. Annu Rev Biomed Eng 2009;11:81–107.
11. Cureton KJ, Collins MA, Hill DW, et al. Muscle hypertrophy in men and women. Med Sci Sports Exerc 1988;20(4):338–44.
12. Abe T, Kearns CF, Fukunaga T. Sex differences in whole body skeletal muscle mass measured by magnetic resonance imaging and its distribution in young Japanese adults. Br J Sports Med 2003; 37(5):436–40.
13. Gallagher D, Visser M, De Meersman RE, et al. Appendicular skeletal muscle mass: effects of age, gender, and ethnicity. J Appl Physiol 1997; 83(1):229–39.
14. Malina RM. Body composition in athletes: assessment and estimated fatness. Clin Sports Med 2007;26(1):37–68.
15. Guenette JA, Witt JD, McKenzie DC, et al. Respiratory mechanics during exercise in endurance-trained men and women. J Physiol 2007;581(Pt 3):1309–22.
16. Gillquist J, Messner K. Anterior cruciate ligament reconstruction and the long-term incidence of gonarthrosis. Sports Med 1999;27(3):143–56.
17. Carter ND, Jenkinson TR, Wilson D, et al. Joint position sense and rehabilitation in the anterior cruciate ligament deficient knee. Br J Sports Med 1997;31(3):209–12.
18. Myklebust G, Bahr R. Return to play guidelines after anterior cruciate ligament surgery. Br J Sports Med 2005;39(3):127–31.
19. Arendt E, Dick R. Knee injury patterns among men and women in collegiate basketball and soccer. NCAA data and review of literature. Am J Sports Med 1995;23(6):694–701.
20. Hughes G, Watkins J. A risk-factor model for anterior cruciate ligament injury. Sports Med 2006;36(5): 411–28.
21. Anderson AF, Dome DC, Gautam S, et al. Correlation of anthropometric measurements, strength, anterior cruciate ligament size, and intercondylar notch characteristics to sex differences in anterior cruciate ligament tear rates. Am J Sports Med 2001;29(1):58–66.
22. Shelbourne KD, Davis TJ, Klootwyk TE. The relationship between intercondylar notch width of the femur and the incidence of anterior cruciate ligament tears. A prospective study. Am J Sports Med 1998;26(3):402–8.
23. Uhorchak JM, Scoville CR, Williams GN, et al. Risk factors associated with noncontact injury of the anterior cruciate ligament: a prospective four-year evaluation of 859 West Point cadets. Am J Sports Med 2003;31(6):831–42.
24. Amis AA, Dawkins GP. Functional anatomy of the anterior cruciate ligament. Fibre bundle actions related to ligament replacements and injuries. J Bone Joint Surg Br 1991;73(2):260–7.

25. Zantop T, Petersen W, Sekiya JK, et al. Anterior cruciate ligament anatomy and function relating to anatomical reconstruction. Knee Surg Sports Traumatol Arthrosc 2006;14(10):982–92.

26. Petersen W, Zantop T. Anatomy of the anterior cruciate ligament with regard to its two bundles. Clin Orthop Relat Res 2007;454:35–47.

27. Petersen W, Zantop T. Partial rupture of the anterior cruciate ligament. Arthroscopy 2006;22(11): 1143–5.

28. Senter C, Hame SL. Biomechanical analysis of tibial torque and knee flexion angle: implications for understanding knee injury. Sports Med 2006; 36(8):635–41.

29. Hewett TE, Myer GD, Ford KR. Decrease in neuromuscular control about the knee with maturation in female athletes. J Bone Joint Surg Am 2004;86(8): 1601–8.

30. Hewett TE, Myer GD, Ford KR, et al. Biomechanical measures of neuromuscular control and valgus loading of the knee predict anterior cruciate ligament injury risk in female athletes: a prospective study. Am J Sports Med 2005;33(4):492–501.

31. Souryal TO, Freeman TR. Intercondylar notch size and anterior cruciate ligament injuries in athletes. A prospective study. Am J Sports Med 1993;21(4): 535–9.

32. LaPrade RF, Burnett QM 2nd. Femoral intercondylar notch stenosis and correlation to anterior cruciate ligament injuries. A prospective study. Am J Sports Med 1994;22(2):198–202 [discussion: 203].

33. Teitz CC, Lind BK, Sacks BM. Symmetry of the femoral notch width index. Am J Sports Med 1997;25(5):687–90.

34. Schickendantz MS, Weiker GG. The predictive value of radiographs in the evaluation of unilateral and bilateral anterior cruciate ligament injuries. Am J Sports Med 1993;21(1):110–3.

35. Colvin AC, West RV. Patellar instability. J Bone Joint Surg Am 2008;90(12):2751–62.

36. Hungerford DS, Barry M. Biomechanics of the patellofemoral joint. Clin Orthop Relat Res 1979; 144:9–15.

37. Ireland ML. The female ACL: why is it more prone to injury? Orthop Clin North Am 2002;33(4): 637–51.

38. Horton MG, Hall TL. Quadriceps femoris muscle angle: normal values and relationships with gender and selected skeletal measures. Phys Ther 1989; 69(11):897–901.

39. Shambaugh JP, Klein A, Herbert JH. Structural measures as predictors of injury basketball players. Med Sci Sports Exerc 1991;23(5):522–7.

40. Barrance PJ, Williams GN, Snyder-Mackler L, et al. Altered knee kinematics in ACL-deficient noncopers: a comparison using dynamic MRI. J Orthop Res 2006;24(2):132–40.

41. Gray J, Taunton JE, McKenzie DC, et al. A survey of injuries to the anterior cruciate ligament of the knee in female basketball players. Int J Sports Med 1985;6(6):314–6.

42. Hewett TE, Myer GD, Ford KR. Anterior cruciate ligament injuries in female athletes: part 1, mechanisms and risk factors. Am J Sports Med 2006;34(2): 299–311.

43. Slauterbeck J, Clevenger C, Lundberg W, et al. Estrogen level alters the failure load of the rabbit anterior cruciate ligament. J Orthop Res 1999;17(3):405–8.

44. Deie M, Sakamaki Y, Sumen Y, et al. Anterior knee laxity in young women varies with their menstrual cycle. Int Orthop 2002;26(3):154–6.

45. Heitz NA, Eisenman PA, Beck CL, et al. Hormonal changes throughout the menstrual cycle and increased anterior cruciate ligament laxity in females. J Athl Train 1999;34(2):144–9.

46. Shultz SJ, Sander TC, Kirk SE, et al. Sex differences in knee joint laxity change across the female menstrual cycle. J Sports Med Phys Fitness 2005; 45(4):594–603.

47. Griffin LY, Albohm MJ, Arendt EA, et al. Understanding and preventing noncontact anterior cruciate ligament injuries: a review of the Hunt Valley II meeting, January 2005. Am J Sports Med 2006;34(9):1512–32.

48. Karageanes SJ, Blackburn K, Vangelos ZA. The association of the menstrual cycle with the laxity of the anterior cruciate ligament in adolescent female athletes. Clin J Sport Med 2000;10(3): 162–8.

49. Belanger MJ, Moore DC, Crisco JJ 3rd, et al. Knee laxity does not vary with the menstrual cycle, before or after exercise. Am J Sports Med 2004; 32(5):1150–7.

50. Moller Nielsen J, Hammar M. Sports injuries and oral contraceptive use. Is there a relationship? Sports Med 1991;12(3):152–60.

51. Arendt EA, Bershadsky B, Agel J. Periodicity of noncontact anterior cruciate ligament injuries during the menstrual cycle. J Gend Specif Med 2002;5(2):19–26.

52. Griffin LY, Agel J, Albohm MJ, et al. Noncontact anterior cruciate ligament injuries: risk factors and prevention strategies. J Am Acad Orthop Surg 2000;8(3):141–50.

53. Myer GD, Ford KR, Hewett TE. The effects of gender on quadriceps muscle activation strategies during a maneuver that mimics a high ACL injury risk position. J Electromyogr Kinesiol 2005;15(2): 181–9.

54. Rozzi SL, Lephart SM, Gear WS, et al. Knee joint laxity and neuromuscular characteristics of male and female soccer and basketball players. Am J Sports Med 1999;27(3):312–9.

55. Gilchrist J, Mandelbaum BR, Melancon H, et al. A randomized controlled trial to prevent noncontact anterior cruciate ligament injury in female collegiate soccer players. Am J Sports Med 2008;36(8): 1476–83.

56. Hutchinson MR, Ireland ML. Knee injuries in female athletes. Sports Med 1995;19(4):288–302.

57. Huston LJ, Greenfield ML, Wojtys EM. Anterior cruciate ligament injuries in the female athlete. Potential risk factors. Clin Orthop Relat Res 2000; 372:50–63.

58. Ford KR, Myer GD, Smith RL, et al. A comparison of dynamic coronal plane excursion between matched male and female athletes when performing single leg landings. Clin Biomech (Bristol, Avon) 2006;21(1):33–40.

59. Boden BP, Dean GS, Feagin JA Jr, et al. Mechanisms of anterior cruciate ligament injury. Orthopedics 2000;23(6):573–8.

60. Emerson RJ. Basketball knee injuries and the anterior cruciate ligament. Clin Sports Med 1993;12(2): 317–28.

61. Zazulak BT, Ponce PL, Straub SJ, et al. Gender comparison of hip muscle activity during single-leg landing. J Orthop Sports Phys Ther 2005;35(5): 292–9.

62. Wojtys EM, Wylie BB, Huston LJ. The effects of muscle fatigue on neuromuscular function and anterior tibial translation in healthy knees. Am J Sports Med 1996;24(5):615–21.

63. Ford KR, Myer GD, Hewett TE. Valgus knee motion during landing in high school female and male basketball players. Med Sci Sports Exerc 2003; 35(10):1745–50.

64. Kirkendall DT, Garrett WE Jr. The anterior cruciate ligament enigma. Injury mechanisms and prevention. Clin Orthop Relat Res 2000;372:64–8.

65. McLean SG, Neal RJ, Myers PT, et al. Knee joint kinematics during the sidestep cutting maneuver: potential for injury in women. Med Sci Sports Exerc 1999;31(7):959–68.

66. Malinzak RA, Colby SM, Kirkendall DT, et al. A comparison of knee joint motion patterns between men and women in selected athletic tasks. Clin Biomech (Bristol, Avon) 2001;16(5):438–45.

67. Fagenbaum R, Darling WG. Jump landing strategies in male and female college athletes and the implications of such strategies for anterior cruciate ligament injury. Am J Sports Med 2003;31(2): 233–40.

68. Boden BP, Griffin LY, Garrett WE Jr. Etiology and prevention of noncontact ACL injury. Phys Sportsmed 2000;28(4):53–60.

69. Ford KR, Myer GD, Toms HE, et al. Gender differences in the kinematics of unanticipated cutting in young athletes. Med Sci Sports Exerc 2005;37(1): 124–9.

70. Loudon JK, Jenkins W, Loudon KL. The relationship between static posture and ACL injury in female athletes. J Orthop Sports Phys Ther 1996;24(2): 91–7.

71. Trimble MH, Bishop MD, Buckley BD, et al. The relationship between clinical measurements of lower extremity posture and tibial translation. Clin Biomech (Bristol, Avon) 2002;17(4):286–90.

72. Allen MK, Glasoe WM. Metrecom measurement of navicular drop in subjects with anterior cruciate ligament injury. J Athl Train 2000;35(4): 403–6.

73. Lephart SM, Ferris CM, Riemann BL, et al. Gender differences in strength and lower extremity kinematics during landing. Clin Orthop Relat Res 2002;401:162–9.

74. Harmon KG, Dick R. The relationship of skill level to anterior cruciate ligament injury. Clin J Sport Med 1998;8(4):260–5.

75. Bjordal JM, Arnly F, Hannestad B, et al. Epidemiology of anterior cruciate ligament injuries in soccer. Am J Sports Med 1997;25(3):341–5.

76. Arendt EA, Agel J, Dick R. Anterior cruciate ligament injury patterns among collegiate men and women. J Athl Train 1999;34(2):86–92.

77. Agel J, Arendt EA, Bershadsky B. Anterior cruciate ligament injury in national collegiate athletic association basketball and soccer: a 13-year review. Am J Sports Med 2005;33(4):524–30.

78. Scranton PE Jr, Whitesel JP, Powell JW, et al. A review of selected noncontact anterior cruciate ligament injuries in the National Football League. Foot Ankle Int 1997;18(12):772–6.

79. Orchard JW, Powell JW. Risk of knee and ankle sprains under various weather conditions in American football. Med Sci Sports Exerc 2003;35(7): 1118–23.

80. Meyers MC, Barnhill BS. Incidence, causes, and severity of high school football injuries on FieldTurf versus natural grass: a 5-year prospective study. Am J Sports Med 2004;32(7):1626–38.

81. Lambson RB, Barnhill BS, Higgins RW. Football cleat design and its effect on anterior cruciate ligament injuries. A three-year prospective study. Am J Sports Med 1996;24(2):155–9.

82. Livesay GA, Reda DR, Nauman EA. Peak torque and rotational stiffness developed at the shoe-surface interface: the effect of shoe type and playing surface. Am J Sports Med 2006;34(3): 415–22.

83. Martinek V, Friederich NF. [To brace or not to brace? How effective are knee braces in rehabilitation?]. Orthopade 1999;28(6):565–70 [in German].

84. Millet CW, Drez DJ Jr. Principles of bracing for the anterior cruciate ligament-deficient knee. Clin Sports Med 1988;7(4):827–33.

85. Houston ME, Goemans PH. Leg muscle performance of athletes with and without knee support braces. Arch Phys Med Rehabil 1982;63(9):431–2.

86. Risberg MA, Holm I, Steen H, et al. The effect of knee bracing after anterior cruciate ligament reconstruction. A prospective, randomized study with two years' follow-up. Am J Sports Med 1999; 27(1):76–83.

87. Fulkerson JP, Arendt EA. The female knee—anterior knee pain. Conn Med 1999;63(11):661–4.

88. Dye SF. The pathophysiology of patellofemoral pain: a tissue homeostasis perspective. Clin Orthop Relat Res 2005;436:100–10.

89. LaBella C. Patellofemoral pain syndrome: evaluation and treatment. Prim Care 2004;31(4):977–1003.

90. Chung CB, Skaf A, Roger B, et al. Patellar tendon-lateral femoral condyle friction syndrome: MR imaging in 42 patients. Skeletal Radiol 2001;30(12):694–7.

91. Cutbill JW, Ladly KO, Bray RC, et al. Anterior knee pain: a review. Clin J Sport Med 1997;7(1):40–5.

92. Baquie P, Brukner P. Injuries presenting to an Australian sports medicine centre: a 12-month study. Clin J Sport Med 1997;7(1):28–31.

93. DeHaven KE, Lintner DM. Athletic injuries: comparison by age, sport, and gender. Am J Sports Med 1986;14(3):218–24.

94. Taunton JE, Ryan MB, Clement DB, et al. A retrospective case-control analysis of 2002 running injuries. Br J Sports Med 2002;36(2): 95–101.

95. Witvrouw E, Lysens R, Bellemans J, et al. Intrinsic risk factors for the development of anterior knee pain in an athletic population. A two-year prospective study. Am J Sports Med 2000;28(4):480–9.

96. Hughston JC. Subluxation of the patella. J Bone Joint Surg Am 1968;50(5):1003–26.

97. Earl JE, Vetter CS. Patellofemoral pain. Phys Med Rehabil Clin N Am 2007;18(3):439–58, viii.

98. Moss RI, Devita P, Dawson ML. A biomechanical analysis of patellofemoral stress syndrome. J Athl Train 1992;27(1):64–9.

99. Hautamaa PV, Fithian DC, Kaufman KR, et al. Medial soft tissue restraints in lateral patellar instability and repair. Clin Orthop Relat Res 1998;349: 174–82.

100. Cowan SM, Bennell KL, Hodges PW. Therapeutic patellar taping changes the timing of vasti muscle activation in people with patellofemoral pain syndrome. Clin J Sport Med 2002;12(6):339–47.

101. Grabiner MD, Koh TJ, Draganich LF. Neuromechanics of the patellofemoral joint. Med Sci Sports Exerc 1994;26(1):10–21.

102. Cowan SM, Hodges PW, Bennell KL, et al. Altered vastii recruitment when people with patellofemoral pain syndrome complete a postural task. Arch Phys Med Rehabil 2002;83(7):989–95.

103. Owings TM, Grabiner MD. Motor control of the vastus medialis oblique and vastus lateralis muscles is disrupted during eccentric contractions in subjects with patellofemoral pain. Am J Sports Med 2002;30(4):483–7.

104. Voight ML, Wieder DL. Comparative reflex response times of vastus medialis obliquus and vastus lateralis in normal subjects and subjects with extensor mechanism dysfunction. An electromyographic study. Am J Sports Med 1991;19(2): 131–7.

105. Gilleard W, McConnell J, Parsons D. The effect of patellar taping on the onset of vastus medialis obliquus and vastus lateralis muscle activity in persons with patellofemoral pain. Phys Ther 1998; 78(1):25–32.

106. Karst GM, Willett GM. Onset timing of electromyographic activity in the vastus medialis oblique and vastus lateralis muscles in subjects with and without patellofemoral pain syndrome. Phys Ther 1995;75(9):813–23.

107. Mohr KJ, Kvitne RS, Pink MM, et al. Electromyography of the quadriceps in patellofemoral pain with patellar subluxation. Clin Orthop Relat Res 2003;415:261–71.

108. Livingston LA. The quadriceps angle: a review of the literature. J Orthop Sports Phys Ther 1998;28(2): 105–9.

109. Fairbank JC, Pynsent PB, van Poortvliet JA, et al. Mechanical factors in the incidence of knee pain in adolescents and young adults. J Bone Joint Surg Br 1984;66(5):685–93.

110. Reikeras O. Patellofemoral characteristics in patients with increased femoral anteversion. Skeletal Radiol 1992;21(5):311–3.

111. Eckhoff DG, Montgomery WK, Kilcoyne RF, et al. Femoral morphometry and anterior knee pain. Clin Orthop Relat Res 1994;302:64–8.

112. Cooke TD, Price N, Fisher B, et al. The inwardly pointing knee. An unrecognized problem of external rotational malalignment. Clin Orthop Relat Res 1990;260:56–60.

113. Tiberio D. The effect of excessive subtalar joint pronation on patellofemoral mechanics: a theoretical model. J Orthop Sports Phys Ther 1987;9(4): 160–5.

114. Johnston LB, Gross MT. Effects of foot orthoses on quality of life for individuals with patellofemoral pain syndrome. J Orthop Sports Phys Ther 2004;34(8): 440–8.

115. Goutallier D, Bernageau J, Lecudonnec B. [The measurement of the tibial tuberosity. Patella groove distanced technique and results (author's transl)]. Rev Chir Orthop Reparatrice Appar Mot 1978;64(5):423–8 [in French].

116. Dejour H, Walch G, Nove-Josserand L, et al. Factors of patellar instability: an anatomic

radiographic study. Knee Surg Sports Traumatol Arthrosc 1994;2(1):19–26.

117. Perry J. Gait analysis in sports medicine. Instr Course Lect 1990;39:319–24.

118. Powers CM. The influence of altered lower-extremity kinematics on patellofemoral joint dysfunction: a theoretical perspective. J Orthop Sports Phys Ther 2003;33(11):639–46.

119. Riegger-Krugh C, Keysor JJ. Skeletal malalignments of the lower quarter: correlated and compensatory motions and postures. J Orthop Sports Phys Ther 1996;23(2):164–70.

120. Patel VV, Hall K, Ries M, et al. Magnetic resonance imaging of patellofemoral kinematics with weight-bearing. J Bone Joint Surg Am 2003;85(12): 2419–24.

121. Powers CM, Ward SR, Fredericson M, et al. Patellofemoral kinematics during weight-bearing and non-weight-bearing knee extension in persons with lateral subluxation of the patella: a preliminary study. J Orthop Sports Phys Ther 2003;33(11): 677–85.

122. Ireland ML, Willson JD, Ballantyne BT, et al. Hip strength in females with and without patellofemoral pain. J Orthop Sports Phys Ther 2003;33(11): 671–6.

123. Paterson I. The torn acetabular labrum; a block to reduction of a dislocated hip. J Bone Joint Surg Br 1957;39(2):306–9.

124. Ferguson SJ, Bryant JT, Ganz R, et al. The influence of the acetabular labrum on hip joint cartilage consolidation: a poroelastic finite element model. J Biomech 2000;33(8):953–60.

125. De Paulis F, Cacchio A, Michelini O, et al. Sports injuries in the pelvis and hip: diagnostic imaging. Eur J Radiol 1998;27(Suppl 1):S49–59.

126. McCarthy JC, Noble PC, Schuck MR, et al. The Otto E. Aufranc Award: the role of labral lesions to development of early degenerative hip disease. Clin Orthop Relat Res 2001;393:25–37.

127. Mason JB. Acetabular labral tears in the athlete. Clin Sports Med 2001;20(4):779–90.

128. Bache CE, Clegg J, Herron M. Risk factors for developmental dysplasia of the hip: ultrasonographic findings in the neonatal period. J Pediatr Orthop B 2002;11(3):212–8.

129. Burnett RS, Della Rocca GJ, Prather H, et al. Clinical presentation of patients with tears of the acetabular labrum. J Bone Joint Surg Am 2006;88(7):1448–57.

130. Dorrell JH, Catterall A. The torn acetabular labrum. J Bone Joint Surg Br 1986;68(3):400–3.

131. Ganz R, Parvizi J, Beck M, et al. Femoroacetabular impingement: a cause for osteoarthritis of the hip. Clin Orthop Relat Res 2003;417:112–20.

132. Fitzgerald RH Jr. Acetabular labrum tears. Diagnosis and treatment. Clin Orthop Relat Res 1995; 311:60–8.

133. Hunt D, Clohisy J, Prather H. Acetabular labral tears of the hip in women. Phys Med Rehabil Clin N Am 2007;18(3):497–520, ix–x.

134. Beck M, Kalhor M, Leunig M, et al. Hip morphology influences the pattern of damage to the acetabular cartilage: femoroacetabular impingement as a cause of early osteoarthritis of the hip. J Bone Joint Surg Br 2005;87(7):1012–8.

135. Ziegert AJ, Blankenbaker DG, De Smet AA, et al. Comparison of standard hip MR arthrographic imaging planes and sequences for detection of arthroscopically proven labral tear. AJR Am J Roentgenol 2009;192(5):1397–400.

136. Faraj AA, Kumaraguru P, Kosygan K. Intra-articular bupivacaine hip injection in differentiation of coxarthrosis from referred thigh pain: a 10 year study. Acta Orthop Belg 2003;69(6):518–21.

137. Otis CL, Drinkwater B, Johnson M, et al. American College of Sports Medicine position stand. The Female Athlete Triad. Med Sci Sports Exerc 1997; 29(5):i–ix.

138. Nattiv A, Loucks AB, Manore MM, et al. American College of Sports Medicine position stand. The female athlete triad. Med Sci Sports Exerc 2007; 39(10):1867–82.

139. Nichols JF, Rauh MJ, Barrack MT, et al. Disordered eating and menstrual irregularity in high school athletes in lean-build and nonlean-build sports. Int J Sport Nutr Exerc Metab 2007;17(4):364–77.

140. Torstveit MK, Rosenvinge JH, Sundgot-Borgen J. Prevalence of eating disorders and the predictive power of risk models in female elite athletes: a controlled study. Scand J Med Sci Sports 2008; 18(1):108–18.

141. Gibson JH, Mitchell A, Reeve J, et al. Treatment of reduced bone mineral density in athletic amenorrhea: a pilot study. Osteoporos Int 1999;10(4): 284–9.

142. Nichols JF, Rauh MJ, Lawson MJ, et al. Prevalence of the female athlete triad syndrome among high school athletes. Arch Pediatr Adolesc Med 2006; 160(2):137–42.

143. Weaver CM, Teegarden D, Lyle RM, et al. Impact of exercise on bone health and contraindication of oral contraceptive use in young women. Med Sci Sports Exerc 2001;33(6):873–80.

144. Hoch AZ, Lal S, Jurva JW, et al. The female athlete triad and cardiovascular dysfunction. Phys Med Rehabil Clin N Am 2007;18(3):385–400, vii–viii.

145. Assessment of fracture risk and its application to screening for postmenopausal osteoporosis. Report of a WHO Study Group. World Health Organ Tech Rep Ser 1994;843:1–129.

146. Drinkwater BL, Nilson K, Chesnut CH 3rd, et al. Bone mineral content of amenorrheic and eumenorrheic athletes. N Engl J Med 1984;311(5): 277–81.

147. Marx RG, Saint-Phard D, Callahan LR, et al. Stress fracture sites related to underlying bone health in athletic females. Clin J Sport Med 2001;11(2): 73–6.

148. Marcus R, Cann C, Madvig P, et al. Menstrual function and bone mass in elite women distance runners. Endocrine and metabolic features. Ann Intern Med 1985;102(2):158–63.

149. Barrow GW, Saha S. Menstrual irregularity and stress fractures in collegiate female distance runners. Am J Sports Med 1988;16(3):209–16.

150. Leib ES, Lewiecki EM, Binkley N, et al. Official positions of the International Society for Clinical Densitometry. J Clin Densitom 2004;7(1):1–6.

151. Torstveit MK, Sundgot-Borgen J. Low bone mineral density is two to three times more prevalent in non-athletic premenopausal women than in elite athletes: a comprehensive controlled study. Br J Sports Med 2005;39(5):282–7 [discussion: 282–7].

152. Hoch AZ, Pajewski NM, Moraski L, et al. Prevalence of the female athlete triad in high school athletes and sedentary students. Clin J Sport Med 2009;19(5):421–8.

153. Chilibeck PD, Sale DG, Webber CE. Exercise and bone mineral density. Sports Med 1995;19(2): 103–22.

154. Nichols DL, Sanborn CF, Essery EV. Bone density and young athletic women. An update. Sports Med 2007;37(11):1001–14.

155. Beals KA, Hill AK. The prevalence of disordered eating, menstrual dysfunction, and low bone mineral density among US collegiate athletes. Int J Sport Nutr Exerc Metab 2006; 16(1):1–23.

156. Feingold D, Hame SL. Female athlete triad and stress fractures. Orthop Clin North Am 2006;37(4): 575–83.

157. Everson-Rose SA, Lewis TT. Psychosocial factors and cardiovascular diseases. Annu Rev Public Health 2005;26:469–500.

158. Beitz R, Doren M. Physical activity and postmenopausal health. J Br Menopause Soc 2004;10(2): 70–4.

159. Layne JE, Nelson ME. The effects of progressive resistance training on bone density: a review. Med Sci Sports Exerc 1999;31(1):25–30.

160. Dugan SA. Exercise for health and wellness at midlife and beyond: balancing benefits and risks. Phys Med Rehabil Clin N Am 2007;18(3):555–75, xi.

161. Vernon-Roberts B, Pirie CJ. Degenerative changes in the intervertebral discs of the lumbar spine and their sequelae. Rheumatol Rehabil 1977;16(1): 13–21.

162. Skinner HB, Barrack RL, Cook SD. Age-related decline in proprioception. Clin Orthop Relat Res 1984;184:208–11.

163. Frontera WR, Hughes VA, Lutz KJ, et al. A cross-sectional study of muscle strength and mass in 45- to 78-yr-old men and women. J Appl Physiol 1991;71(2):644–50.

164. Gleeson PB, Protas EJ, LeBlanc AD, et al. Effects of weight lifting on bone mineral density in premenopausal women. J Bone Miner Res 1990;5(2): 153–8.

165. Dalsky GP, Stocke KS, Ehsani AA, et al. Weight-bearing exercise training and lumbar bone mineral content in postmenopausal women. Ann Intern Med 1988;108(6):824–8.

166. Sinaki M. Critical appraisal of physical rehabilitation measures after osteoporotic vertebral fracture. Osteoporos Int 2003;14(9):773–9.

167. Sinaki M, Itoi E, Wahner HW, et al. Stronger back muscles reduce the incidence of vertebral fractures: a prospective 10 year follow-up of postmenopausal women. Bone 2002;30(6):836–41.

168. Huddleston AL, Rockwell D, Kulund DN, et al. Bone mass in lifetime tennis athletes. JAMA 1980;244(10): 1107–9.

169. Ducher G, Courteix D, Meme S, et al. Bone geometry in response to long-term tennis playing and its relationship with muscle volume: a quantitative magnetic resonance imaging study in tennis players. Bone 2005;37(4):457–66.

170. Block JE, Genant HK, Black D. Greater vertebral bone mineral mass in exercising young men. West J Med 1986;145(1):39–42.

171. Fehling PC, Alekel L, Clasey J, et al. A comparison of bone mineral densities among female athletes in impact loading and active loading sports. Bone 1995;17(3):205–10.

172. Smith EL, Gilligan C. Dose-response relationship between physical loading and mechanical competence of bone. Bone 1996;18(Suppl 1):455–505.

173. Shields BJ, Smith GA. Cheerleading-related injuries to children 5 to 18 years of age: United States, 1990-2002. Pediatrics 2006;117(1):122–9.

174. Hutchinson MR. Cheerleading injuries: patterns, prevention, case reports. Phys Sportsmed 1997; 25(9):83–96.

175. Marshall SW, Covassin T, Dick R, et al. Descriptive epidemiology of collegiate women's gymnastics injuries: National Collegiate Athletic Association Injury Surveillance System, 1988-1989 through 2003-2004. J Athl Train 2007;42(2):234–40.

176. Goldstein JD, Berger PE, Windler GE, et al. Spine injuries in gymnasts and swimmers. An epidemiologic investigation. Am J Sports Med 1991;19(5): 463–8.

177. Sward L, Hellstrom M, Jacobsson B, et al. Disc degeneration and associated abnormalities of the spine in elite gymnasts. A magnetic resonance imaging study. Spine (Phila Pa 1976) 1991;16(4): 437–43.

178. Wiltse LL. The etiology of spondylolisthesis. J Bone Joint Surg Am 1962;44:539–60.

179. Dugan SA, Weber KM. Stress fractures and rehabilitation. Phys Med Rehabil Clin N Am 2007;18(3):401–16, viii.

180. Loud KJ, Gordon CM, Micheli LJ, et al. Correlates of stress fractures among preadolescent and adolescent girls. Pediatrics 2005;115(4):e399–406.

181. Covassin T, Swanik CB, Sachs ML. Sex differences and the incidence of concussions among collegiate athletes. J Athl Train 2003;38(3):238–44.

182. Janda DH, Wojtys EM, Hankin FM, et al. A three-phase analysis of the prevention of recreational softball injuries. Am J Sports Med 1990;18(6):632–5.

183. Werner SL, Jones DG, Guido JA Jr, et al. Kinematics and kinetics of elite windmill softball pitching. Am J Sports Med 2006;34(4):597–603.

184. Sandow MJ, Ilic J. Suprascapular nerve rotator cuff compression syndrome in volleyball players. J Shoulder Elbow Surg 1998;7(5):516–21.

185. Witvrouw E, Cools A, Lysens R, et al. Suprascapular neuropathy in volleyball players. Br J Sports Med 2000;34(3):174–80.

Index

Note: Page numbers of article titles are in **boldface** type.

Radiol Clin N Am 48 (2010) 1267–1274
doi:10.1016/S0033-8389(10)00217-4
0033-8389/10/$ – see front matter © 2010 Elsevier Inc. All rights reserved.

United States Postal Service

Statement of Ownership, Management, and Circulation
(All Periodicals Publications Except Requestor Publications)

1. Publication Title	2. Publication Number		3. Filing Date
Radiologic Clinics of North America	5 9 6 - 5 1 0		9/15/10

4. Issue Frequency	5. Number of Issues Published Annually	6. Annual Subscription Price
Jan, Mar, May, Jul, Sep, Nov	6	$361.00

7. Complete Mailing Address of Known Office of Publication (*Not printer*) (*Street, city, county, state, and ZIP+4®*)

Elsevier Inc.
360 Park Avenue South
New York, NY 10010-1710

Contact Person
Stephen Bushing
Telephone (Include area code)
215-239-3688

8. Complete Mailing Address of Headquarters or General Business Office of Publisher (*Not printer*)

Elsevier Inc., 360 Park Avenue South, New York, NY 10010-1710

9. Full Names and Complete Mailing Addresses of Publisher, Editor, and Managing Editor (*Do not leave blank*)

Publisher (*Name and complete mailing address*)

Kim Murphy, Elsevier, Inc., 1600 John F. Kennedy Blvd. Suite 1800, Philadelphia, PA 19103-2899

Editor (*Name and complete mailing address*)

Barton Dudlick, Elsevier, Inc., 1600 John F. Kennedy Blvd. Suite 1800, Philadelphia, PA 19103-2899

Managing Editor (*Name and complete mailing address*)

Catherine Bewick, Elsevier, Inc., 1600 John F. Kennedy Blvd. Suite 1800, Philadelphia, PA 19103-2899

10. Owner (*Do not leave blank. If the publication is owned by a corporation, give the name and address of the corporation immediately followed by the names and addresses of all stockholders owning or holding 1 percent or more of the total amount of stock. If not owned by a corporation, give the names and addresses of the individual owners. If owned by a partnership or other unincorporated firm, give its name and address as well as those of each individual owner. If the publication is published by a nonprofit organization, give its name and address.*)

Full Name	Complete Mailing Address
Wholly owned subsidiary of	4520 East-West Highway
Reed/Elsevier, US holdings	Bethesda, MD 20814

11. Known Bondholders, Mortgagees, and Other Security Holders Owning or Holding 1 Percent or More of Total Amount of Bonds, Mortgages, or Other Securities. If none, check box ▸ ☐ None

Full Name	Complete Mailing Address
N/A	

12. Tax Status (*For completion by nonprofit organizations authorized to mail at nonprofit rates*) (*Check one*)
The purpose, function, and nonprofit status of this organization and the exempt status for federal income tax purposes:
☐ Has Not Changed During Preceding 12 Months
☐ Has Changed During Preceding 12 Months (*Publisher must submit explanation of change with this statement*)

PS Form 3526, September 2007 (Page 1 of 3 (Instructions Page 3)) PSN 7530-01-000-9931 **PRIVACY NOTICE:** See our Privacy policy in www.usps.com

---

13. Publication Title	14. Issue Date for Circulation Data Below
Radiologic Clinics of North America	July 2010

15. Extent and Nature of Circulation			Average No. Copies Each Issue During Preceding 12 Months	No. Copies of Single Issue Published Nearest to Filing Date
a. Total Number of Copies (*Net press run*)			5442	5250
b. Paid Circulation (By Mail and Outside the Mail)	(1)	Mailed Outside-County Paid Subscriptions Stated on PS Form 3541. (*Include paid distribution above nominal rate, advertiser's proof copies, and exchange copies*)	2475	2286
	(2)	Mailed In-County Paid Subscriptions Stated on PS Form 3541 (*Include paid distribution above nominal rate, advertiser's proof copies, and exchange copies*)		
	(3)	Paid Distribution Outside the Mails Including Sales Through Dealers and Carriers, Street Vendors, Counter Sales, and Other Paid Distribution Outside USPS®	1423	1396
	(4)	Paid Distribution by Other Classes Mailed Through the USPS (*e.g. First-Class Mail®*)		
c. Total Paid Distribution (*Sum of 15b (1), (2), (3), and (4)*)		▸	3898	3682
d. Free or Nominal Rate Distribution (By Mail and Outside the Mail)	(1)	Free or Nominal Rate Outside-County Copies Included on PS Form 3541	180	112
	(2)	Free or Nominal Rate In-County Copies Included on PS Form 3541		
	(3)	Free or Nominal Rate Copies Mailed at Other Classes Through the USPS (e.g. First-Class Mail)		
	(4)	Free or Nominal Rate Distribution Outside the Mail (Carriers or other means)		
e. Total Free or Nominal Rate Distribution (*Sum of 15d (1), (2), (3) and (4)*)		▸	180	112
f. Total Distribution (*Sum of 15c and 15e*)		▸	4078	3794
g. Copies not Distributed (*See instructions to publishers #4 (page #3)*)		▸	1364	1456
h. Total (*Sum of 15f and g*)		▸	5442	5250
i. Percent Paid (*15c divided by 15f times 100*)			95.59%	97.05%

16. Publication of Statement of Ownership
If the publication is a general publication, publication of this statement is required. Will be printed
in the November 2010 issue of this publication. ☐ Publication not required

17. Signature and Title of Editor, Publisher, Business Manager, or Owner

[signature]

Stephen R. Bushing – Fulfillment/Inventory Specialist

Date
September 15, 2010

I certify that all information furnished on this form is true and complete. I understand that anyone who furnishes false or misleading information on this form or who omits material or information requested on the form may be subject to criminal sanctions (including fines and imprisonment) and/or civil sanctions (including civil penalties).

PS Form 3526, September 2007 (Page 2 of 3)

Moving?

Make sure your subscription moves with you!

To notify us of your new address, find your **Clinics Account Number** (located on your mailing label above your name), and contact customer service at:

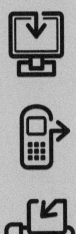

Email: journalscustomerservice-usa@elsevier.com

800-654-2452 (subscribers in the U.S. & Canada)
314-447-8871 (subscribers outside of the U.S. & Canada)

Fax number: 314-447-8029

Elsevier Health Sciences Division
Subscription Customer Service
3251 Riverport Lane
Maryland Heights, MO 63043

*To ensure uninterrupted delivery of your subscription, please notify us at least 4 weeks in advance of move.

Printed and bound by CPI Group (UK) Ltd, Croydon, CR0 4YY

08/06/2025

01896875-0016